LEADING INTERPROFESSIONAL TEAMS IN HEALTH AND SOCIAL CARE

This book presents compelling narrative case studies of a variety of interprofessional teams and explores how teams work in three key and interrelated areas: creating and implementing change, team working and leadership. Each case study is followed by an analysis in which creative approaches to interprofessional working and examples of best practice are identified. This book shows that there are many different new forms of leadership and demonstrates tensions between traditional models and emerging models. It also looks at how theory and policy are translated into practice and how service change may benefit service users.

The wide range of examples of practice in complex settings make this book essential reading for all students in health, nursing and social care, at undergraduate, postgraduate and professional levels.

Vivien Martin is Head of the Centre for Collaborative Programmes in University College Chichester. She contributed to development of the NHSU and has held posts in the Open University and in the NHS. Her previous publications include *Leading Change in Health and Social Care*, *Managing Projects in Health and Social Care* and *Managing in Health and Social Care* (co-authored with Euan Henderson), all published by Routledge.

Anita Rogers is an educator in human resource development, leadership and management. She is a lecturer at the Open University, School of Health and Social Welfare, and co-ordinator of management skills development for Master's level students at the University of Wales, Aberystwyth. She is also a non-executive board member for the Ceredigion and Mid Wales NHS trust.

Health and Social Care

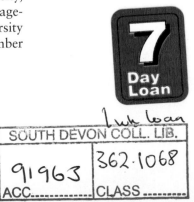

LEADING INTERPROFESSIONAL TEAMS IN HEALTH AND SOCIAL CARE

Vivien Martin and Anita Rogers

Routledge
Taylor & Francis Group
NEW YORK AND LONDON

First published 2004 by Routledge
2 Park Square, Milton Park, Abingdon, Oxon OX14 4RN

Simultaneously published in the USA and Canada
by Routledge
270 Madison Avenue, New York, NY 10016

Routledge is an imprint of the Taylor & Francis Group

© 2004 Vivien Martin and Anita Rogers

Typeset in Great Britain by Peter Powell Origination & Print Limited
Printed and bound in Great Britain by
TJ International Ltd, Padstow, Cornwall

British Library Cataloguing in Publication Data
A catalogue record for this book is available from the British Library

Library of Congress Cataloging in Publication Data

ISBN 0-415-30793-7 (hbk)
ISBN 0-415-30794-5 (pbk)

CONTENTS

FIGURES

EXAMPLES

PERSPECTIVES ON CHANGE IN HEALTH AND SOCIAL CARE

PERSPECTIVES ON TEAMWORKING

PERSPECTIVES ON LEADERSHIP

PREFACE:
OVERVIEW OF THE BOOK

This book is organised in three parts. Part 1 offers an introduction to the context, Part 2 presents the case studies and Part 3 reviews the extent to which the practice described in the case studies reflects or challenges theoretical perspectives on change, leadership and teamworking.

PART 1 – INTRODUCTION

This gives an overview of the health and care context from which the issues raised in the book have emerged.

PART 2 – CASE STUDIES

Part 2 of this book presents five case studies that illustrate the issues of leading and teamworking in the interprofessional, interdisciplinary and interagency environments that are emerging in health and social care.

Each case study presents an account from some team members describing their work and their views. This is followed by a number of examples drawn from these interviews but presented as perspectives offered by the team on change in health and social care, teamworking and leadership. These examples are not attributed to particular members of the team but used to indicate the issues that have arisen in that particular context.

Each case study concludes with a short section suggesting some ways in which readers might learn from the case studies to improve their own understanding of emerging issues in these complex interprofessional, multidisciplinary and interagency environments. The case studies are as follows.

Virtual Multidisciplinary Team

This team includes members of cancer service teams in a number of geographically remote settings who meet regularly through use of a video conference. Issues raised include difficulties in changing perspectives from former hierarchical relationships, formal and informal teamworking, introduction of new technology and frustrations over lack of funding.

Assertive Outreach Mental Health Team

This team includes staff from health and social care and focuses on working in the community with people who have serious mental health problems. Issues raised include tensions between this innovative service and traditional hospital services, inclusive teamworking with qualified and non-qualified staff, and difficulties in working within a regulatory framework that was developed for traditional provision.

Outpatients Referral Team

This is a widely dispersed team represented by a hospital manager, a service user representative and a General Practitioner. Issues raised include political and service user involvement in service development, tensions over funding priorities and the extent to which centres of excellence develop around expert staff rather than in response to local planning priorities.

Cancer Collaborative Network

This team are all members of this local collaborative arrangement but also of different service delivery teams. They are all working within a framework for improvement developed nationally by the Modernisation Agency within the Department of Health. Issues raised include use of facilitation, tools and techniques for effective continuous improvement within service provision, transition from traditional structures to partnership working and development of new flexible roles.

Reablement for Homecare Team

This team includes both social care and health staff and works in the community to support people who have been discharged from hospital, often with a reduction in ability, to care for themselves at home. Issues raised include strong views on the dangers of disempowering service users, practical difficulties in providing assistance when it is needed and tensions arising from balance of work in using expert and generic skills.

PART 3 – THEORY AND PRACTICE

Part 3 takes a wider view of the issues raised in the case studies and considers the extent to which existing theory can be applied to help us to understand change, leadership and teamworking in these complex settings. It concludes with some suggestions of areas in which it would be helpful to focus new research.

ACKNOWLEDGEMENTS

This book would not have been possible without the generosity of all the people who took part in the discussions and interviews reported. Although we cannot name people or organisations we thank all those who helped to produce this book. We hope that the book contributes to improvement of health and care services to benefit service users and the dedicated staff whose voices we hear in these case studies.

PART 1
INTRODUCTION

CHAPTER 1

LEADING INTERPROFESSIONAL TEAMS IN HEALTH AND SOCIAL CARE

Health and care services in the United Kingdom are delivered through a range of organisations, each of which operates with a degree of interdependence within a local healthcare economy. Service users want timely and effective services that improve their quality of life, organised in ways that make them easy to use. When these services are delivered by a number of different providers, people find themselves having to go to a series of different organisations and individuals, explaining their needs to each one and giving a range of personal information time after time. The focus of change in public services is on 'joining up' services to enable smooth pathways for service users. Barriers to working across agencies, across disciplines and across professions must be overcome. Leadership and teamworking are essential in order to design and develop new service configurations and new ways of working.

The goodwill and co-operation of the staff who work directly with patients and service users at a local level have reduced some of the barriers to seamless care. The best efforts of patient-focused staff, however, are frustrated by the hierarchical structures and bureaucratic processes that have contributed historically to the organisation and control of statutory public bodies in the United Kingdom. Attempts to improve public services seek to address this problem by encouraging the integration of previously separated services. The 'joining up' of public services is part of the political drive to modernise service provision.

The overriding aim of modernisation of public services is to reduce deprivation and social inequality in order to improve the health of individuals and of society as a whole. Instead of aiming to treat problems when they become apparent, a preventative approach seeks to improve the conditions in which people live so that ill-health and social need are reduced and, as far as possible, prevented.

If services are examined from the perspective of service users, the need for more seamless service provision becomes all too apparent. Both health and social care services have traditionally been provided by a variety of different public, private and voluntary agencies. The providing organisations differ considerably in size, capability, funding arrangements and the extent to which they are subject to public accountability. Whilst a number of these agencies operate under the overall umbrella of local government, many lie outside their jurisdiction, including National Health Service provision and the wide range of voluntary organisations. As a result, the allocation and disposition of resources to each of the contributory areas of service provision is subject to the accountability frameworks, funding regimes and operating practices of each of the 'providing' organisations. These features may be very different. It may require a great deal of leadership and teamwork to bring systems and processes together sufficiently closely to enable joint or partnership working to produce real benefits for the service user.

Demand for more coherence has been fuelled by highly publicised service failures, particularly incidents involving abuse of children or elderly people. In many of these cases, investigation revealed a need to cope with problems that exceeded the capacity of any one organisation or profession. Policy changes have contributed to increasing the need for care in the community through closure of the old-fashioned mental health institutional hospitals.

Health and care services are now required to consult more widely with citizens and to be more inclusive in involving local people in development of local services. This increasing involvement in decision-making has raised expectations of wider choice for service users. Alongside these developments, however, the increase in demand on resources threatens spiralling costs. Attempts to control costs inevitably include consideration of different approaches to managing service provision.

Modernising Social Services (Department of Health, 1998) detailed service failings in social care and set out an agenda that was intended to bring services up to the standards required. The paper emphasised the need to improve protection and services for children alongside improvement of workforce standards, partnership working and improvement of delivery and efficiency of service. The NHS Plan (Department of Health, 2000) detailed the government's plan for investment and reform that was intended to lead to staff working differently with more decision-making located in local health and care communities. It acknowledged that structural and cultural change would be required to align responsibilities at the local level and to enable resources to be devolved. The Health Act (Department of Health, 1999) took away legal obstacles for joint working across health and care public services by pooling budgets, supporting commissioning arrangements for partnership agencies and merging some services to provide a 'one-stop package of care'. Development of Primary Care Trusts provided for closer working at the most usual first point of contact for service users. Funding was targeted at improvement of quality and efficiency of care through development of services including rapid-response teams, intensive rehabilitation services, recuperation services, one-stop services for older people and integrated home care teams. Joint commissioning for mental health and services for older people was introduced to bring those services closer together.

The drive to modernise these services has placed particular emphasis on changing the ways in which services are configured. Reconfiguration involves linking service areas and different organisations to create easier access and smoother pathways for service users. When care provision crosses these traditional boundaries there are often difficulties in establishing new systems. These can result from a wide range of factors, including differences in pay scales, overhead charges, methods of calculating workloads and formal agreements over work practice. Different performance indicators may be in use leading partners to value (or have valued for them) different measures of what might be considered successful outcomes. In addition, professions in the health and care environment have different approaches to provision of care. There are often differences in cultures, values or in focus of service provision that make it difficult to make progress in partnership until enough common understanding and agreement has been established.

Social workers expect to engage in interagency working as a normal activity when they collaborate with others to achieve objectives for service users. Health professionals often focus on direct personal care or on delivery of a high-quality specialist service, even if this will only address one area of a service user's needs. There is, however, always a tension between maintaining the specialisms and developing a more holistic approach by accommodating the strengths brought by other professions.

Development of interprofessional education has attempted to address changing expectations:

> Interprofessional education has developed over the years ... It has worked to restore equilibrium as working relationships have been destabilised, the unquestioned authority once enjoyed by the established professions challenged, hierarchies flattened and demarcations blurred, as new professions have grown in influence, consumers have gained power and a better informed public has expected more.
>
> (Barr, 2002, pp.13–14)

Unfortunately, there is often a gap between the aspirations of a holistic and interprofessional approach to care developed in educational environments and the reality experienced by students in work placements. The workplace experience is often of a service under extreme pressure to deliver and without time or energy to be able to work in anything other than familiar and well-understood ways.

Ultimately, it is people, not organisations, that work together. People make partnerships work. Organisational leaders set the direction within which organisational partnerships can be formed.

Leaders and staff at all levels develop the interpersonal relationships that enable collaborative working. If people are to think and work in different ways they need to learn to do things differently. Government policies have acknowledged the need for learning throughout working lives (*Working Together, Learning Together*, Department of Health, 2001). This approach to lifelong learning was also supported by a Human Resource programme (Department of Health, 2002) which focused upon improving workforce planning, modernisation of training and education, modernisation of services and enhancement of staff skills to enable them to work differently. In order to achieve so much change, leadership is crucial:

> Leaders work with others to visualise how change could make an improvement, they create a climate in which the plans for change are developed and widely accepted and they stimulate action to achieve the change. Leaders who can work with others to achieve improvements are needed at all levels of health and care services. Leaders are needed to make the small day-to-day changes that ensure services continue to meet the changing needs of the communities they serve. Leaders are also needed to achieve the more dramatic step changes that have to be accomplished to change the direction or focus of services when new approaches are introduced.
>
> (Martin, 2003, p. 5)

Leaders are required to set a proactive agenda. They have a key role in developing a shared and compelling vision of better services and then aligning this vision with the direction and objectives of the organisation to clarify purpose and to enable strategies to be developed so that the desired change can be achieved. Leaders can develop the capacity of organisations to change and to work in partnership by negotiating to find ways of working across barriers.

Nothing now stands still for very long. Both theory and practice are constantly changing. Theory becomes out of date as new ideas and discoveries replace older theories. Practice also changes as new procedures and processes replace older ones in response to development in knowledge about the impact of people's actions. Individuals also have to change and develop practice to accommodate new technology and processes. The knowledge that informed actions five years ago might no longer be a sound basis for decisions today. In health and social care, professionals, clinicians and others, whose work is informed by traditional bodies of knowledge, are increasingly aware of the need for continuous personal development. High-quality services cannot be sustained unless health and care staff are consistently engaged in learning, individually and together.

PART 2
CASE STUDIES

CHAPTER 2

VIRTUAL MULTIDISCIPLINARY TEAM

INTRODUCTION

The Virtual Multidisciplinary Team has been established for about three years. It began as a project looking at the feasibility of using new technology to connect rural Trusts with other Trusts to overcome clinical and physical isolation.

This team was developed to conform with new guidelines for multidisciplinary teams for each type of cancer. The team uses video links to connect them to other organisations and to specialist centres. As the Trust deals with a wide range of referrals for cancer, other teams have developed in a similar fashion, often including some of the same staff but each with a lead clinician.

The use of this technology as a way of developing a multidisciplinary team has also provided the opportunity for the Trust to engage at a distance in conferences. Some of the team members comment on the potential they see for wider use of similar technology to improve services in future.

How the team works

The team has developed ways of working that facilitate decision-making in the meetings and have invested time in improving their practice. Most of the team members' activities take place in their normal practice teams and setting. Members of the virtual team are selected because of their roles and the view that this enables them to bring to the discussions.

Meetings are scheduled and the participating individuals prepare to ensure that time is not wasted. Sometimes quite a large number of people are involved. In this small rural Trust, the team usually meets in a room that is large enough to accommodate everybody physically but not large enough to allow the video camera to relay all of the participants visually. This results in the lead consultants appearing to communicate directly with other consultants and other members of the team claiming a presence only as voices if they contribute at all.

Many of the members of this team acknowledge that the use of video has brought advantages in various ways. There are, however, many frustrations and concerns amongst the participants. These are rarely connected with the use of technology, but almost always about how the ways of working within the Trust enable the specialist teams and this multidisciplinary team to provide a high quality of service. Many of the participants have experience in other settings and comment on the difficulties of moving from traditional service delivery into any new ways of working.

PERSPECTIVES FROM THE TEAM

Strategic planner

When I first came here the Trust was new and we had to develop a mission statement, a vision for the Trust and write our first strategic plan. So I was involved in all of that and became strategic planner so that included projects and funding.

My first involvement was as the project manager looking at the feasibility of using new technology in rural Trusts like ours to reach out to other Trusts in the UK to overcome geographic and clinical isolation. At the same time a new way of working was being introduced for cancer care. For every type of cancer, and they identified ten types, you had to have a multidisciplinary team within each Trust to collectively review every new patient referred to it. That was new for us because our teams don't just concentrate on one type of cancer. We link into specialist centres but to get people from those different sites to come together was virtually impossible. But it was a requirement, so we had to find a way to overcome it. The use of video conferencing was ideal for a place like this. We had commitment from the clinicians at both sites because they could see it was a practical solution to their problems. So my main involvement was finalising the local study, but then, at the end of it, there was no funding to implement all these wonderful ideas that we had.

Everybody began to feel quite let down, so we decided that we would write business cases and that was where I came in, writing them. We identified possible sources of funding and eventually caught the attention of a cancer and scanner appeal. They funded our equipment and somewhere to connect to. So that's how it started.

There was a set of minimum standards we had to follow and the first one was to set up a multidisciplinary team and to identify a lead clinician for that particular cancer type. So they became the nominated leader of each team but we also have an overall clinician responsible for cancer. We decided that we had the most referrals for three types of cancer, which were lung, colon/rectal and breast. So we established those teams first. The meetings just took off really. We went live, didn't test it. My involvement was making sure that the equipment was set up, that it worked on the day and that people knew how to use it. Also I had to work with members of the teams to sort of set up the etiquette of the meetings to make sure that people didn't interrupt each other, that the room was set out correctly and that everybody had a say on the day.

In a meeting like that certain people always dominate and often people interrupt each other. Because of the very slight delay in the video link, so fractional it's almost imperceptible, but if someone butts in they do take over. So we had to talk through where people were going wrong. The senior consultant was good too as he told members of the team off if they weren't acting correctly. Like a coaching session.

We have these sessions every so often because people tend to lapse into their old ways of working like everyone does, so have to be reminded of how to conduct the meeting. Often it is when we have an outsider watching or observing – like today when we had a link with a conference in London. There'll be hundreds of people there watching us and the senior clinician wants to make a good impression so he'll be there today to make sure. Straight afterwards we'll stay in the same room and we'll talk through how we thought we did.

Lots of the etiquette, as I call it, is about how the equipment is used. We now have a format. The lead clinicans should prepare a case history of each patient. Everybody has a list of the patients so we follow them through in the same order, everyone knows exactly who we're discussing so there should be no controversy. It follows a pattern where the lead clinician describes the patient's condition and the background. Then the pathologist talks about the histology and the radiologist talks about the X-rays and their findings. Then the members of the team will add what they've found. It's facilitated really by the members of the team. People just jump in usually. The camera should be a lot further away so they can see the whole team. It's often the specialist nurses who have a lot to say. It depends on personality. There's one nurse who's very confident and self-assured and always speaks up on behalf of the patient. Often she contradicts what the consultant said. She's very direct but he values her opinion – that's one of the benefits of this type of working.

One of the downsides is the time meetings take. They're booked through the year but if there aren't many patients referred they can cancel a meeting because they are frequent. Preparing for the meeting takes time. Often referrals come in a day or two before, so somebody, usually a medical secretary, formulates the list to give to a consultant the day before summarising the case histories, which puts pressure on the secretary. Then they have to make sure that the histology reports are ready. The pathologist tends to do this himself, going through all the slides to make reports and so do the radiologists.

Some people might feel it's not worth the time it takes because before a consultant would just have picked the phone up and spoken to someone in another hospital. But frequently the patient used to have to travel between the two sites. They'd go to a consultant there, who'd write a letter, then our consultant would review that and write a letter. So the patient suffered really because in a period of their life when they were quite ill they had to travel. They don't have to now as all the information can be transferred electronically, unless they need treatments we don't do here.

The composition of the teams has changed. With changing technology you get different people becoming important in the team. We have just introduced a new system here for radiology, digital imaging, and we have someone who started as a secretary who is now the manager. She can operate the computer and video conferencing equipment herself, so doesn't need a radiologist there. She draws the images from the network and displays them and can talk through what the report says.

We'll end up with more teams. There are more types of cancer that we're not covering at the moment. We have general practitioners coming into the hospital to provide those services. They need to have links with specialist centres as well, and they work in their surgeries, so that's another extension of this technology.

I like this work, new technology, setting up projects and new ways of working. On technical stuff they always come to me. They seem to depend on me but they know what to do. I find they communicate very well with me, they always make sure that I'm made aware of everything. Not just their problems, but what's going well. They know they can always call on me. People come to me because I can often get them the funding to expand their service. I've just managed to secure about eight thousand pounds for a new microscope and another camera for our postgraduate centre.

Radiologist

The team started before I came. The senior consultant inspired it – he went to America and saw this happening. I got interested because of applications of telemedicine in radiology – that will happen in a big way in a year or two.

Video conferencing could always be done better. You shouldn't meet people for the first time on video – you should eyeball people first, it's not ideal on a television screen. You get to know them by seeing them every week on the square box but it would be better to travel down there to meet the first time. It works reasonably well. Improves the quality of the meeting because you have folks there you wouldn't normally have. All the people in the room probably meet every day in the coffee room or we would see them in the corridor, talk about cases – you know those people well.

If I was talking about an investigation I might say all the evidence is here, we know what to do, or I might say shouldn't we be doing this or that. It's not my role to make any decisions. These meetings are to make decisions about patient management. The person with responsibility should make the decisions.

I think video conferencing is a good thing – though people say that it doesn't really alter very much about what they're going to do because the next course is fairly obvious. So why are we doing this politically correct thing, sitting round consulting with everybody when we know what we're going to do anyway? I think the patients would probably be reassured if they knew. The decisions are taken seriously and thought about. On the whole, although people groan about it, it is a good thing. Part of it is playing the game but partly also because they know it's quite a good thing. A few technical things would make it snappier and smoother. More time to prepare, more dynamic in some way.

I worry about patients who don't want to be fitted into this system. The people managing the health service want to be in charge. To take over from medical people and control them more. They think it can be better managed, more value for money. The people who are most resistant will retire, so these ideas will have to gain more purchase as new people come in. I think a lot of things are quite positive. We treat patients much better than we used to but because of the costs, the whole system is not being pushed in the right direction. Change is constant, change is accelerating. In the NHS you can't assume that everyone will agree with your ideas or assume good will – or it will almost always all end in tears – you somehow have to be prepared for that change.

I once sat for ages on a committee that looked at medical complaints and the most striking thing about it, so constant it was unbelievable – it was to redress a sense of grievance. Always about not being told, not knowing to expect something. Most people did not want money. Most said that if it could possibly be avoided, I don't want this repeated. Staff are not daft, they know things are changing and things will be different. They accept that. What they don't accept is that no-one will talk to them about it. It's easy to say but not easy to do.

Chemotherapy nurse

I haven't got a degree but don't have burning issues about it being needed. In clinical work, how you perform is how you learn and improve on yourself. Working as a team you get a chance to learn from colleagues on a clinical basis.

When I worked in London it was very much more relaxed, we were seen as equals, were seen as a team, introduced ourselves as a team, nurses, doctors, occupational therapists, physiotherapists. Patients would be with us for twelve months or so. They would get to know us as nurses, as doctors, the whole team. We had a family environment and carers wanted to be seen as part of that family. Doctors were called by their first names, nurses were all called by their first names. It was the first time I came across a consultant who said, 'I'm Jack', not Doctor something. It was a multidisciplinary team where we'd have an afternoon each week and talk about individual people. Our plans, our fears, how we were going to deal with it ourselves, how the families were going to deal with it, where we'd go from there, who else we'd need to involve, whatever.

I came here and we've tried to have multidisciplinary meetings but it hasn't been successful due to time constraints, lack of resources. I wondered whether it was because we're a small unit, only the one consultant. However, with the video link it has taken off. People are making more of an effort. Consultants are there and find it quite comforting, reassuring, to have a colleague on the other side of the link that they can talk to.

For me personally, it's made people aware of me and who I am, the chemo nurse. I know that people know who to phone. Before I don't think people were aware. I like the fact that I know all the consultants and can phone them up myself. I know deep down that if I were to phone one and say we have a problem with one of the patients, they'd take me seriously and deal with it. I phoned one this morning and he came immediately. He knows me, he trusts my judgement and we're more on the same level. The barriers that have been built up over the years between nurses and doctors are going. The older I get there will be consultants the same age as me, that helps. You feel more like a contemporary, remember the same things, schools, holidays.

In the multidisciplinary team the consultant knows that if he's not there I'm there and will pick up the referrals and plan. It's very helpful when it works well. What doesn't work is that sometimes we discuss people when we're not ready to discuss them – but they're just administration problems really. We can be a bit too keen to decide treatments – treatments that haven't been discussed with the patient.

What I do find a bit annoying is that with one group I go to we discuss the patients with one hospital but they get referred to another. So I get no benefit because I don't know what treatment that person's going to have, so we waste time and discuss things that aren't appropriate. The consultant writes and says this is what I advise, the next one discusses it with another, so we're going round and round in circles. Once the referrals are made we don't need to discuss it all again in the multidisciplinary team.

The consultants quite like to chat, it's like going to a conference for them. But for me it's valuable time, time that I'm taken off giving treatments. I haven't got anybody to fill my shoes in, I can't cancel clinics. I have to build this into my daily work. We're a nurse led unit. The consultant is here as support but when he's away he doesn't have someone to deputise for him. We have to be confident in what we do, knowledgeable in what we do. We have to give patients support and for them to have faith in us.

But innovations, there's lots of them, it's nice to see people that are still innovative. It's nice to go to conferences, see people. There's lots of ideas but it's finding the time, the energy to do it. You come in and do more than your paid hours each day, then it's difficult to build new things up. We like to be seen as a happening kind of place. We do our bit. One of the nurses does aromatherapy and she and the art therapist have set up a group that look at alternative therapies and how they can be of help and benefit to people in the community. Hoping to get any patient, or carers, who might benefit to try. Things have been a bit slow getting off the ground but that would be an innovation.

Sometimes I find the multidisciplinary team meetings quite useless because we don't come to a decision. If I give two hours every fortnight I want a decision – not all that wasted chit chat. I'd rather be back on the shop floor doing some good. You can't waste time in meetings all day, sounding boards for people to talk, talk, talk. Life's not like that any more. The NHS has changed. It's hard. We haven't got this time, we are pushed for beds, patients coming in all the time, out of our ears …

Consultant surgeon

I lead a team in cancer management. The thing that I find, certainly in terms of the multidisciplinary side of things, is that you generally divide the decision-making, almost as though there is strength in numbers. I think that's not necessarily a good thing – at some point, someone's got to say, thanks for this, thanks for that, what we're going to do is that.

There might be a patient who is not of sufficient performance status to have a particular form of chemotherapy. That decision might have been made, but alternatively, that decision might have been made in the referral clinic. So the team makes a collective decision. But I would have referred this patient for their opinions before treatment. It is checks and balances, but against that you have to put the time involved in doing it. The patient care I've no objection to at all, but I find complying with the administration absolutely irritating. For example, all patients have to be considered – that's not a problem. All multidisciplinary team decisions have to be written in the notes, but then when you have to audit it to find your evidence there's a problem. There's a tail to all the lists that's extremely annoying. If you then base your hospital comparitors essentially on the administrative criteria, there's no clinical outcome measure, which I find extraordinary. There are administrative outcome measures, but no clinical outcome measures. I'd be looking for survival and quality of life – but these seem to be purely administrative standards.

This multidisciplinary team really just puts into a managerial context what I've been doing for a long time. This way of working is fine as long as you've got everybody believing in it, everybody participating. I have no-one to discuss things with surgically, no histologists, but we use protocols so that everybody with these particular conditions gets these things. It would be nice to have colleagues to say think about this or look at this. Whether it's a good interchange of ideas I'm not absolutely sure. Whether it's putting patients on a production line. But the resource cost of having a proper meeting would be enormous. If you take the hospital as a hub and the various spokes there would be a lot of meetings. I think that it is wrong to discuss every patient, I think you should discuss exceptions. I think that these standards should be looked at again from what's happening. This presupposes that in the old days we didn't have meetings – we did. This undercuts and standardises. How would I do it better? The first thing I would do is discuss patients by exception. Many are routine. There are one or two a month perhaps where there would be benefit. If I led the team I'd say there's no need to discuss the others. We should look much more at the technical priorities. Breast-screening, for example. Most people who look critically at the literature say that it's a complete waste of money. But women vote, no politician is going to stop it. You should screen for bowel cancer to find pre-cancerous conditions.

I can just battle on until someone takes notice. I think that the command model of the army works much better than NHS. My personal satisfaction is in the clinical side – I should be left to get on with it. It would be good if someone came and said you had a problem in theatre yesterday, how can I help? This won't happen. It's resources. They're so terrified of the possible waste of resources that they won't allow people to make decisions. Multidisciplinary teams spread the decision collectively so they can't be wrong. It would be difficult to sue the whole team. It's a comfort zone – everyone shares the blame.

A while ago our audio-visual system was awful. I decided to get it upgraded – I just did it. We got half the money from the postgraduate dean then the Trust paid for the other half. They didn't like it but it got done. I also made the decision to get operating lights here and went out and raised money – the Trust agreed to pay to have them fitted if I paid for them. It just wasn't a priority for them.

The boundaries are very blurry. I always get the impression that the management is an obstacle, albeit not for their own fault. To me it is a complete anachronism that there are not enough nurses. We don't pay enough. I said, 'Get a crèche.' They said, 'There's nowhere to put it and you'd have to get someone in qualified to manage it.' I gave up on that – choose your battle! Be prepared to make yourself such a nuisance that it's easier to agree with you than not to.

Macmillan nurse

When we first started as Macmillan nurses they saw us as able to do anything. The difference I found was the community side. The multidisciplinary meetings have brought the team much closer, helped to build relationships. Prior to those meetings we didn't have any regular contact.

It meant the consultant having to shift his work schedule round to come earlier to fit in this meeting so that he could do his clinic and then have the meeting. Those meetings were good, we all got to talk a lot more because with the technology the background noise means you can hear what's going on so you have to be very quiet. A lot of the early video ones people would say they couldn't hear. We've had lots of feedback with people going and sitting in at the other end. It's bad enough just with the traffic. In both cases, they have delivery lorries and on many occasions we've heard lorries backing. Also it has to be very rapid, you have to get through a large number of people at a time, so it had to be honed as much as possible. I don't feel as though I should be giving any sort of opinion – it feels like information-gathering.

The team leaders are each of the lead clinicians from each cancer type. They set the agenda. It's about direction rather than day to day or a particular meeting. A sort of agreed agenda, taking you along. On the team there are the chemo nurses and consultant, the surgical team, consultant and the stoma nurse. She gets us involved very much earlier because she feels she hasn't got the counselling skills for social problems, how they'll get home, etc. We lack direction at the moment – everyone's doing their own little bit, no-one's pulling it together. We've got to keep reminding people that we're here. I like to think that I can get certain things sorted out for patients, make things better for them.

Clinical trials nurse

I'm a research nurse, but because I'm the only one here and they wanted to develop the clinical trials area here, I was given this title. I've been here seven months. I used to work for a charity with general practice research. Coming back to hospitals was quite a shock. Leadership had changed. The multidisciplinary team – I had no idea what it was until I came here. In the loose sense of the word, we all work in multidisciplinary teams, with different grades of staff and different disciplines, we learn to do that anyway, but to have a set multidisciplinary team that meets regularly and communicates with other hospitals was new. I think it's better, because you know who everybody is and what their roles are, much more organised.

The purpose of video conferencing is for the consultants to discuss cases. It's the way it's always been. Consultants have a case load of patients and take responsibility for them. Sometimes people feel that we meet as a matter of keeping up targets and keeping up figures. We have multidisciplinary team meetings with the main regional hospital every week, then with others every other Friday and Tuesday. Some people feel that it's doing it for the sake of doing it, to keep the powers that be happy. I find it quite useful because I work on my own and don't have anybody to talk things through with. You also get a sense of what happens to the patients that you'd miss if you didn't have the meeting. I am a little bit out from the rest of the team, although I liaise with them. The rest of the team treat the patient, I don't. But if I get to hear, in the multidisciplinary team, of a patient receiving treatment who might be suitable for a trial, I approach them.

I like talking to patients, doing paperwork and mixing with others in the hospital. I miss working as part of a research team. I read but if you can talk it through with someone you understand it better. I learn about new treatments from journals – but you can't buy a journal every week.

PERSPECTIVES ON CHANGE IN HEALTH AND SOCIAL CARE

We have extracted from the individual interviews some of the team's views on change in health and care, teamworking and leadership to discuss in this and the following sections.

This team came together through use of new communications technology that enabled video conferencing. This team see themselves as pioneering use of this technology and are particularly aware of changes that new technology might bring to service delivery. They are also very much aware of the difficulties of introducing such change. In this range of perspectives about change in health and social care they raise a wide range of issues, few of which are related to learning how to use new technology. Although recognising advantages that new technology might bring, this team has a strong sense of historical tradition and its potential to smother change.

In Example 2.1 some of the vision for use of technology in service improvement is expressed, together with disappointment that adequate funding is not necessarily provided to enable such innovations to be introduced.

Example 2.1
How new technology can enable change in service delivery

The use of new technology has been recognised now so appears in every policy document. With a small amount of money we could restructure to change the way the A&E department works. The equipment we need costs about forty thousand pounds, which really isn't a huge amount. That would mean we could take calls from all the peripheral community hospitals with minor injury units, to review cases before they're transferred here to see if we can provide advice and guidance instead of transferring patients here physically. They may not need to be admitted here then. Likewise we could then link with our specialist centre for head injuries before we transfer patients. Video technology again.

I have this vision about how we could change the whole way in which the hospital works. We'd have to have enough input financially and then a change in attitude, particularly in some of the older consultants. We're moving towards it anyway because we have this new digital imaging system being installed this month that means that people will be able to view X-rays on their desk-top. So if we convince all consultants that it's worthwhile in their consulting rooms, they wouldn't have to wait for a written report about an X-ray. They'd be able to have it on their screen with the report alongside and show the patient. Involve the patient in discussion about their treatment options instead of telling them what they've decided. That's a big change.

It takes time and focused attention to develop a workforce able to make effective use of new technology. Although there is so much potential for use of new technology to enable improvement in service delivery, some staff only see it as a personal tool that they might choose not to use. In Example 2.2 we are reminded that many senior professionals have not necessarily learnt to be comfortable and confident in using computers.

Example 2.2
Attitudes and skills in using technology

The technology offers the opportunity for instant results and to include the patient. That's the key, otherwise we're just using technology to speed things up for staff, for their convenience. For example, the radiologist accesses things from home. But some of the consultants don't want these computers. They still dictate letters and give them to their secretary and write a list of points for a secretary to deal with. They don't take any responsibility to do these things themselves.

There is also a fear that in rapid change, some of the good practice that has built up over years will be lost. There is a perceived tension between the need to provide cost-effective services without forcing service users into predetermined slots through stereotyping. This is discussed in Example 2.3.

Example 2.3
Everyone is different

I think that we're losing the element of wise counsel really, part of treating people in the right way. Each person is absolutely unique, so they don't fit well into systems. Everyone is different. What is appropriate treatment for one person might be completely wrong for the next person. Medicine run by ever stricter protocols has its limitations. We've made huge strides in treating people, but don't start stereotyping.

Attempts to standardise services so that service users can expect similar treatments wherever they happen to live may make it more difficult to respond to the essentially personal and individual nature of heath and illness. This theme emerges in various accounts, but Example 2.4 comments on the nature of change but also raises issues about the relationship between education and practice. The suggestion is that if a new generation of practitioners are developed with expectations of new types of roles, these will quickly become the norm in practice settings. Professional education is only partially provided in academic settings and practice is developed within contemporary practice settings. If the philosophies, values and attitudes do not align, student professionals will be very much aware of that through their reflection on experience. It is unlikely that significant change can be achieved without the full engagement of those working in the service workplace.

Example 2.4
Change of power structure

The power structure that was totally outrageous in the past is being dismantled slowly in the NHS, so that doctors are being taken right off the top of the pyramid. They are becoming more specialised. Increasingly patients are slotted into a particular straitjacket – if you have a stroke, this is the way that strokes are managed. It's not a case of individual medical opinion which could be capricious at the best of times. Everything is done more to protocol. There's much more involvement of nurses. Probably doctors will be far less highly trained, nurses better trained – all changes hugely resisted by medical people, but people who train in that new system won't know anything else.

Roles in health and social care have frequently changed. Many new professions and specialisms have been developed. Although expertise is important, service users often need to use a sequence of service provision and expect much of that provision to be geographically close to their homes. Even in densely populated urban areas it is not easy to appoint staff with an appropriate mix of specialised and generic skills. Recent initiatives to introduce more flexible roles and workers with more flexible skills have raised a number of issues, some of which are discussed in Example 2.5.

Example 2.5
Change in roles

The role of nursing staff is developing and in all of the other professions you're having changes. For example, radiography are now taking on an enhanced role. There are fewer radiologists because they're so specialised. So the radiographer's role is changing as a result. They're taking on a lot of things because there's no radiologist. And below that we're having new levels of staff coming in with different supporting skills and often with interdisciplinary skills as well. Usually support workers support more than one area – radiography assistants don't only have to just work in radiography, they can work across different disciplines. Therapies too – occupational therapy helpers can also do physiotherapy and speech therapy, a bit of everything. A good interdisciplinary worker needs initiative, and an 'OK' attitude. Sometimes people hide behind their profession as though it's their whole identity – I'm a radiographer, I'm a nurse – but it's starting to blur.

There is a possibility that in developing more flexible roles for health professionals they become less involved in using their expert skills. In Example 2.6 a nurse comments on how the nursing role has changed and how she thinks this has impacted on the quality of patient care. She is particularly concerned that nurses are not in close enough contact with patients to use their specialist skills. This example raises questions about the extent to which we want nurses to have generic and flexible skills and which expert skills they should have.

Example 2.6
What do we want nurses to do?

When I trained as a nurse, we were trained to take care of people. Nowadays, nurses go to university and learn how to write about how to look after people, not the hands-on stuff about how to do it. You look around here and the trained nurses don't do any of the physical care. They're running around with drugs lists and care plans but you don't see one doing a bed bath. The care assistants do the caring now. I'm not saying they don't give good care, they do. But they're not trained to notice certain things, like a bit of facial droop.

In Example 2.7 another nurse is concerned about the impact that changes in both nurse education and practice have had on aspects of the service. She suggests that the wider education necessary for nurses to be able to take more specialised roles has created a gap in the practical activity of giving care to patients when they are unable to care for themselves.

Example 2.7
Quality of care

I think patients are probably getting less care than they did. I had a private operation a few years ago and the care was fantastic. When I trained that was the care that everyone was entitled to. When you've had an op you want to get out of the gown that has blood on it – in the NHS you don't get that now. You have to wait for a relative to come in and change you. A friend I trained with did a return to nursing course. We assumed you'd update skills and and treatments, but all she did was learn about hospital policies. Then people get on the wards, find they can't do it and leave.

When new roles are introduced, there may be difficulties in using new specialist skills to work differently if the ways in which work is organised are not reviewed. Example 2.8 comments on the strength of old traditions in describing how an exclusive team could be built around an individual consultant.

Example 2.8

Who do nurses 'belong' to?

There was a feeling that you're a specialist nurse with that consultant, his handmaiden. So you go and work with his patients and don't have anything to do with other patients even if they desperately needed our skills. We needed to break down those old taboos. Macmillan nurses were always intended to be available for any palliative condition throughout the Trust. We belonged as much to the General Practitioners as to any consultant.

Some new roles have been developed with the intention of contributing specialist skills wherever they are needed. An example of this type of role is the Macmillan nurse, whose skills are in palliative care and intended to support any individuals with a terminal illness and their carers. It is not always easy to introduce this type of service into existing frameworks where each service area feels ownership of its own patients. Example 2.9 gives an account of one type of problem encountered.

Example 2.9

Making new services available to service users

We've had problems getting patients referred to us early enough. The ward and chemo nurses felt that they didn't need us earlier, that there was nothing of value we could put in. We felt that we were picking up pieces too far down the line. That wasn't good for the patient themselves but was particularly hard when you were supporting a bereaved person afterwards because they felt that there were so many unresolved issues, lots of things that hadn't been discussed.

Some members of staff thought that we should be involved earlier, but one senior person was vetoing them. She couldn't justify why she was keeping ownership of her patients and not handing them on and eventually backed down. She said that the patients didn't ask for the service, so there wasn't any need. But we should be offering the service, not waiting for them to ask for a service they probably don't know exists. When that was put to her she suddenly realised that she had got a role in referring patients to us. We still have the odd hiccup but most of the time now, it's fine.

Many of the new specialist roles that nurses are taking are proving very successful, but there is still often difficulty in finding appropriate funding to resource different types of staff. Example 2.10 describes how specialist nurses can provide effective leadership and management to take on a very senior role.

Example 2.10
New types of nurses

We're constantly fighting for resources for new types of nurses, so they can take on these specialised roles. We have hospital practitioners who really run things at night. They're really more skilled than junior doctors. They work with all disciplines within the hospital and liaise with GPs and the ambulance service too. They have a huge role and they are leaders in their own right. Their authority must come from the respect they command. We work long shifts and then hand over to them. I can go home and don't have to worry at all. I used to take lots of calls from junior staff because they had no-one else to refer to. Hospital practitioners feel that they are in command. They are the most senior operational manager on site and if they have a problem they go straight to the executive team.

Nurses may also find themselves directly involved with trying to secure resources to support their area of service. In Example 2.11 a nurse explains her involvement in fund-raising. We might be concerned about how much of a nurse's time should be spent in securing the funding to provide premises and equipment.

Example 2.11
A nurse-led improvement

We've put in a bid for some money to have the two portacabins out in the car park knocked down and have our own palliative care building there. We went to a session where people from the Opportunities Fund were describing what this money was and what it could be used for. We kept thinking we can't apply for this – we don't fulfil their criteria. It was all about refurbishing things that you'd already got – but our portacabin wasn't fit to be refurbished. It leaks and you can't get a wheelchair in there, so it just wasn't feasible.

We set up a meeting. We've got an art therapist and an occupational therapist and invited one of the chemo girls and the ward sister, so brought them on board and the consultant. We talked about what we actually want, what is feasible and whether we could apply. One of the managers knew how to set about tackling the bid, how to put it in the right language and set it out. The head of works in the Trust also came to a session. We heard last week that we've got the money! And just through a chance phone call the local Rotary Club are raising money to equip that building. A lot of our work now is going out and promoting this.

In Example 2.12 there is a discussion about how change can be carried out. It is acknowledged that change can be enforced, but it is suggested that if people understand the need for change they will co-operate much more readily.

Example 2.12
It works because people want it to

This team works because everyone, by and large, wants it to. Things either work because they're enforced through totalitarian structures or because people want them to. Consultants have traditionally been totally independent. Traditionally you couldn't push them into any straitjacket, you could only coax and lead and get their assent to do things. It is less so now. The coaxing and encouraging is still necessary – particularly about the need to consult. The structures are all worked out but it still relies on people seeing the need and wanting to do it.

When a number of specialists are involved in contributing to decisions about treatment, as in a multidisciplinary team, the decision is no longer made by one consultant in isolation. Different or conflicting views may be expressed and opinions are potentially open to challenge. This is a very different environment for those used to taking decisions without wider discussion. Example 2.13 comments that it is helpful to review each case on the basis of the evidence that is presented because different views can be shared in reaching a decision.

Example 2.13
Evidence as a basis for decision-making

It's becoming less common now, but someone from the old school type wouldn't want to hear any other opinion. They would just make the decisions whatever anyone else said or whatever the circumstances. But it's a much tougher world out there now and people are wanting to share the burden more, to receive ideas and other people's opinions as well as their own to make decisions. Although there are different opinions, it seems to gel fairly quickly and having seen the evidence people almost always agree.

An evidence-based approach to decision-making facilitates consideration of more than one perspective. In Example 2.14 there is agreement that the multidisciplinary approach can improve the experience of service users but a suggestion that the benefits may only provide an improvement in the experience of treatment but not in the outcomes. When there is a strong policy drive to change practice in order to achieve proposed benefits, it is important to ensure that appropriate measures are in place to confirm whether or not the new ways of working are bringing the anticipated benefits.

Example 2.14 ▬▬▬▬▬▬▬▬▬▬▬▬▬▬▬▬▬
Process and outcomes

We're more aware of what we each do in the clinical management of these patients, so it does improve standards. My general impression is that it does improve quality of life. Patients may feel a hell of a lot better, but may not survive longer. This is something that we want to look at, but there's no way of doing this at the moment within the multidisciplinary team system. Clinical outcome is very difficult to measure – it is easier to look at how many times, etc. We should be making the important things measurable, not just measuring what is easy.

When staff are working in multidisciplinary teams it is difficult for them to contribute if they feel subordinate to others who they believe, or are expected to believe, have a greater right to voice an opinion. In Example 2.15 a nurse explains how she has experienced changes that have brought her greater respect.

Example 2.15 ▬▬▬▬▬▬▬▬▬▬▬▬▬▬▬▬▬
Hierarchies and equality

Years ago when I first started nursing, nurses were here, doctors, even junior doctors, were above. The ethos was very much nurses would run around after a doctor, set trolley, do everything for them, even wipe their noses. Throughout my training I thought, OK, this is how life is going to be. But as I became older, more confident, knew more, I thought this isn't how I want to be treated, or to treat them. They were predominantly men. There were a few of us at the time, young nurses who were qualifying and getting sisters' posts. Things changed. We fought to be seen as an equal.

Changes of attitude do not necessarily happen quickly or involve everyone at the same time in any particular context. Not everyone believes that multidisciplinary team approaches have made a difference. One of the nurses commented, 'The buck does stop with the consultant. At the end of the day, the consultant will say that's what I want and he'll find someone else to do it if necessary.' So that even if a nurse challenges a consultant the concern might be ignored or overridden.

We have heard about the increasing range of roles that some staff are encouraged to take. We have also heard about the increase in monitoring, recording and other administrative systems. Many staff experience an increasing workload and sometimes feel overwhelmed by pressure of work. Some staff feel exhausted and have no energy to innovate or engage in change. In Example 2.16 one of this team explains how she feels.

Example 2.16 ▬▬▬▬▬▬▬▬
No energy to be innovative

I always used to think I was innovative, but the unfortunate thing now is pressure of work seems to have sucked out every spare bit of energy I have. I feel so demoralised, and I think a lot of my colleagues feel the same. I want more staff, a better unit. We're dealing with a hundred people a month in that small room and trying to give a good service to people who are suffering terribly. That's my experience. We do work very hard but we're expected to work with such constraints that it's unfair. And you know that there aren't going to be any changes however loud you shout or stamp your feet, so you do sometimes lose a bit of hope, faith, whatever.

PERSPECTIVES ON TEAMWORKING

In Example 2.17 one of the key benefits of working in a multidisciplinary team is described as the potential to take a holistic view of the patient. To consider an individual with a personality and a lifestyle rather than treating a condition as though bodies are all the same.

Example 2.17 ▬▬▬▬▬▬▬▬
Building the holistic approach

It works well when each patient being discussed is known. Consultants need to know their age, diagnosis, past history, the scan, histology results. We also need to know how the person feels. That's where the nurse comes in. The doctors might steam ahead and say that's surgery, or agree, yes that's a chemotherapy regime. We might say, hold on a bit here, she's not quite ready, there are family problems, or he's elderly, they're weak or cannot cope. That's the part we contribute to, so we have a whole picture, see it holistically.

Over the years we haven't been seeing people as a whole, especially doctors. They have seen people in beds. They haven't been thinking of the family, their social or financial background, their networks, that kind of thing. We are starting to see the person as a whole and thinking, chemo, radiotherapy, surgery? Is that the best? As specialist nurses you know that if you speak out you're going to have some support from somewhere. With doctors you do get some who're gung-ho but you'll have someone who'll say let's slow things down a bit, consider this type of treatment. So you get the best.

Those who are used to making decisions alone, however, may find it frustrating to be asked to consider other opinions. In Example 2.18 we hear from a team member who thinks that taking time to consider a range of opinions has the potential to cause damage by delaying treatment.

Example 2.18 ■━━━━━━━━━━━━━━━━━━━━━━━━━━━━
Decision-making in a multidisciplinary team

One problem with multidiscipline is that although it contributes a lot of different opinions it will still take someone to make the required decision. This may dilute the surgeon's role, which has, by necessity, to be relatively decisive. This is one of the drawbacks because although you have the reassurance of a multidisciplinary team it takes the decision-making out of your hands. If you use the multidisciplinary team as a decision-making forum, then you can, by definition, delay treatment.

If the multidisciplinary team does not have the ability to make decisions together it is difficult to see what benefits could be gained. In Example 2.19 a team member explains how the process challenges decisions that might have been made by a consultant who is prejudiced against or favours particular types of intervention.

Example 2.19 ■━━━━━━━━━━━━━━━━━━━━━━━━━━━━
Consideration of a wider range of options

One advantage of the multidisciplinary team is that the safety net is much bigger. There's less chance that you might forget to refer patients on and it gives you protocols and guidelines to work to. So it would stop a surgeon who would never refer patients to chemotherapy or radiotherapy because they didn't believe it was beneficial or effective. Within the multidisciplinary team that's less likely to occur.

We might hope that evidence of successful clinical outcomes also influences judgements about treatment. This raises issues about how staff in isolated settings can keep up to date. The interdisciplinary team meetings offer an opportunity for peer review that is not usually possible in smaller, isolated organisations. As we see in Example 2.20 the review of each case does raise the question of which treatment is currently considered to be most effective. As there are different costs involved in different treatments, this discussion may also raise difficult issues regarding what is valued when we use the term 'value for money'.

Example 2.20 ■━━━━━━━━━━━━━━━━━━━━━━━━━━━━
The benefits of peer review

They may cast doubts about what each other should or should not have done. It's very rare to hear doctors challenging in front of other people. One of our consultants was criticised for choosing a low-cost treatment option. They were horrified that we would consider cost as a factor. Our consultants said it was value for money as the treatment's well tried and tested. They said that there are far better treatment options, although at a cost. The patient's outcome is of paramount importance so they changed the treatment. The consultant is usually very pleased. He'll change his practice because of that. It's like peer review really – it would never have happened before.

One of the nurses confirmed in Example 2.21 that she saw a particular benefit for consultants in the peer review aspects of the team because nurses tend to already have those benefits in teamworking in their everyday areas of practice.

Example 2.21
Working in peer groups

Sometimes consultants feel quite isolated here. For nurses it's different. We've got a huge team, we're used to that kind of camaraderie, support, saying I'm out on a limb here, I don't know what I'm doing, can you help? I think consultants don't like to say hey, I don't know what to do. However, they've got a compatriot down there and they find it useful. Doctors find it more useful than I do personally.

Another nurse talked in Example 2.22 about how she constantly learnt through teamworking – but in her professional groups rather than in the multidisciplinary team. It is also interesting in this example that she mentions including the patient in discussing treatment options. Although there is an increasing emphasis in national policy on including service users in decision-making about their own use of services and development of services, this has rarely been mentioned in connection with this multidisciplinary team's activities.

Example 2.22
Learning in practice

Sharing experience, that is how we learn, that is how we improve. If something's not happening, I stop and I do it another way. If there's something I don't know I read up, I discuss it with colleagues, I phone colleagues. Having meetings is important, discussing with contemporaries is important, keeping updated is important. If somebody is having a treatment and I thought it wasn't doing them any favours, we'd discuss it with the other nurses and then we'd go to the consultant and he'd come along and we'd make a decision with the patient being involved.

The virtual meeting arrangements involve a number of people sitting around a table with their video connection to one or more other Trusts. The equipment and lay-out only allow, however, for a small number of people to be visible on the video link. The people who are always visible are the consultants. The nurses are never visible although their voices can be heard if they speak. In Example 2.23 one of the nurses commented that she felt this was disempowering.

Example 2.23 ▬▬▬▬▬▬▬▬▬▬▬▬▬▬▬▬▬▬▬▬
The power of visibility

Nurses don't count you see. I didn't say that. Historically consultants have always been god, have taken the lead. It's our fault in a way. Nurses don't sit in front of the camera in the multidisciplinary team. The three chairs that are for the surgeons, the consultants who sit at the top of the table, so the rest of us don't get seen. What is there to say? The kinds of thing that we as nurses would say about a patient would not be very interesting to the consultant on the other end of the video. He's not going to want to know if the patient is happy with their treatment or if the patient's got problems at home, or things like that. They just want to treat people, don't they? They're not interested in the whole person like nurses are.

In Example 2.24 one of the nurses comments that they do contribute to the team meetings, but only when the discussion touches either on their specialist areas or concerns a patient with whom they are working.

Example 2.24 ▬▬▬▬▬▬▬▬▬▬▬▬▬▬▬▬▬▬▬▬
When we contribute to the team

There are times when we feel like we're probably closer to the patients. Things will crop up that are particularly about palliative care and we can take a lead in those. The chemo girls will put in their bit about chemo. When it impinges on us or the patients we're seeing then we will say.

The extent to which visibility empowers or disempowers individuals may be less important than attitude. In Example 2.25 a medical secretary, who might in a hierarchical setting be considered as having less of a voice than a health professional, is able to make challenging contributions whilst others disengage themselves from the proceedings.

Example 2.25 ▬▬▬▬▬▬▬▬▬▬▬▬▬▬▬▬▬▬▬▬
Choosing to be involved

The medical secretaries are always invited to the meetings. There's one medical secretary who will always speak out. She'll say, 'I spoke to that lady on the phone and she didn't tell me that,' so she'll certainly contradict people. Another secretary says she falls asleep, it's so boring for her.

One aspect of developing a team involves sharing humour. In Example 2.26 a problem is presented as a joke. In services that focus on delivering one particular type of treatment there is a danger that everything will be seen from that single perspective. This might lead to the possibility of other causes or other conditions being overlooked.

Example 2.26
Some truth in an old joke

There's an old joke that the worst place to get appendicitis is in a hospital, on the wrong ward, because nobody will think of it. They'll go off on the condition they're focused on because it's getting much more specialised and concentrating more on the specifics of an illness, without the causes of illness. The mental and spiritual, the cultural causes; there's a massive number of things related to why people get sick or are perceived to be sick.

Jokes of this type can be a difficult issue in a multidisciplinary setting as each contributing discipline or professional group may have different attitudes towards what they consider to be humorous. In very stressful work, which includes many areas of work in health and social care, teams sometimes use 'black' humour to find a funny side to tragic conditions that might otherwise overwhelm them. This sort of humour is often tolerated within a team because its therapeutic purpose is understood and shared, but it can be considered offensive to anyone whose work area is different. In Example 2.27 this type of humour is cited as a reason for not involving patients in the meetings when they are being discussed.

Example 2.27
Talking about patients

We still haven't involved patients directly in the meetings. It wouldn't really be right because they're being discussed in detail. Each of the teams has its own individual character and they all operate in slightly different ways. Sometimes they become quite light hearted which I find quite offensive really, when they could be joking about patients with cancer – but it's part of the way that they deal with things.

With increasing emphasis on involvement of service users in decisions about their treatment and about service development, we might expect consideration to be given to use of this type of technology to include individual patients in a conference at appropriate times, even if that does mean that black humour has to be avoided.

Some practical suggestions to consider if virtual multidisciplinary teamworking is to be effective are outlined in Example 2.28.

Example 2.28
Factors that facilitate virtual multidisciplinary teamworking

You definitely need a focal point. For clinical teams you need a clinical champion who will support the whole process and not let go, always be there. To motivate people, bring them together, co-ordinate and control the whole clinical side of things. You don't need IT support because it's just communications and anybody can learn how to use it. You need a trainer and troubleshooter. But you need someone to be a catalyst. To make sure that it, and the equipment, is up and running. You also need someone with the authority to get people into the room.

PERSPECTIVES ON LEADERSHIP

Several members of this team commented on both leadership and management, implying different types of activity. In Example 2.29, leading is seen as being senior amongst professional colleagues rather than engaging with the systems of the organisation as a manager would be expected to do.

Example 2.29
Leading and managing

They all say, 'I'm a nurse, I'm not a manager.' There is resistance to becoming managers. They seem to like the concept of leading rather than managing. They're leading their colleagues rather than managing resources. They don't want to manage money and budgets. They want to treat patients and use their nursing skills.

More perspectives on the differences between what leaders do and what managers do are given in Example 2.30. The control, monitoring and co-ordination roles usually associated with management are mentioned as examples of leadership along with giving support and direction.

Example 2.30
Aspects of leadership

I think any area or any place that you work there has to be an element of leadership. When I work on the ward I give directions, but not in this role. In this unit I take the leadership role because I'm the one that's here full-time, I go to the multidisciplinary team, I see the patient through their journey. However, as far as telling my colleagues what to do, that's not necessary because we're all practitioners in our own right, we know what to do and how to do it. I don't give instructions and tell them this is what you're meant to be doing today. We know what's to be done and we just do it. But you do need someone to take overall charge, leadership, control, coordination. How everything fits together.

Leadership means someone to take control, to co-ordinate and support. Not somebody who is yes, follow me, gung-ho, that sort of type. Somebody who can give direction, give a solid basis to your daily work. I give direction to myself. I know what I'm doing, when I walk to work I work it out, what I'm going to do that day, when I go home I set it up for the next day. I've always done it for myself. I tend to look to myself for leadership and so give that as well.

In Example 2.31, professional leadership is aligned with the management roles of allocating work and delegating. Clarity about how work is allocated is valued.

Example 2.31
Leading in a managerial way

A good leader in a managerial way was one of the ward sisters. We knew what we had to do on a daily basis. She would allocate and delegate. She wasn't democratic though, she was quite autocratic and a lot of people didn't like that, but it suited me. At least she got things done and they were done well. She'd look to me clinically to look at people and see if there were any improvements needed. She didn't lead well that way because her clinical skills weren't that good. Things like looking after a patient, dealing with them psychologically, she'd look to me. We ran a tight ship, but it was a good one.

A view of leadership that is more differentiated from management is offered in Example 2.32. In this example the ability to build on strengths is valued.

Example 2.32
Working with strengths

She was a good leader on all sorts of levels. She was very dynamic but was good at using people's strengths. She was very perceptive about what people's strengths and weaknesses were.

Example 2.33 gives an account of the discomfort of working with a manager who tried to control and enforce through criticism. Although this manager worked very long hours, this was not considered to be beneficial and there is an implication that this put an expectation on others to work unpaid overtime.

Example 2.33
Not a leader

I'd had quite a rough time with a male charge nurse whose first ward it was, who didn't know how to run a ward, couldn't let go. He was very hands-on. Instead of arriving at half past seven he'd be there for six o'clock. Instead of going home at three thirty he'd go home at eight in the evening. He'd come in on his holidays. We used to joke amongst ourselves because we had to be strong, but he had to find ten things wrong with you or with your performance before you could get on with your work. He just didn't know how to handle people.

The difference between use of force and use of support and encouragement is discussed in Example 2.34. It suggests that it can be very powerful if people realise the need for change sufficiently to wonder why they hadn't already thought about it for themselves.

Example 2.34
Push and pull of leadership

Leadership should be persuading people to follow you. It's the baddies that push people into straitjackets. If people think, maybe I should have been doing this for myself, then they'll follow. People are pushed into things by massive interests outside themselves, like corporate interests, that might seem glittery and seductive and the right way to go. But people who resist that only bring out in us what was there already, perhaps explain to us why it's not right, why we should resist. Articulate it.

Another aspect of leadership is described in Example 2.35 where it is associated with offering guidance without taking over control. It is suggested that authority is gained through being knowledgeable.

Example 2.35
Leader as guide

Leadership to me means guidance. It would be someone to steer the ship through stormy waters, not necessarily to take control but to steer. In my last job my leader was a medic as well, most of the time they have been. Everybody's expected to be a leader which is alright in one way, to lead yourself and to lead colleagues who work for you – but I think it's gone a bit far. You have to be quite strong minded because there are some difficult people, including consultants. If you're going to lead nurses you have to be strong minded, knowledgeable and know what you're talking about.

In Example 2.36 the term 'covert' leadership is used to describe how a leader can encourage and steer, sometimes push, in the desired direction.

Example 2.36
Covert leadership

In these meetings someone's pushing the thing and running it and keeping it up to scratch, but you don't know that because everyone else is tacitly happy with that situation. They've put their own bit of effort into it and it's working well. If it doesn't work, someone stands up and says so. Allowing the players to play. Command and control – forget it, everyone would get cross.

Another aspect of leadership in this team (Example 2.37) seemed to be a rather parental role in keeping order. Several members of the team mentioned that there are often 'difficult' people and it seems that leaders are associated with the authority to settle differences. We might expect team members to want to develop skills that enable them to find resolutions for themselves in these circumstances instead of looking for a senior figure to intervene.

Example 2.37
Leadership and keeping order

The senior consultant would ensure we all had our say and actually come up with some sort of agreement about how we would work after that. Because we're all nurses and he's a doctor – we all sort of think of ourselves as being three equal groups and unless he gets on board things are difficult to resolve. He doesn't stand any nonsense if he feels that things are getting too emotional or tied up in little things that we shouldn't be worrying about. We've got some very strong personalities that clash badly at times so it gets very personal.

One of the nurses commented in Example 2.38 on the parental role that the leader sometimes took in the multidisciplinary team meetings. She seems conscious of the parent/child relationships that seem to have developed, but although she is willing to offer support to the leader, she seems unable to influence the meeting to ensure that it makes good use of her time.

Example 2.38
Frustrations in meetings

If there is a leader there things run a bit better. If there is any dilly-dallying he'll say let's get back on track. But sometimes it depends how he feels. Sometimes he gets exasperated. He must get tired of doing it too. I know how I'd feel if I had to say it at a meeting with nurses, I'd wonder what they'd think of me. Sometimes we'll come out and say well, that was a waste of time. Or we'll come out and laugh and say how awful it was. Sometimes I'll try and catch his eye so he'll think he's got a bit of support when it's awful and say something.

In Example 2.39 one of the team members is aware of her strengths but thought her need to think things through before voicing an opinion made her unsuitable as a candidate for leadership.

Example 2.39
I don't sound like a leader

I'm not a natural leader. I think they'd be more able to voice their opinion. I wish I could think more quickly and come up with pat remarks. I'm one of these people who like to take things back and mull them over. I'm more analytical, not quick. My skills are useful though, because I'm a bit of a perfectionist, dotting all the 'i's and crossing all the 't's.

Another team member mentioned that there seemed to be an expectation in the Trust of a particular type of person as a leader. This was not necessarily the same sort of person as patients might choose: 'The Trust is looking for a figurehead – the patients are looking for someone who can get things done on an individual basis.' Another mentioned 'getting things done by fluttering your eyelashes', which is probably not how the Trust intends decisions to be made.

One particular aspect of leadership was suggested as important in the context of rapid change in health services. This is the ability to understand the potential impact of change on all of those who work in the context. Example 2.40 outlines this idea of the leader's role in anticipating and planning for impact of change.

Example 2.40
Anticipating the effect on others

The easiest thing to miss is how much the folks around you are being affected, particularly the non-medical staff. Things are changing around them rapidly all the time. If you're not careful, no-one considers them until there's a big outbreak of anger or something. We've all got to look out for each other more. The old patterns and relationships are changing and some are breaking down. Not necessarily a good or bad thing, but it affects everyone. The leaders will be those who anticipate that, the effect on other people. Most of us rush around dealing with problems that have got out of hand. The really clever thing would be to anticipate the effects on other people.

There are also some examples of shared leadership in this team. In Examples 2.36 and 2.38 we heard accounts of how the person chairing the meeting was frustrated by the behaviour of team members. Interestingly, it was one of the team members who took the lead in finding a way to address the issues (Example 2.41).

Example 2.41
Shared leadership

If something went drastically wrong or seemed to be not up to standard, he'd get angry. Though he didn't show his anger, you could sense his frustration. He'd say to me after, 'That was not how we should conduct these meetings.' So I'd make a list of all the things I'd noticed that we could correct and we'd go through those points with the members of the team. Not particular people, but behaviours. Though some people would jump to conclusions and defend themselves strongly even if they weren't at fault!

LEARNING FROM THIS CASE STUDY

This multidisciplinary team was formed to comply with policy guidelines intended to shape improvements in cancer services. Team members give a range of perspectives on change, leadership and the value of formalised teamworking through interprofessional meetings.

The subject of meeting etiquette flags up a number of important issues about ways of working, models of service, losses and gains within the transition and change process. The change that has enabled them to work in a virtual conference has itself opened wider potential for use of computer and communications technology to improve services.

Implicit throughout the case study is a question – what does it mean to be a professional? Professionalism has traditionally been associated with expertise. There is concern now that being a professional is much more diffuse. For example, you might think about what would happen if all of the participants were visible on screen in a video conference and whether this would have implications for expertise and power.

Consider the processes of developing a 'meeting etiquette' and the impact on ways of working. You might find it helpful to refer back to the strategic planner narrative who refers specifically to meeting etiquette. Examples 2.21 to 2.26 are particularly relevant. You may find it useful too, to consult the earlier examples in Perspectives on Teamworking and the discussion about teamworking in Part 3. Reflect on the following questions:

- How might an evolving meeting etiquette impact service provision?
- How might it impact ways of thinking, leadership and teamworking?
- What advice might you give this group about effective teamworking?
- How might a member of this team lead development of a service improvement that made use of the experience the team has in use of new technology?

What insights have you gained from considering the case study and how might you apply them to your own situation?

CHAPTER 3

ASSERTIVE OUTREACH MENTAL HEALTH TEAM

INTRODUCTION

The Assertive Outreach Mental Health Team was established to improve the service offered to those in the community with identified long-term serious mental health problems, including schizophrenia, bi-polar disorder and psychosis. In particular, the outreach approach is intended to extend the service to people who, for whatever reason, do not use the more traditional services that are delivered in health and care organisations.

The Assertive Outreach Mental Health Team was the first to be established in the area and started eighteen months ago when the team leader was appointed. The government set the National Service Framework for Mental Health Care and a Policy Implementation Guide which provided criteria for the composition of the team. While there is flexibility to adapt the team to local need, the guidance is prescriptive about essential personnel. These include a consultant psychiatrist, a certain number of nurses and social workers per population, a psychologist, community psychiatric nurses, an occupational therapist and support workers. It is a fully multidisciplinary and interprofessional team.

The government policy states that all patients with a mental health problem should have a care plan approach. Most teams work with individual clients and patients on a one-to-one basis, each qualified professional having a personal case load. This team is different in that although it uses care co-ordination it does so through a team approach. The theory is that all the people in the team will have working knowledge and a day-to-day relationship with each client.

The team was initially jointly funded by the National Health Service Trust, the Social Services Department and the Drug Action Team. These management structures have now merged with one direct manager and one source of funding.

How the team works

The team works from nine to five Monday to Friday but also, due to locality needs and constraints on numbers, the team members work flexibly to cover evenings and weekends. The team operates in deprived areas and tries to address social inclusion because people with mental health problems are often isolated and less likely to go out and have a social life. For example, on Bonfire Night team members went with clients and patients to a local pub for a meal and then held a party to help to enmesh participants into the local community. The team differs from other teams in the informality of its approach, trying to work on people's strengths to increase their independence and coping skills.

Each qualified member of staff is expected to have approximately ten clients. Every morning staff have a risk and allocation meeting, mentioning every patient by name. Certain work is ongoing but some work is more therapy oriented. For example, occupational therapists might meet to work on independence and self-care. Nurses might have fixed time to work on voices or delusional symptoms. The team also, however, have to respond to day-to-day crises.

PERSPECTIVES FROM THE TEAM

Team leader

I'm a nurse by profession and have done a variety of nursing jobs. This is the first time I've managed a multidisciplinary team. I'm from a health and social care perspective and the two, through government and politics, have been very much separate entities. I've got very frustrated over the years at how people have to go through lots and lots of paperwork and assessments to get holistic care. This post is certainly a leadership challenge, with lots of issues of diversity and rights and personal differences.

The team was the first to be established in this area. This is probably why it has had a lot of profile and people were aware of us. Our general manager was very passionate about leadership and developing staff, saw this job as evolution and was successful in getting the drivers along with her, of which I'm one. This is what I've always wanted to do.

I think that teams evolve and have had a lot of freedom in how they evolve. It's very positive in that we have looked at what was missing in this locality. We knew that there were less community staff per population in this area and nobody worked weekends or evenings, so nothing for people in crisis, people who were very needy. It was very easy for me to appoint, because I had new monies, new offices, people who wanted to work here chose to come here – nobody's been reconfigured. People are here because they want to be here. So leadershipwise, a doddle. Very challenging, lots of ideas, not always easy to manage, but easy stuff to lead.

I'd worked in the locality for fourteen years. So I had strong beliefs about what the needs were and I wanted to fill that gap. I thought I knew a lot about social care until I worked with social workers and realised that my knowledge is very limited. I think learning in the team takes a lot of time. This team has a smaller case load than in the rest of the service. We have a lot more time for the clients. We have a lot more time to learn with each other and with the clients.

We try to approach people who wouldn't go out without us, some people would get out anyway. So we focus on people who would be sat at home alone and try to get them out and to mingle in society. So we do quite a lot of things, go to the pictures, go bowling, play pool, whatever they are interested in – go horse-riding, do some quite interesting things with some people. So that's why we are different from other teams. We don't sit in a room. We don't work on people's problems but try to work on people's strengths to increase their independence and their coping. If they were to come to us it would be different. We had three people come to us this morning and for assertive outreach that's brilliant because normally they don't want to see us. We're a year in now and have developed quite good relationships, but they're difficult to engage. We do structured work with them in our interview room, but a lot of our work is informal and done in informal settings. We go to them. Which a lot of community teams do, but I guess we have more flexibility.

As they know more about us some of the clients know who can solve their problems quickest. A guy came in with debt problems and asked for a social worker because they know the phone numbers, who to ask and they're quicker. One of the ways of addressing the issue was to get the unqualified workers. It's been the biggest success of the team. They are, perhaps, the most important members of the team, including running errands and leaving qualified people free, but that's brought about a challenge in itself. Of the two support workers we've got, one's going away to do his training next month, so we've developed him. Training is quite important to me. Learning and being flexible. We've had three 'away days' in the year and we've changed our policies each time, to adapt. Our clients are always changing as well, of course; their needs are changing.

We have quite a few informal team-building days – and nights, drinking nights – as well. There is an acceptance that we're all very different in how we carry our personal lives, but there is respect. There are times when I get it wrong. For example, I've felt very removed from the team recently, there's been so much demand from above. This week's been better. I realised that I've got to look after them. The top's got to wait for a while. There are times when I don't perform but there are times when I've got to let them see how it goes without me. We do have a delegation model.

It's the best job I've ever had in my career. I would have left a while ago. What worries me is that there's been so much research done about this service saying that retention of staff is very difficult. Burn out is very high and team leaders often work for two or three years and then move on. I think, for me, that needs to be addressed. It needs to be looked at day to day. I've got a youngish team, pregnancies, babies, marriages and that's quite important. You need to look at where people are in their lives. Your biggest resource is your staff.

Community psychiatric nurse

I'm qualified as a mental health nurse and have been in the team for eighteen months. I've worked in acute wards and I feel quite privileged to have got a job in the team. In teams I've worked in before it's been just nurses. I've carried quite a large case load of about thirty clients on my own and had sole responsibility for those clients. Whereas in this team we have smaller case loads so we have the flexibility to see the patients more often and everybody sees all the patients.

We work with quite a challenging client group. The clients I was seeing before were primarily primary care clients with anxiety and depressive disorders whereas this is the other end of the spectrum and it's a much more intense kind of job. So although I've got a smaller case load it's actually a much more stressful job.

We're all fairly senior clinicians really. We've all reached a certain level and all got a lot of experience and all paid a similar amount of money and all on similar terms and conditions. Everybody's committed to this type of work and everybody respects everybody else. I think the team leader's quite skilled at picking people who are able to get on with each other but, more importantly, able to get on with the clients.

There were high expectations placed on the service at the beginning, before things were in place. We're expected to see a certain number of patients per month and in reality, we just can't do that safely. There's pressure on us to take on certain patients that are maybe not appropriate. Maybe that's about numbers. Boxes have got to be ticked and patients have got to be seen regardless of how effective that is. Time is the biggest constraint because we just don't have the time to do the job we're expected to do. We are doing positive work but then people say you're only seeing forty patients and it should be ninety patients. There is quite a lot of criticism of the team. Then they'll say, 'Oh, which pub are you going to today?' We're seen as the team that takes people out and does all these nice things, but they don't see the hard work that we do.

I really think that we could put this passion that we've got over to other staff, because I've seen all the other staff on the wards and they're really burnt out. If we could say that the patients are real people and educate about what we do, it would be really nice. People still don't know what Assertive Outreach is. They've got certain perceptions and it's up to us to put those perceptions right. It's about having time to do it – you still have all these other things to do. Patients have got to be the priority. Maybe we have to prioritise that now though because it's affecting the way the patients are being treated when they have to go on the wards.

There have been hard, hard times when we have really struggled. We've done remarkably well to put up with the criticism that we've had and to put up with the pressure we've had from other services to take people off them. We need to look at saying no to things. Staffing is the big thing. We're nearly up to full strength now. We've been so keen to prove ourselves that we've taken on more than we should have done. It only takes a couple of people to be off sick or on holiday and you really notice it.

It's been really tough because it's not only this pressure but we're seeing a very demanding client group. Often it's a thankless task. You feel so deskilled. But you can say I don't know what to do and maybe someone will take some of the work off you. If it wasn't for other members of the team I'd have walked off ages ago. You need that with this client group. They're just so demanding. We had a client who died unexpectedly. That was very traumatic. We've had violent incidents against staff. These sorts of things you need to pull together.

We've all learnt to be realistic. Not expecting clients to be going to work or living a wonderful lifestyle, but looking at the small changes that you've helped them achieve. If someone's just managed to reduce their drug intake by a small amount each day. Seeing changes and realising this is a real bonus. We were talking about a patient today who is really poorly at the moment but instead of just going off and wandering into the fields to walk as he used to, he came in here and said, 'Can you help me?' We've not stopped him becoming ill but we've managed to get him to come here and say he's ill. Others are still being admitted, but maybe it's only for a few days now and not for weeks. We try to say something positive about what we've done at each team meeting.

The team is an exemplar in some ways – we need to hear that more. The team leader is very good at selling what we do. She is so passionate about it. Having a positive leader makes such a difference.

Health care assistant

My role is as a support worker. We work alongside the trained staff, sort of like the buffer between the trained staff and the clients. We're more friendly, they can relate to us a lot better. We look more towards engagement, social inclusion, medication and benefits issues. So we're more like friends. Possibly because they find that we're not judging. They're not talking to us about reducing medication, side effects. We do talk to them about that, but not to such an extent.

A lot of people we deal with have no social network, they don't have many friends to talk to. They're coming in just to talk to you because they've got nobody else. Just about everyday mundane things. Someone to say yes, that's a good idea, or no. You find that you get a lot of one-word answers and you're digging around to try and find some common ground to work your way in.

You often find with your dinner break that when you're having your dinner you're having it with clients or that's the time to get your notes written up. Everyone's so passionate. It's not a case of everything stops because we've got to have a dinner, we've got to start at this time or got to finish at this time. We're willing to be flexible because we're so passionate. If someone comes in at five o'clock we can be ten o'clock at night just because they want you there.

Before, in a traditional in-service team, if you needed to see someone you had to wait and book them up. We're all accessible and we've all got a voice. If we don't particularly agree with somebody else's diagnosis or somebody else's thoughts on a particular person, it's healthy that we can all have a discussion. You can see why, for example, an occupational therapist wants to go down this particular way of thinking. So you've got social workers talking about the social aspects, the occupational therapist talking about the home environment, your community psychiatric nurses and medication issues, the support workers on social inclusion issues, so we've all got a say. But if you've got someone who's got a drugs- or drink-related problem it's no good sending them to a social worker or an occupational therapist. We've got a dual diagnosis specialist, it's their speciality. Overall the team leader has to take the call and say yes or no and take the consequences. The total package, I think, is very good. It's the best service I've ever worked in.

I feel as valued as the consultant, because my point of view is taken on board. I feel that in the team I'm not lower down the ladder but equivalent. For me it's a plus because before it was, 'What do you know, you're only a support worker'. Now it's a good point because support workers get more contact with the client.

For me the downside is that you've got different disciplines on different pay and different hours. For me it's not an issue because we chose to come here. Social workers get more money and they get more holidays and community psychiatric nurses don't, they get less. But there's no animosity, no malice – we all accept it. It would be nice to be under one umbrella, but a lot of the time you're rewarded for passing particular courses but the course doesn't necessarily make you any better. For a nurse or social worker, it's experience, hands on, that makes you better so there's no particular way to assess you on that.

With any new service, there are people looking to see if it's ready for a fall. People who want to knock because they don't understand. We actively encourage anybody and everybody, from the wards, from different disciplines, from upstairs – the rehab service, the generic services, the elderly services, to spend a day with us to see how we work. Because we're a new service and we're teamworking, people are unsure. They don't know what to expect, they don't know what our expectations are. With any new service it's got to be established and, I suppose, show a success that people can measure.

Because it's a new service and there have been no other ones on line, we've been certified, forensic, elderly, crisis treatment – we've been all treatments. These services are coming on line now, but we were getting everything. We were thinking, until these services come on line should we step in and help? We could offer a little bit more than other services could at the time, but we weren't ideal.

Dual diagnosis nurse

I used to work in a high-security hospital with sex offender treatment of personality disordered patients. I'd always been interested in drugs and alcohol, professionally I mean! I've only for the last six to nine months actually felt that I've been doing the job I applied for. When I first started there were very few members of the team. We all had to muck in with anything and everything. We didn't have support workers to do some of the more practical day-to-day tasks. It's since the team expanded and we've got more staff that I've been able to move into my role, which is dual diagnosis: individuals with severe and enduring mental health problems including substance misuse, drugs and alcohol.

Research shows that a large proportion of psychiatric patients, up to fifty per cent, at some point in their lives have a substance misuse problem. So it's a big problem. Although it's a specialist role, it's quite a wide population, really. The process is to identify the folk that have those two problems (although they have a hundred and two generally), assess the needs of those patients and then advise the rest of the team as to what, from a dual diagnosis point of view, I think should happen. So that might include detoxing people from various substances. It might include health education, minimising harm that people do to themselves through using substances. These are often chaotic, transient kinds of people living on the streets. It's quite an achievement to track someone down and talk to them.

I think the team are doing extremely well. Although I'm on my own in the sense that there's only me in the team doing my sort of job, the rest of the team are very supportive. I couldn't do all the interventions myself because there wouldn't be the time and I'm just not qualified in certain areas. My role is more advisory. If you're involved by yourself for a long time with patients of this sort you can very easily become disillusioned, burnt out, burdened with it all. It's very useful to have the rest of the team to give bits of that person's care too.

The multidisciplinary element in the team is a big help in enabling that to happen. The occupational therapist, for example in the team, can speak very knowledgeably about her subject and the other people in the team probably don't have a great understanding of that but are prepared to listen and learn. So we're always educating one another about what we do and how we do it. I think this openness of opinion has evolved from that. You need to know that people are up to speed with what's happening, know what the potential problems are and know what the plan is if something were to go wrong or a certain situation were to develop. With the client group that we work with, you definitely need people you can trust.

It comes back to people's opinions being valued, the honesty. People are passionate about things and that comes over in the way they communicate about things – I'm going to tell you what I think and I'll tell you in the way I think you need to be told. In some instances, in some teams, that can cause a problem because people are viewed as aggressive or over-opinionated or whatever, but I don't think that's happened in this team.

We have a meeting every morning to discuss every patient. Even if you're not directly involved with that patient, for that particular part of their care, if something happened later on that day that you had to deal with, you'd have a broad outline of what was going on in that person's care. You could comment on it knowledgeably, you could give an opinion about that because you would have a broad overview. There would be people that you'd be very definitely involved with and you'd pass that information on to other people so that they could do the same if you weren't around. I think communication is the most important part of what we do. At every level, between ourselves, us and our clients, us and other professionals, it's the key to keeping people safe.

In my particular role, I'm given a certain amount of autonomy purely due to my experience, knowledge, the specialism that I'm in. Which is a good thing because there are times when you need to make decisions there and then and you can't refer back to someone else.

Personally, I would like to be given more responsibility for developing that area of work but there are constraints. But day to day, I don't feel constrained at all. If I needed to go and do something and I was confident to do that, there wouldn't be any constraints placed on me.

PERSPECTIVES ON CHANGE IN HEALTH AND SOCIAL CARE

The examples in this and the following sections are drawn from the interviews with team members and illustrate issues related to change, teamworking and leadership.

This team frequently compared their way of working with traditional models to indicate how much had been changed to enable this different way of working. In Example 3.1 a comparison is made with the traditional hierarchy in which all other disciplines defer to consultants and in which senior staff do not expect their actions or judgement to be questioned by those junior to them.

Example 3.1
Traditional hierarchy and teamworking

Before I worked in a team where the staff nurses, and especially the consultants, wouldn't want to be questioned. What they said went. People do act differently if there's a medic about, if they think they're being watched, being judged. In past cultures they knew best, which isn't always the case. In this team, from the student observing support workers to the occupational therapists, we all see things differently, like a big jigsaw. Everybody's thoughts are taken on board, whether they're right or wrong. You're not condemned for speaking out of turn because something relevant may not have been picked up.

Everyone in health and social care services has experience of change but not everyone finds it easy to adapt. In Example 3.2 one of the team described how staff in one area of work were openly hostile to change. She suggested that this resistance was partly because people were not aware of the potential benefits of delivering services in different ways and partly because they resisted being forced to change.

Example 3.2
People don't want change

When there was talk about the Assertive Outreach team being set up some staff said, 'Why the hell do we need that? Things are OK. What do we need that for? Here we go again. Change for change's sake.' That attitude really does pervade through. I think that's why we need to be selling the positive result of that change. There is an attitude, 'We'll stay as we are, thank you very much.' People don't like to think that change is being forced upon them.

Resistance to change is also often associated with not recognising the need for change. If people believe that change is necessary they are less likely to resist it. Several members of the team mention that they think it is important to convince staff in other services that the approach used in Assertive Outreach is more successful for some clients than traditional service delivery. Institutionally based mental health services changed dramatically when many of the institutions were closed and replaced by care in the community. The community-based approaches used by this team may not have been appropriate before these policy changes.

The flow of funding for mental health services has also changed to focus on resourcing service delivery in the community. Many health and care staff are very aware of resource constraints although budgets are usually only held by managers and team leaders. In Example 3.3 a nurse explains why she thinks it is difficult for nurses and other professionals to be successful in gaining funding for innovation. The traditions that helped nursing to develop into a profession may also be holding the profession back from engaging fully in service development.

Example 3.3
We're supposed to be humble

Historically we nurses are very bad at singing our own praises because we're supposed to be humble. In nursing, particularly in this country, we're still being Florence Nightingale. It's still the female occupation. What we haven't realised is that if we do sing our praises, we'll get more resources. The Trust is being inspected in January – it would be so simple to stomp around and criticise. But if we succeed, we get increased funding. And if we could spend that on service users, job done! There's a lot of cynicism about change and nurses are no different. I think we've been our own worst enemies.

There have also been long-standing tensions between different professional roles. Members of the team described tensions between social workers and psychiatric nurses related to overlapping roles and different priorities in approaches taken in different areas of practice. These differences also caused tensions between services delivered within institutions and this new service delivered in the community, particularly as described in Example 3.4 when a patient might need to be admitted temporarily to a ward.

Example 3.4
Tensions between services

Sometimes patients are admitted to an inpatient ward and we get quite a lot of hostility from the ward staff. It was affecting the way I deal with clients and the way I deal with other staff. There's a lot of bad feeling about this team because it's new and needs to prove itself, two hundred per cent perhaps. We're completely different. It's a whole new, creative and flexible way of working. Until we can see real positive results people aren't going to believe in it, but these results aren't going to come up overnight. They've got to be a little patient with us really.

Much of the tension in this case seemed to arise because of different models of care. Services that develop with a philosophy that differs from the traditional hierarchical, institutionally based services often need to develop new ways of working. This is where leadership is usually considered important, as the ability to set a new direction rather than the management role of monitoring and controlling an existing area of work. In Example 3.5 the distinction between leadership and management is discussed but it is proposed that this is not an easy distinction to make in health and care because change for improvement is a constant feature.

Example 3.5 ▬▬▬▬▬▬▬▬▬▬▬▬
Leadership as keeping a balance

I consider myself a leader and not a manager. When you manage something it doesn't move easily or grow easily, you're usually managing something so that it is contained. Health and social care cannot be contained – it's growing every day as we learn and progress, so it is a bit different. Some things have to be managed to be kept safe, risk issues and problem-solving. Also fifteen people with very different ideas. Unless you manage that you've got chaos. How do I do that? Balancing, lots of good supervision and stepping out. Good training for myself and learning. Most important for me has been to learn and to listen.

In Example 3.6 the team leader comments on how her experience helped to pave the way for development of a new service area.

Example 3.6 ▬▬▬▬▬▬▬▬▬▬▬▬
Leading in health and care

The vision at the top is that health and social care will have to work together. Although I'm a nurse, I'm passionate also about change and truly working together. I think they thought that I'd bring people together and do that. There is passion there and determination. I've been given the freedom of having budgets. Also, I've been around a long time and know people and I think that helps. When something has worked they trust you next time. But even if things have gone wrong, we've owned up to it and said next time we'd do it differently, so it's being genuine and honest.

PERSPECTIVES ON TEAMWORKING

The approach of this team is based on a philosophy that is significantly different from the underlying philosophy of traditional service provision for mental health. Example 3.7 outlines the difference between the traditional 'medical model' and the new and more holistic 'bio-psychosocial model'.

Example 3.7 ▬▬▬▬▬▬▬▬▬▬▬▬
Conflicting philosophies of care and treatment

The philosophy of the team is to try and maintain people in their own homes, in their own environment. Basically to improve their standard of living and quality of life, rather than to treat them medically. Before, I worked to the medical model, just nurse led and consultant led. Whereas in this team the consultant is part of the team and we work to the bio-psychosocial model, so it's not just about medication and jabbing people.

So when you say what do we actually do, sometimes it can feel like it's just about medicine but we also visit people in their own homes and it's

much more of a supportive role than in my previous jobs. It's much more
on the same level as the patients, it sounds a bit corny, but being a friend.
Actually looking at what they want, their needs and their strengths. Trying
to see patients grow and develop rather than just going and treating their
illness.

This new service model demands that professionals relate to service users in a different way. Developing this new type of relationship
is not always easy for people who developed their practice in traditional services. As a nurse commented: 'Before, I was almost a therapist type. Now one of the patients said you're my friend, you're my
family. I think a lot of traditional services would be a bit edgy about
this but it works for her and that's what patients want.' This change
of attitude towards patient-centred services is unlikely to develop
unless services themselves change. Service delivery that involves
patients and clients may need to look and feel very different from
services delivered by experts to treat conditions rather than people.
In Example 3.8 one of the team explains the importance of sharing
a vision of how the service should work.

Example 3.8
Sharing a vision

Certain things are a base line. A foundation of what we're trying to
achieve. A common vision that we want to see anybody who walks
through this door in control of their care. Being able to articulate what
they do and don't want. Able to minimise their distress and maximise
their potential. It's our core philosophy and every discipline has got that.

The vision describes the aspiration for this new service approach
but different ways of working are necessary in order to achieve these
outcomes. Example 3.9 explains the difference between how this
team works and how staff usually work in more traditional services.

Example 3.9
Working as a team

The difference between this team and others you compare it with is that
this one works as a team. The government policy is that all patients with
a mental health problem should have a care plan approach. Other services work with one qualified professional with a case load. So if the professional is off sick, someone else in the team will have to open their case
files and read them. In our team we do still use care co-ordination, but
it's a team approach. The theory is that all the people in the team will
have a working knowledge and a day-to-day relationship with the client.

This team put considerable emphasis on bringing their various strengths to bear on meeting the needs of their clients. Example 3.10 describes the benefits to be gained from this approach.

Example 3.10
Meeting clients' needs

The team works together well because we're all passionate and we're all client orientated. We're all looking for what clients need. From the lowest-paid support worker or student up to the highest-paid consultant, we've all got a voice, we've all got a say in this person's care. We can all see things from a different perspective and we are all client focused. We've all got strengths in certain areas and we've all got weaknesses in certain areas so we all compensate for each other and we all look after each other.

Although this way of working together brings benefits that the team value, people sometimes feel that their professional contribution is less visible than in traditional services. In Example 3.11 a nurse discusses some of her feelings and the importance of developing a shared evidence base to underpin practice in these new settings.

Example 3.11
Roles in the team

The other nurse and I have had this ongoing conversation about how other members of the team have quite specific roles. The occupational therapist does the occupational therapy and the social workers will deal with sections and benefits but what does the psychiatric nurse do? Sometimes it feels like we're just mopping up what other people don't do. Like medication. Like being the injection nurse – everybody else does the nice psychological therapies and things like that and we give the injections. It means that your relationship with a client is basically different because you're seen as the person who gives them the nasty injection. It's sounding very negative really, but that's the reality. We've had to do some self-analysis to forge our roles in the team as specialist workers like everybody else. I'd like to do some of the psychological work. I'm on a course at the moment on psychosocial interventions for people with psychosis. Theoretically, at the end of that I'll be able to look at things like cognitive behavioural therapy for people with psychosis and do much more in-depth assessments. It's really about having an evidence base for what you do, being able to say what you do in a structured way.

Many professionals in health and care have a strong personal identity with their profession. When their role is wider than the normal professional one, particularly if their activities seem sometimes not to include a professional contribution, people can feel a loss of identity. This is discussed in Example 3.12.

Example 3.12
Personal and professional identity

One of the challenges of the team is because it's more mixed, with a lot of evidence and research to build on. In the eighties they tried this, made what we called a community mental health team. You ended up with groups of staff quite concerned about their profession and where their profession sat in a multidisciplinary team if they became generic workers. They lost their professional identity and their skills and their ability to be confident in their profession and where it sat. A lot of hostility and anxiety was caused.

I think the challenge is to ensure that people are able to take up what they wanted to do when they became a social worker or a nurse or whatever, but at the same time, to meet the needs of the team. And that is a day-to-day challenge, especially if you have less staff. If you're short, people start feeling very deskilled. One of my nurses said, 'I'm just an injection nurse', and she's much more than that, but that's what she'd become that day. So that is a challenge as a team and it's how it differs from other teams. It is because we're multidisciplinary.

In a team that consists of professionals and trainees from many different disciplines the differences in education and experience can create difficulties for individuals in learning to work with the team. The team leader is not always the most senior member of staff but usually takes responsibility for developing teamwork. In Example 3.13 this team leader discusses some of the issues she faced.

Example 3.13
Developing teamworking

It's a challenge to manage people who are more academically qualified than myself and who get paid more. The psychologist very much wants to be part of the team and his core values are about teamwork. He's come from a similar environment and is quite passionate about it. He's certainly a genuine team player but has clear beliefs as a psychologist of what his role will be. That's brilliant, because he's there for the team but very much a team player.

The consultant to the team has been around for many years and probably had (by his own admission) the least idea of what teamworking's about, but he's really been sold the team model. It works and he feels valued. He has learnt to accept the support workers – they may not have all the qualifications but they see the world more through the client's eyes than any of us. He's started to value that.

A good team player feels able to do their bit and understands their role within that team, but, at the same time, values every other player. It's like a game of football. The striker can never score goals on his own and the goalkeeper can't stop them without all those people in the middle. It's vitally important that those people communicate and respect each other. If one person in that team's ignored, then you've got a weak link.

Although the professional roles in the team are important in bringing the necessary knowledge and skills to deliver the service, the personalities in the team are important in enabling staff to work together. In Example 3.14 the importance of humour is mentioned as one way of helping individuals to deal with stress and occasional traumatic events.

Example 3.14
Personalities in the team

We're all fairly good at recognising when somebody gets stressed and saying, hang on a minute, calm down. We share a similar sense of humour. You have to have quite a sick sense of humour. These things matter. You have to be able to laugh. Some of the things you see are quite traumatic and we've had some quite difficult times lately with patients. So to be able to go off and have a laugh and debrief informally. There's a good mix of personalities too. There's a couple of people who are quite loud and a couple who are fairly quiet and the whole thing seems to meld together quite well. We've all got quite strong personalities too, all quite assertive. That comes from passion for the job, I think.

In this team the approach to service delivery makes it essential to be close to the patient as an individual. This close relationship necessarily involves the emotions of staff in responding to individual patients. The nature of the service means that many of the service users are very distressed and this can sometimes be overwhelming for members of the team. In Example 3.15 one of the team's rituals is mentioned as one way in which the team try to give themselves a supportive environment.

Example 3.15
Team rituals that help

We have a little handover each morning, a little team meeting and whoever's in first makes everyone else a cup of tea. These little rituals – you need a bit of grounding in these sorts of things really. If you think about the job you do, sometimes it can blow your mind, so many really troubled and distressed people that you see. We're very good at supporting each other.

Emotional support is not the only type of support team members need from each other. Some of the team's patients and clients are dangerous to themselves and to others. Example 3.16 describes an occasion when the team made a decision to refuse to accept the transfer of a patient from an inpatient service to their community-based service.

Example 3.16
Staying safe as a team

Historically there's been a quick burn out because of demands made on staff. For example, we had somebody referred to us because they can't be managed on the ward. It's taking seven or eight staff to control this person on the ward. What good is it sending them home and asking us to visit them as lone workers or pairs? What good could two people do in one person's home when they're struggling with seven or eight people on the ward? We did have to take a team decision. Although we're all passionate about it and we like the job and do want to be here, it is just a job and we all want to go home safe.

The degree of risk faced by the team demands that the team members have considerable trust in each other. In Example 3.17 one of the support workers discusses how this degree of trust has to extend to all members of the team, regardless of their role or qualifications.

Example 3.17
Trust in the team

The foundation of trust was built by the people who were here at the beginning and that has sort of rubbed off on the people who've come since. With the type of clients we are dealing with you have to trust the people you are working with and you have to trust their opinion, regardless of your role or qualification. The support workers are often viewed as the unqualified staff, but in lots of situations their opinion is often the most important because they have the most day-to-day contact with someone. Therefore I would trust their opinion implicitly, not over anyone else's, but due to the amount of contact they would have with someone. So I think trust is a very big part because you've got to feel that you can say what you want without being made to feel inferior or inexperienced or that your opinion isn't valued.

As a new team, it was inevitable that their practice as a team would be shaped, to some extent, by their experience. Sometimes useful learning came from making mistakes. Example 3.18 describes how the team learnt to build more careful planning into their routines.

Example 3.18
The need for planning

When we first opened, we saw clients who were all new to us. They all carry an element of risk in terms of their health and injury to themselves or others. We'd decided who could go and visit people but there wasn't a particular structure. Then people visited a client on Monday and two different people went on Tuesday. There was no continuity. This caused an incident that was quite risky because we hadn't had feedback from the people who visited on Monday. On Tuesday the client was quite frustrated and said he'd told our colleagues these things yesterday, so we found ourselves quite at risk. We had quite a heated debate about that as there was no plan before we went to see that client of what we would do as a pair. There was no planning basically. It was very early on in the team's development.

After that we met as a team and changed our procedure for visiting clients to make sure there is continuity with all our clients. We listened to clients too and made them more in control of who they see. We did that initially by problem-solving, evaluating what happened, learning from it. Then identifying areas for training and certain people are on a course now because of it. We've adapted our behaviour as a team.

Openness to learning seems to be an important feature of this team. The trust that they have in each other enables individuals to admit errors and to accept that they need to learn. In Example 3.19 we are offered an insight into how one of the senior professionals in the team felt when being open about mistakes.

Example 3.19
Developing together

I can think of things I've done that weren't the wisest things. I would like to think that the staff in there would tell me. I certainly think they would and that they feel able to and that I could tell them. There have been a couple of times when the risk was quite high, times when it was quite dangerous and we've all had to learn from that. I think that the fact that I can hold my hand up and say that I've got a lot to learn here has enabled others to say, 'OK, if she can say it, I can say I did that wrong.' It's a learning philosophy and it's OK as we evolve and grow to keep refining that.

In Example 3.20 one of the team proposes that turbulent relationships are only symptoms of the commitment that the team feel to the service delivery model. The team have respect for each other that transcends day-to-day difficulties.

Example 3.20
Tensions and the glue that holds the team together

There've been lots and lots of battles. Traditionally there's always been this thing about social workers versus psychiatric nurses. This all goes on in our office but it's light hearted. I think the fact that we've got lots of people who are quite dedicated to the model that we use helps. This team is fantastic because of personalities in it. But it has the potential to be blown apart if one person were to come in and not be committed to the model. We find that because everyone's passionate about what they're doing means that we all have respect for each other.

The importance of the model of service delivery is frequently mentioned by team members. The team leader expanded on this in Example 3.21, explaining why she thought it important that team members and service users should know something about the origins of the philosophy guiding the team and the evidence base that supports their practice. This example is interesting in demonstrating how local service delivery can be directly informed by initiatives in other countries. It gives an example of the growing importance of considering models of health and care in an international context.

Example 3.21
Learning from other countries

It's very important when you get a new member of the team to say that the biggest change in mental health is the closure of institutions. So rather than just saying this new team's developing here, let them know the model's developing nationally. Say it's an American model, it's a Canadian model and it's a New Zealand model.

A patient came to a bring and share session and said, 'Do you know, the first team was from America?' The boost I got from one of my clients telling me and the group that this came from America was fantastic and her excitement at knowing this. It made us all look at what happened. Why was it set up in America? Why have we adopted it in England? What's different? The latest thing wasn't working in England and why was that? In England we've made it national policy but in America it still isn't national policy.

So it's not just about giving information, it's about getting them to think about it, asking them questions and then personalising it to here. What's working here, what isn't. My job is, when something's going well, to tell them, they need to know that.

In a team where learning and development are important it is interesting to hear in Example 3.22 of the experience one of the team had in a previous area of health services and in this team. There are both practical and personal aspects to learning and the attitude of workplace colleagues can help or hinder.

Example 3.22
What helped and hindered my learning

When I joined the health service my qualifications weren't very good and I opted for an access course. There were some obstacles put in my way. For example, the course was on one particular night every week and I was often on the wrong shift. It would have been easy to work out for me but I had to do a lot of swapping and shifting myself although I was after getting on nurse training.

In this job, I told my manager that that's what I was after ultimately and she actively encourages me. Which is nice if I need extra time off for studying. I'm being seconded which means I'll get paid to train and have a job waiting for me. I'm on the student rate so it's the light at the end of the tunnel and I'll be getting paid.

For the interview for nurse training at college I was advised about what to say, what not to say, what to show and what not to show. I'd started at college before and when I came for this job I asked if our hours meant that I'd have to miss college work because you don't want to miss. I was told that if I needed the time I could have the time.

I was constantly asked how I'm doing. When I passed there were congratulations, everybody was pleased for me. It's helpful. Help with any assignments, anything. Even now if I'm struggling or want a chat about the way I'm working with particular clients – if I think it's working or if it's good or bad – I can ask any member of the team and they'll give me advice. It is also nice to be asked for advice as well – it's not just a one-way street where you're constantly asking and no-one's asking you.

This team are not alone in being established to develop new ways of working. As more new teams are established to develop new services, new mechanisms will be needed to link these teams together and to provide links into the other services provided by the host organisation or the local health economy. In Example 3.23 the team leader comments on the need to share information and experience openly rather than allow replacement 'silos' of practice to develop. There is a danger that the strength of passion and vision that fuels development of new services may lead to reluctance to consider other, possibly potential alternative, ways of working. She suggests that host organisations may have a role to play in helping to develop opportunities for discourse related to service development.

Example 3.23
Linking teams within the organisation

I think it is important that we have the connection of threads, of all these teams. People became very proud to say they were part of this team and we had a lot of conflict from other services. It was very easy for some of us to do the 'them and us'. But that was just repeating what we've always had, just new silos. I think what we need to do is to genuinely look out of the box. There's another new team just started this week, equally as passionate as we were. They all want to come for induction. We will listen to what they want and their beliefs and let them tell us what they think is good and what's bad. We have a lot of vision ourselves and we need to think about their vision and how we fit in that vision.

PERSPECTIVES ON LEADERSHIP

Some of the team members had very definite ideas about what makes a good leader. In Example 3.24 we have a description of a leader whose priority is to work in and with the team, acting as a personal example.

Example 3.24
A team leader

Someone who is a team player, enthusiastic, accessible. Not someone who's shut away in an ivory tower so you never see them. If you know that your team leader is ready to put the same hours in as you or more, you have nothing but respect because it rubs off.

For another team member, the leader's role is described in Example 3.25 as about developing direction in a way that involves the team and shares responsibility.

Example 3.25
Leading by developing direction

To me a good leader would be someone who offers direction. Somebody who will make decisions, who looks after their staff and their needs, but also who is willing to enable their staff to develop and to take on part of that leadership role. Leadership to me is about direction but not in a pre-scriptive way. Guiding people towards a vision. The leaders I've not respected in the past have said you will do this or that. The ones I respect are more ready to allow people to come to their own decisions.

It is not surprising in this team that the vision and direction are closely aligned with their practice. The team leader sets out her approach to leadership in Example 3.26, reflecting their model of practice.

Example 3.26
A psychosocial model of leadership

There's a theory of psychosocial intervention and I'd like to adapt that to management and leadership. It's no different – working on people's strengths, minimising their weaknesses, giving them independence, giving them control – you can adapt all of that to staff. That's my philosophy in leadership. The best day in my office will be when I'm redundant because they're doing it all.

People do not always want to have to be independent and responsible in a fully democratic environment. There are occasions when the leader's role is seen as being the decision maker and taking the ultimate responsibility on behalf of the team. Some of the tensions between a democratic and autocratic leadership style are discussed in Example 3.27.

Example 3.27
Democratic and autocratic leadership styles

I think the effective leader is in the main democratic but sometimes autocratic. Certainly in times of emergency a leader needs to make those tough decisions, stick by them and rationalise why they've made them. If everything is democratic, there's an implied sense of shared leadership. But a team like ours, with the client group we deal with, needs a strong leader. It needs someone who is prepared to fight the corner of the team if necessary, and to be fairly secure in their own convictions. It would be patronising to be told everything you had to do. I don't think that would make an effective leader.

There is also some personal frustration if individuals hope that their leader will take up an issue on their behalf rather than support them to solve the problem themselves. The comment in Example 3.28 links this frustration with difficulty in managing personal emotions about the situation.

Example 3.28
Try to solve it yourself

I found it frustrating. She said, try to solve it yourself. A big part of me would like her to say, 'I will do that for you as your manager.' She always says she's a leader, not a manager, so I can see where she's coming from on that, but it was very frustrating at the time. I was aware that if I was to go and address this issue my own feelings could have come to the fore. It was something that was really grinding me down. I could see her rationale for doing it, but it was quite frustrating.

This discussion about personal responsibility and decision-making appears to have been an open one within the team as the team leader makes a point of explaining, in Example 3.29, why, on one particular occasion, she made and enforced a decision.

Example 3.29
It has to be my decision

Sometimes you have to make decisions and to own it, the decision. Risk is a good example. There's a gentleman that a note says on no circumstances is anyone to visit this person. There was a query about whether he'd got a gun. One of the staff said she was quite happy to go in there, but I said no, end of story, because if anything were to happen I'd be carrying that to the end of my professional career. So I've made the decision that nobody visits until that's sorted. There are times now when I'll say no, that's not going to happen.

Leaders also have expectations of those who lead and inspire them. In Example 3.30 the team leader comments on how inspiration can come from both senior and junior staff.

Example 3.30
Sources of inspiration

For me as a leader it's vitally important that I have somebody to inspire me, to give me vision. I can think of who those people are straight away. You need people who you believe mean what they say at the top but you also need equals and people below you who will inspire you. There's one of the unqualified staff here now whose core beliefs, values and passion to learn has reinvested me.

Inspiration can also come from people who are able to demonstrate effective models of practice and share their enthusiasm with others. In Example 3.31 we hear more about how one clinician's enthusiasm prompted development of the Assertive Outreach model in England.

Example 3.31
Inspiration for service development

Assertive Outreach is an American model and we've got very strong. The Americans come to us and we go to them. I was inspired by the passion of a clinician who set up the National Forum. She passionately believes that this benefits clients. So it was her own vision, her own style of leading Assertive Outreach into this country. She met with two or three who were trying to do similar things here and it's now a national organisation. For me it's the best network, grass roots, led from the bottom up, with very small funding but led by clinicians for clinicians and with the people we care for. So she really inspired me, the whole philosophy.

In this country, if you've got a psychosis it's the end of your life. You're on benefits for ever, you'll never work again and your family will desert you. If you go to America, it's very different. You don't automatically get benefits or lose your family. Clients over there seem to have this belief, the American way, to think things can get better and I've got to be strong and fight this. That's what gets it going here. As we've seen clients grow and get better, that's what inspires us.

There are also some practical aspects to leadership that the team have noted. In Example 3.32 the team's practice of taking it in turn to chair meetings demonstrates how this has enabled individuals to develop leadership skills and recognise these strengths in others.

Example 3.32
Chairing a meeting

In our meetings we always have a roving chair, a different person each week. I'm not the best. What makes him the best? His style I think. He's quite boxlike, quite structured, but keeps things moving. He'll say enough and move on, but everyone has a chance to speak.

In Example 3.33 we see how one team member took a leadership role in offering a development opportunity to another.

Example 3.33
Leading the development of others

He's a support worker and came along with very little experience of mental health and he had one client who was acting quite dangerously with bi-polar disorder. So the qualified nurse sent him off to read all about manic depression and low arousal techniques. So the qualified nurse was able to use her skills in setting the care plan but also got a lot of reward after teaching this unqualified person how to deal with that client.

This team frequently mention their need to explain and demonstrate their work within their organisation to gain wider understanding of what they do and why they believe it is a good service. In this context, the role of the leader in influencing opinion is important. Example 3.34 offers an example of how this leader used her influence and sought to involve senior staff in the work of the team.

Example 3.34
Influencing up the organisation

The chair of the Trust came here for a day. He's a very busy man but he spent the whole morning here. The team said that if he's coming here, he wants to see what we do. No pomp and circumstance – we sent him an email telling him to dress down. Then he met patients, real patients. He met someone who was stuck on heroin, someone who was injecting. Sadly, one of the people he met that day has died. I next saw the chair at a conference and I wanted him to know that this client had died and I wanted him to know how that had affected the team. And I wanted the team to know that he knew that.

What can he, as the chair of the Trust, do to stop that happening again? It's about linking the hierarchy together. From the bottom up. I'd like to believe, for once in my life, that support workers can inform the chief executive.

There is an emphasis in this team on developing leadership at all levels. In Example 3.35 the team leader explains how she offered the opportunity for someone else in the team to deputise in her role while she was on holiday. This appears to have been done in full knowledge that his preferred style was different and in the expectation that this would be helpful rather than something that might undermine her authority.

Example 3.35
Delegating the lead

When I took my holiday I invited someone to develop their leadership and management skills by acting up in my absence. His style of leadership is quite different to mine but there's something quite challenging about that. He's quite autocratic. He's from Social Services and used to be a manager, quite clear about direction. More likely to say, 'That's your role, get on with it and if it goes wrong come and see me.' He's taught me things about management and decision-making – at times I can sit on the fence. Whereas he's very quick to make decisions. We complement each other.

This team also appear to feel free to challenge each other, including the formally appointed team leader. In Example 3.36 style of leadership is important as both the issue that provoked the challenge and the means of addressing the problem.

Example 3.36
Challenge to leadership

I was challenged about my behaviour with the client by one of the team. I think that was quite interesting as there were quite a lot of challenges then about style of leadership. He challenged me somewhat harshly and publicly. I dealt with it by speaking to him in private and saying it wasn't appropriate and don't do it again. He came back and apologised and said he was quite passionate about it because it was his client's care. Then I said some of the things he'd said had been quite right, just not how he'd delivered them.

The notion of leadership at all levels is essentially concerned with how people find themselves able to take the lead. Flexibility is often important in enabling people to take the initiative. As the team leader commented, the degree of financial flexibility varies: 'Social Services are a lot more flexible – you have a pot of money called "service user monies", and they're much more flexible, less dominant. So I have a pot of money so that if I want to take the clients out for a day, I can. If I see an urgent thing that I think needs doing, I can get it done. I'm more able to respond to crisis and I love that because that's what this team's about.'

In other cases, flexibility is required in the interpretation of regulations, particularly if they were designed for a significantly different working context. In Example 3.37 a number of issues are raised relating to interpretation of what constitutes health and safety risk and who might have the authority to approve activities that might appear to flout the regulations. In this example, there are two reasons given for paying service users to do decoration and repairs to rooms used by the service. The team member argues that it is beneficial to clients to pay them for the work if they need the money, implying that some clients would be grateful to be employed in this capacity and that it would enhance their self-images. There is a budget aspect in that she implies that it is cheaper to pay for casual labour than to bring in the Trust's estates department. A further dimension is that the team member felt that the chair informally supported the idea of involving patients in decorating the team premises.

Example 3.37
Flexibility in context

Some of the decorating and odd jobs here have been done by clients. The chair of the Trust said to me, 'We get so heated up about health and safety policy, but if you're telling me we can get patients to paint the rooms'. It's a lot cheaper to give clients money for food and debts than to get the estates department. Lots of middle managers were saying you can't do that because of policies, but because the top had told me I could, I scrapped the middle bit. And it worked.

In this case, this approach worked, but what would have happened if there had been an accident? Risk assessment would have considered the extent to which involving patients in carrying out improvements to buildings would bring unnecessary risks. Risk, however, is always a matter of judgement about balancing potential benefits against the potential risks. Risks can often be minimised without reducing the potential benefits. In this case, advice might have been sought about how to carry out this work as a community activity supported by the team. In a team where activities include supporting clients to carry out normal domestic and social activities, are odd jobs and decorating very different?

Perhaps there is risk to the team, however, if they are perceived to ignore the organisation's regulations and the managers who have to ensure compliance. The team members often mention their concern about gaining support and understanding for their innovative approach. Innovation usually involves challenge to the existing ways of doing things and this may include challenge to individuals whose roles involve maintaining order, often through use of rules and regulations. There is always a tension between the urge to disregard the established system in order to take swift action and the benefits of working with the system to create the changes that would enable different ways of working to fit within the regulations.

Example 3.38 explains how risk-taking is encouraged but within the boundaries of policies and procedures.

Example 3.38
Boundaries to risk

Our chief executive says make decisions, try something out. Take a risk. If it goes wrong, own it, look at it. If something does go wrong and you're honest about it and can justify it, that's OK. Certainly a rule's in place that if you can't justify it you're out on your ear. That's fine by me. I get excited about that ability to bring about change. The boundaries are the policies and procedures.

There are several features of this team that facilitated shared leadership. Although it is a big team it operates without a pyramid hierarchy and individuals take substantial personal responsibility for the overall operation of the service. The degree of respect that team members hold for each other is frequently mentioned, along with the importance of listening to each other. One of the team members explains in Example 3.39 how each member of the team takes a leadership role over particular issues.

Example 3.39
Clinical leadership in the team

I'm taking a clinical leadership role as opposed to a managerial one. There are several levels of leadership in this team. There's the kind of organisational leadership which is above us. Then there's the managerial and micro-organisational role that the team leader holds. Then individual team members from myself through the other nurses, support workers, occupational therapist, all have leadership roles clinically. In the team leader's absence, if she's not here to deal with certain things, there are some things we'd feel competent enough to deal with. Some of that leadership would be passed on. One person stays in the office and deals with any crisis calls, emergency calls or unplanned visits. The role of that person is to co-ordinate the rest of the team. Finding out where people are physically, allocating whoever to that particular job. That's another element of leadership. So I don't think there's one type of leadership in the team, I think there's numerous different types.

One type of leadership identified by a team member was leadership in discussions. In Example 3.40 this is discussed in the context of the value that the team places on the contribution of each member.

Example 3.40
Leadership in discussions

Different situations need different styles of leadership. We all participate in leadership in team discussions. No-one's opinion is less valuable than anyone else's, regardless of role, qualifications, experience. The strength of that is that the team is able to communicate more effectively if everyone feels valued. A good leader would step back from that and allow it to happen as opposed to imposing it. It's almost evolved naturally in this team that everybody does have a say and that what they say is valid and will be taken into account. We're able to give opinions and have that recognised.

I think leadership is fairly evenly distributed within the team. Staff initiate debates about the way we work. We're all capable of saying this is how we think things should be done. We all feel responsible enough to do that and accountable for the care that we're giving. The team leader has fostered this atmosphere of respect, said that we're all responsible for our own actions. Others in the team, particularly the support workers, have said, 'I'm not used to being asked my opinion.' I just take it for granted that we would ask.

People coming in now remind me of the fact that this is unusual.

Example 3.41 explains how the way in which the team works and the emphasis they place on discussing their work together enables them to develop a bigger picture for themselves and their clients.

Example 3.41
The team develops a bigger picture

Obviously there are certain clients that you deal with more than others. When you spend time with clients they'll discuss and open up different avenues. So you could possibly be able to pick up on the issues and bring them to the attention of everybody else, particularly if it's not been discussed before or it's not been thought of as an issue. In one way, the more people who are involved in seeing the client, the expanded social networks, they're not just seeing a worker – the team is thought of as a whole. You just get a bigger picture.

In spite of the apparent openness of the team there are sometimes difficulties that they do not find easy to resolve. In Example 3.42 the team leader explains how she helped the team to resolve an issue that had been developing into a problem.

Example 3.42
Dealing with problems in the team

There is high emotion at times. Of course we all have our professional conduct, but the team has to set standards as well about what's acceptable to the team. Individuals will tell me about things that are annoying them and ask me not to do anything about it, but I'll say, how can I not do now that you've told me. So what I try to do then is to pass it back to them about how can they solve it, because it would be much better if they can sort it out. I try to make them feel empowered enough to do it themselves. If two or three of them come to me with similar problems then I'll resolve that in terms of a staff meeting.

Two or three people mentioned to me that it was really annoying that one person was always late. For me as the team leader, that person gives me a hundred and fifty per cent when she's there. She gets here late and she lives a long way away. But I look at what she does in the team – she's the one that was here until three o'clock one morning. She stays late, always has, until a thing's done, and she works hard. So for me as the leader, how can I resolve this? Without offending her too much, but addressing the needs of the team. Eventually, I said at the team meeting that there are issues about everyone getting here at nine and shall we change the team meeting to quarter past? I said that some of us aren't great at mornings, me being one of them.

Afterwards, one of those who'd complained said, 'I really liked how you dealt with that because you owned it too. You were one of those who was sometimes late but I didn't tell you.' Well, it's true because I like to see my boys off to school. This has worked for a while and if there is a problem again with any member of the team they know that I'll deal with it.

Much has been said by this team about the problems faced in their work and how long it takes to achieve successful outcomes for most of their clients. In Example 3.43 we are reminded that it is very important for individuals and for the team as a collective to have their work recognised.

Example 3.43
Sharing success

It used to be if you've done a bad job you get told about it but if you've done a good job it's just taken as read. Here the leader's so enthusiastic that a pat on the back works wonders for anybody. If you've done a good job, you're told you've done a good job and it's shared with everybody else. So it does make you feel great. Because we're a team, if someone's done a good job it's shared, we've all contributed something to it.

LEARNING FROM THIS CASE STUDY

A number of themes emerged in the narrative accounts. The team has a high profile because it was the first to be established in the area. It is a large team, but flat in regard to qualifications and structure and members describe it as a respectful environment where everyone has a voice. They attribute this working environment to two factors, the person in the lead and the strong personalities of the team members. The team is united by a common vision and philosophy and shares a passionate belief in the model of service offered. There is a shared sense of humour but open conflict is not unusual and is often resolved by the camaraderie established through various processes and shared rituals built over their time together. There is an ethos of learning, a willingness to take responsibility and to share leadership.

Like some other teams we have encountered in the case studies, this team sees itself taking a lead in new ways of working, new approaches to service. Members of the team experience both struggle and pride as they uphold their shared vision. They refer to the 'high emotion' of dealing with a high risk client group. Their internal group relationships and communication sometimes mirror that high emotion and the team has developed ways and means to handle this.

The case study highlights too a number of other significant issues, the boundaries between leadership and management, the role of learning and development and the influence of leadership approaches in the larger organisational context.

Consider Example 3.37. Do you think this was an example of effective leadership within the team? Within the Trust? How might the team have worked with the middle managers instead of apparently ignoring their concerns? How do we move from people using their energy to 'fight' the system to involving them in developing a better system? Can you apply these ideas to your own situation?

In reading and reflecting upon the case studies and the range of examples you may find it useful to consider the following questions:

- How does the team handle emotional encounters?
- In what ways does a learning and development ethos relate to leadership approaches described here?
- How do the varying demands of leadership and management get reconciled?
- What aspects of the case study are relevant to your own experiences of working in teams?
- What would you consider changing in your own situation as a result of working with this case study?
- List the three most significant things you have learned from this case study and why they are significant to you.

You may find certain sections of Part 3 helpful, including the section on emotional intelligence. Can the various models of leadership help you to identify what 'leadership frameworks' the team uses to implement its unique service?

CHAPTER 4

OUTPATIENTS REFERRAL TEAM

INTRODUCTION

Members of this team contribute to provision of an Outpatients Referral system in a rural area. The only full-time member of this team is the manager of the service, who co-ordinates referrals. There are a number of other people who might be considered part of the team. Here we include perspectives brought by a service user representative and a general practitioner.

How the team works

Their general practitioner refers patients who need specialist services to an appropriate consultant, usually in their local hospital Trust. Once the referral is received, the Trust contacts the patient to arrange an appointment with the specialist. Patients remain as outpatients unless, during their treatment, it is necessary for them to stay in a ward as inpatients. Although the general practitioner refers the patient to a consultant, they continue to communicate with each other until the patient no longer needs the specialist services.

In this area there is a Community Health Council which represents the interests of health service users (these have been replaced by other mechanisms in many areas of the UK). In this case study, the chief officer of the Community Health Council explains how she contributes to the Outpatients Referral service to ensure that service users' concerns are considered.

The full team meet infrequently but much of the collaboration is carried out through informal processes. Although there have been improvements in the services provided by the Trust, the system for referrals can be affected by many factors that are not within the immediate control of the Trust, including the availability of specialist staff.

PERSPECTIVES FROM THE TEAM

Outpatients manager

I don't see myself as a leader – it's more of a co-ordinating role. I receive information, decide what to do with it and put in place the actions to do it. There's very little delegation.

The problem of having a little Outpatients User Group is that there's a danger of diluting things, of having too many grass roots people involved to make decisions. Within limited funding the Outpatients User Group can make decisions on the funding we've been allocated. But to make more fundamental change it's quite a lengthy process to get executive support plus the Trust Board, to go upward to get support for major change that needs more funding.

The Innovations in Care Board are a partnership chaired by an executive member of the Trust and including local authority and community representation. I think it needs to be at a high level, chief executive level, then you can drive it forward. You're then looking at professional managers running the show rather than health professions – but if you want to make change you have to have appropriate means.

At the moment I sort of lead the process, but have to input the process as well, which isn't very helpful at times. You know what needs to be done at the basic level, but no-one volunteers to do the work. Some people seem to want to meet about everything but I think that's a waste of time. I'll get on and do the work and if there are any problems I'll ask people. I consult as I go through the process. If I need to talk to a colleague, I'll talk to a colleague. If I need to talk to the boss, I'll talk to the boss. If I need to talk to files, I'll talk to files. If I need to talk to a nurse, I'll talk to a nurse. That to me is good. In terms of chairing and leading the process forward, if you can have that sort of dialogue and process, that's fine.

I have tried to get executive-level managers on the group. The impact has a monetary risk if you're looking at the cost of risks. There's nothing that this project doesn't touch on. That's where you have problems. It started with just the Outpatients but we need to change the Information Department and other departments. We focus on achieving targets but we don't focus on strategic improvement.

Some people work with just determination and guts. Certain people on the Board can move things on. Fortunately things that I ask for tend to get through. You need allies, powerful people.

Chief officer of the Community Health Council

I have a patient watchdog type of role. I got into it totally by accident. I'm a biochemist by profession, always having worked in a lab. I took a career break and then when the children started school looked around for some part-time work, but I was constrained by living in a rural area. I was using skills that I'd picked up doing voluntary work and then this job. I've been ten years now. The job has evolved as my situation has evolved – now it's full time.

Most of the job is to service the Council. Basic administration, organising the meetings and taking minutes and taking forward whatever the members want me to take. Writing letters. Lobbying Parliament or whatever. Trying to take the members' vision forward. If there is a lack of dentistry or whatever, perhaps ambulance problems, I forward this to other domains. That's a very main part of the Community Health Council role. Another very significant part of my role is helping people who have complaints about the NHS. This takes about a third of my time and it can be quite stressful. There's an awful lot of pain out there. A lot of counselling as well as going with people to reviews and consultants, holding their hands through things and on to the ombudsman. There are also visits, making sure the reports go to the right people and that the reports are followed up. I also train staff and members, in the wider region. It is like a leadership role without being the power behind the throne. It's the chairman who is the face of the Community Health Council, but I like to think I support him very strongly.

At first you do what has been done before, but you soon put your own stamp on it, have a view of how things should be developing. You get to know how things work. Working with politicians and Members of Parliament you get to know their thinking. In my position I've got to speak up for the lay person. I am a lay person. I'm a patient. My Mum is elderly. I've got kids. I just try to be honest and say this is the type of service I'd like us to have here and play it with a straight bat.

We meet for a couple of hours at lunchtime when there is something for us all to discuss and meanwhile the manager is beavering away. He brings us up to speed and asks for opinions. Everyone comes from a different position and represents a particular viewpoint. Our sphere of influence is very, very wide. Everyone wants to get into public consultation, public involvement, which is not an easy nut to crack. It does put pressure because you can never get it right. You're often faced in public meetings with stony silence. You meet a lot of people and a lot of different public bodies.

I'm very good at switching off. I think it's very important. I take a lot of work home, do a lot of reading, but I switch off in that if I've had a particularly difficult day or difficult complainant, I try not to take baggage home. You have to be flexible over timing though.

General Practitioner

The referral process depends largely upon the expectations and beliefs of the patient. They may or may not be expecting to be referred. Or might expect referral to a specific doctor or site. There are huge differences in referral patterns for very complicated reasons. You can have somebody doing more referrals to a specialist because that person knows more about the condition. For example, an expert in attention deficit disorder may do more referrals onto a tertiary centre. On the other hand someone may do more referrals because they know very little about it and don't have the skills to deal with the problem. Our practice very rarely do any paediatric referrals because we are all quite experienced and qualified paediatric general practioners, so we deal with most of it in house. A person may have a special interest in an area therefore keep the patient to deal with themselves. The analysis of referral patterns is a complicated issue because there are at least four or five variables. Referral patterns are very interesting and complicated, with what the patient brings to the process and what the practitioner adds to the process. Complicated as in where you refer and why.

Referrals fall into several categories in my head. I've got one that's 'urgent and important'. It has to be important before it ever becomes urgent. That's why you set up 'safe havens' for referrals like suspected cancers or incredibly serious things that need to be acted upon swiftly. There is a time scale that has to be met for the welfare of the patient. So for suspected breast cancer, suspected bowel cancer, things that need urgent action, it is crucial to set up a place where referrals are genuinely important.

Change is usually clinically driven. Obviously it's a clinical drive to improve and to standardise quality. You really want a standardised quality of referral letter and a standardised response. You want people seen appropriately to their need. Unfortunately it still probably relies an awful lot on the old boys' or girls' club. Over periods of time, decades, surgeons will have got to know various general practitioners personally, not as friends but in terms of their clinical functions. If a paediatrician I know gets a referral letter off me they wake up because they will know it is something unusual. Alternatively, we could have a situation where a particular surgeon gets a lot of referral letters off me but through postgraduate education and personal contact knows that every letter he gets off me will need surgical input because we still have access to imaging at our surgery. Therefore, a lot of our knee referrals, we know they're broke. The orthopaedic surgeons love getting those referral letters because they know what they are going to do.

On top of that you have your managerial drives. You have waiting lists and the Patient Charter. It's alleged that waiting lists are being closed for political reasons or financial reasons. So there is a managerial and financial impact on referral patterns. Some hospitals have been known to shut their waiting lists altogether so that they don't breach the charter. Paradox. It is interesting when you listen to people speaking who have an overview from above, a complicated understanding of a very large institution. Often people forget that something is the way it is usually for very good reasons.

How complicated it does become. I might refer a patient to a new team because of their clinical skills. Sometimes people don't need more surgery. Maybe I'll save someone from having another operation, because that clinician will say whether someone does or does not need an operation with confidence and ability. You are aware, though, that making that decision has a ramification on your local provider unit because you're not using it. Referral can change the pattern of provision. The service quality in the local provider unit has to be good enough to continue to refer people to it. With additional specialists, interest and commitment, it could change completely.

Speaking about the NHS on a grand scale, it affects referral patterns. If someone said my patients' hips could be done in the south of France, go for six weeks and come back fixed, but these options are not available. If they do become available we would have quite an iconoclastic population base. They'll travel. There are practical advantages to having a local provider unit, but I think there is a rapidly changing perception that it is not necessary for routine surgery. It's totally different when you are ill. When you are acutely ill you want to be where your family is. It has a real knock-on effect to your recovery chances. Again, standards have got to be adequate.

PERSPECTIVES ON CHANGE IN HEALTH AND SOCIAL CARE

In this and the following sections we consider some of the issues raised by individuals in the team. We have grouped these into perspectives on change, on teamworking and on leadership.

This team are very conscious of the political drive for change. As discussed in Example 4.1, the nature of political power tends to encourage support for initiatives that can be expected to show improvements in a short time. This approach to change is not always in the interests of service users.

Example 4.1
Political and patient agendas

I think it would be nice to have a period of stability. Whenever we have new structures they say it will be cost effective and save money, but I've yet to see that. A patient isn't interested in administration and structures, they just want a hospital and a service when they need it. So I do feel that there's perhaps a bit more reorganisation than is really wanted. A politician's agenda wants to be able to say, 'I've set up this', when 'this' probably didn't need to be set up. They set up projects that run for two years then want to set up new ones, not give money to the ones that have just started working and could do with another two years. The pot is only for new projects. I think, oh dear! We can see this, most people can, but we can't influence it. Politicians don't want to hear 'just keep it the same', particularly if it was set up by a previous administration. Democracy has a price, but maybe it isn't as democratic as we think it is. Patients don't want all this change. They want a service.

Funding is often a fundamental problem for those trying to improve the connections between services, particularly in health and social care where the funding systems are significantly different. In Example 4.2 some of these difficulties are discussed, together with implications of political involvement.

Example 4.2
Barriers to joint working

It's been going on for years, wanting the divide between health and social care more seamless, but it never works. Social care is often means tested and health isn't. There's been talk about putting social care into health, but it is difficult. There's a vision to work together but local councils say they haven't got the money and they'd have to increase the rates – no politician wants to do that. So even if they want to do good work, they can't capitulate over this one because they wouldn't get in again to do the good work.

Some initiatives gain funding to pilot a scheme but not enough to achieve sustainable change. In Example 4.3 this problem is described, but in this case the change was sustained by funding from a different source.

Example 4.3
Need for sustainable development

There was a scheme set up initially with money from Social Services, an intensive care at home package for people who had been discharged from hospital but who needed a bit of nursing input. It worked really well. Was able to unblock beds, helped patients, but then was threatened because the money ran out. Health put some money into it then, because they realised there were such advantages, but it was limping along, trying to find enough money. Another initiative has come up now that does much the same but it went through another pot of money and can now carry on the same sort of work.

Example 4.4 discusses a particular frustration over lack of investment in the infrastructure that supports service delivery and mentions some of the areas that would benefit from being able to make use of computers.

Example 4.4
Long-term gains

There's a whole range of things that without investment won't be possible. People are used not to having these things. They think that we've done it this way for ages and don't see a saving to be made. They see it as a drain on resources. They don't see the gain over a long time. If we actually put whizz-bang new computers in every room, complete with bar-code scanner, that's a cost of about fifty thousand pounds. But they don't then see the saving over five or six years in admin time, time in clerical costs, in the way in which we manage our case notes. Savings in all of the systematic changes that support the whole process of improving services.

Example 4.5 outlines another potential improvement that has been delayed by lack of funding for computers.

Example 4.5
Need to plan investment

There is a joint assessment plan between Social Services and Health. Joint assessments of need. That's being held up because none of the district nurses have direct access to a computer terminal. The Trust can't afford to buy them. There is talk about using charitable funds to support the system. We're strapped for cash.

Example 4.6 comments on how increasing use of computers has brought the possibility of changing the system of referrals to offer more direct access to consultants' lists by general practitioners. This type of change, however, is also easily disrupted if staff do not have sufficient access to equipment.

Example 4.6
Potential improvements in referrals

The mechanics have changed with the computerisation of the practice. The paper is disappearing. We are looking forward, possibly, to direct access to waiting lists. That would mean instead of seeing the surgeon, a simple hernia might go straight to the operating waiting list. So a general practitioner would be able to refer directly to the waiting list. You would need to have a great deal of trust between the clinicians involved. You'd obviously have to have occasional meetings and agree protocols and pathways.

There was an attempt to have a computerised referral for prostate problems recently. Including the referral form. But it didn't work. It was almost comical. The computer that was on the Trust site wasn't in the Outpatients department so they couldn't use it often. There are technical things like that. It doesn't all happen immediately. It needs a critical mass of change and then it will happen.

Increasing use of computers has streamlined referral systems to some extent, as described in Example 4.7, but wider access to information has also led to a better-informed public with some knowledge about which centres have the best records of success in treatments. As this team member explains, comparisons are not always made from similar base lines. As records of this nature become more available, they will not be meaningful unless the assumptions underlying the data are made clear and those using such data are helped to understand how to interpret the information.

Example 4.7
Informed patients influencing the referral process

Breast lumps are a relatively simple referral pattern. With a breast lump you'll get a secondary referral to a Breast Centre, hopefully a dedicated treatment assessment centre. You need, as a practitioner, to have confidence in the clinical ability of your referral centre. So more and more of our breast referrals are going now to another county. Patients don't even go to, the local hospital. The time when people accepted a referral to the local hospital purely because it was the local hospital is fading. Publicity about the difference in outcome, depending on the ability of the unit you go to, makes people more aware, particularly at the higher socioeconomic level, of differences in quality. Between doctors and between hospitals. Ten years ago, people saw a doctor as a doctor and didn't perceive differences.

Patients have every right to influence where they are referred to. I think the government league tables, albeit crude, in terms of waiting times and outcomes has influenced this. Outcomes have been criticised. This has not gone down well with the profession because of the very complicated nature of outcome. If you look at a tertiary liver referral unit the outcomes are appalling because you get people who are usually going to die. So the outcomes actually may be remarkably good. If you are a super specialist, you take on the more difficult cases. It's the same thing for cardiac surgeons. The best surgeons do the most difficult cases. It would be very easy for a good surgeon to have an almost perfect record if they always picked easy valve replacements. So league tables are complicated. It should be possible to grade people going in and grade them coming out.

Example 4.8 suggests that decision-making power has shifted from consultants to politicians because of increasing public demand for information and high-quality services.

Example 4.8
Who has the power?

I used to think that consultants thought they had the power. But times have changed and they're realising that their little domain is not as powerful as they might want. I think the power actually comes from the politicians because Trusts have to dance to the politicians' tunes, have to return various returns every month, have to deliver to the politicians' agendas. The politicians are listening to the people and saying what they want.

Political interventions have set targets as an attempt to improve services and to ensure a more even quality across geographical areas. This is not always successful when resource limitations also have to be overcome. Example 4.9 comments on how the political attempts to reduce waiting lists to improve the quality of services may sometimes reduce quality for individuals by taking decisions about allocation of scarce resources away from the clinical staff.

Example 4.9
Attempts to force improvements don't always work

You've got the 'need to be done soon' conditions. Like hernia and hips. The problem with hips is that they go to a waiting list. The waiting list initiatives and the time initiatives are detrimental to patient care. Someone who goes onto a waiting list to have their hip replaced may still be walking around, perfectly well, managing. But you may have someone else crash onto the waiting list with a very rapidly deteriorating hip who within a month can't walk. You can't skip the person who can walk on this list to treat the more serious one first. There is a managerial force pushing the clinical need down, and the waiting list up in terms of importance. Time is now being given a more important status than the quality of a person's life. You have a new factor in the referral pathway that never existed before.

Standards and targets can cause other difficulties when funding is not available to meet new requirements. In Example 4.10 some of the issues that may arise when organisations attempt to meet new standards are discussed. There are not only funding problems but also muddles over estimating changes in staffing needs.

Example 4.10
Muddles and manipulation

One of the standards is that everyone who has a heart attack should see a cardiologist within twenty-four hours. There's a very weak clinical evidence base for that. It's weak research. No real evidence behind it whatsoever. It's a political statement but it's deemed a good standard of care.

So you try to find a coronary specialist to meet that standard locally. You obviously need the infrastructure around that person to allow them to function. A dedicated coronary care area is a standard of practice. And you ain't got it. So, in a political arena, the money is found to build one. Then you've got nobody to run it.

Then you get involved in this very complicated area that I think needs to be sorted out behind closed doors. At the moment, say you have ten people in a day who have had a heart attack. There are nurses looking after them, they are in beds and they have monitors. It's disingenuous of an organisation then to make a business plan that staffs the unit from scratch. Which clearly doesn't take into account that the drugs are already paid for, the nursing staff are there, the beds are already there, the monitoring is already being done. There is an upgrading cost undoubtedly. But it's not a staffing from scratch cost.

There are also often difficulties in finding highly qualified staff to lead areas of clinical expertise. As we see in Example 4.11 the arrival of a specialist in a particular locality may lead a Trust to take a rather opportunistic approach to establishment of a specialist centre.

Example 4.11
Who should the funding follow?

Let's say a well-known consultant married a girl from this area and moved here. The hospital would say, 'Yes, come and work here.' The people who are already working here on the surgical wards would be enthralled, enthused and committed (which they probably already are). Suddenly it's all turn around. Now a General Practitioner has the advantage of a surgeon you want your people to see, with the abilities to do the level of scanning that needs to be done and with a chemotherapy team on site, on the patient's doorstep. One man could make the difference. There is knock-on effect to the management structure. You have to resource the surgery. Then you need to look at where the money goes. That money needs to follow the patient. Which it doesn't at the moment.

From this account, some people might think that money seems to follow the personal location choices of specialists. We might consider how the situation described in Example 4.12 would change if resourcing decisions were made with due consideration of both the evidence base and the existing local infrastructures.

Example 4.12
One way of creating centres of clinical expertise

It's very interesting that when you have a clinician with a special interest land somewhere, they will create a clinical team and go out and canvass referrals. Most hospital consultants when they arrive will go around and introduce themselves to clinicians and even have postgraduate evenings so that we know what is happening. Even Trusts will send out flyers – it's routine practice. The new consultants come around and tell you what their interests are: 'Hello I'm Joe Bloggs. I'm interested in stomachs.' I say, 'OK, I'll refer stomachs to you then.' So if somebody gives very good care in gastroenterology, suddenly, gastroenterology referrals go through the roof.

The autonomy of consultants has often been presented as one of the barriers to change in healthcare. Example 4.13 suggests that more recently trained and appointed consultants may be more ready to engage in wider service improvement.

Example 4.13
They take their toys away

There are certain consultants who want to do things their own way. They have their own lists and they want to do them as they've always done them and they're not going to change for any politician. So they take their soldiers and just don't play. So getting them onto the system tends to be done behind the scenes, not actually in this group. So there's a lot of smoothing. Change is hard and some feel that they don't want appointments to go centrally. They think, 'I want them to go through my secretary,' so they have control and don't want the control to go. But I think we now have most of them on board. As the older ones leave and the new ones come in there is a new ethos, I feel.

The increasing emphasis on consultation and involvement of service users in co-development of services is also contributing to improvement. A local initiative is described in Example 4.14.

Example 4.14
Local improvements

We did an initiative about food in hospitals. We were getting a lot of grumbles, food was cold, etc. So we went to the hospitals, asked if we could we do a little survey on this and they agreed. So we compiled a questionnaire. Volunteers went up and had meals in the hospitals. That resulted in a slight change in meal times to allow later suppers and more variation in menus, so a few changes. Also things like heated trolley and covers on plates – some little things that we managed to get on board. The patients are the people we want information from but the hospital has to be involved as well. We needed the catering department and the Chief Executive to be willing.

As organisations gain more experience of consultation with service users it often becomes apparent that special efforts have to be made if all potential service users are to be included. Example 4.15 explains how an approach was made to young people.

Example 4.15
Wider consultation

It worried me for a while that when we consult people we tend to go to middle-aged, white and middle-class people. Where are the children? So we went out to a primary school with a school governor and talked to the children about what was important to them in the health service and took that back to the hospital. One issue was sexual health, for example, having a little clinic for the teenagers so that they don't have to see their own family General Practitioner.

PERSPECTIVES ON TEAMWORKING

Much of this team's work is carried out in large meetings. Example 4.16 outlines some of the issues that arise in these meetings.

Example 4.16
Herding cattle

Clinical networks are groups of consultants – ophthamology, general surgery, radiology, dental, all sorts, and lay members. Their purpose is to co-work across these areas to cover each other, perhaps to specify. Perhaps they can do more hips in one place than another. Clinical governance is another topic. They need to train together, so instead of saying this is my domain, they have to work together. The chair is a very good co-ordinator. He doesn't lead strongly but gets everybody inputting and does lots of smoothing and pouring oil on troubled waters, getting them all to work together – a bit like a sheepdog, like herding cattle. Everybody is equal but the person who actually leads has to have a lot of social skills and credibility because it needs a lot of people skills to draw people together.

In large meetings the behaviour of participants can create difficulties for others present. Example 4.17 describes some of the feelings raised for one participant when others seem not to share an understanding about protocols of behaviour in meetings.

Example 4.17
Behaviour in meetings

An example was in a Primary Care Board. We got the General Practitioners on the Board and went through a big organisational development plan. We got them functioning as a Board. You don't all butt in, you address through the chair. Basic common sense about meetings. Then there's the responsibilities of Board members, because General Practitioners can, of course, go out and say whatever they want as individuals, but as members of the Board they can't, they have to toe the Board line.

That basic stuff about how to behave in meetings isn't known very well and it becomes very important, for example, when you're discussing with professionals. Especially nurses, because nurses don't really know how to behave in meetings. They're butting in, they're talking. The idea is that you pick up on body language, so you know when people are pausing naturally or when people have stopped and finished what they're saying.

Example 4.18 describes a situation in which it is possible to disagree but still to maintain a good working relationship.

Example 4.18
Maintaining good relationships

You have to build up relationships with people. It can be difficult. There are times when you have to criticise the Trust and sometimes you are not going to see eye to eye and that's the end of it – you have to agree to disagree. But you've got to be careful about the relationship. Sometimes things have gone terribly wrong and you have to say this is something different and we actually want to do that . . . there's an interplay . . . give and take.

Example 4.19 describes some improvements that this team has made and some of the ways that they overcame difficulties.

Example 4.19
Service improvement

The team is about innovations and care. Waiting lists are always a big issue. You have to think how can we make it easy for people who don't intend to cancel and that type of thing. So from the patient's point of view, you go to your doctor and you're told yes, I'll refer you to so and so, but then you're left at home and you have no idea how long this is going to take, a month or six months – you're left in limbo. So it occurred to us that if a patient had more information, they'd be able to plan. So if you're told it will be so many months you'd be able to think, well yes, I can go on holiday, I needn't think about this yet. We thought that there are lots more things that could be made more patient friendly.

So now when people go to their General Practitioner they will say 'I'm referring you to so and so', and they can flick it up on the screen and see that the waiting list is about five months. Then they'll say, 'You'll get a letter from the hospital to say that I've referred you. What will happen then is that a month before the appointment is due the hospital will get in touch and make an appointment.' So people have more choice, can make the appointment that suits them. More people turn up because they won't be at work or moved away. The 'do not attend' rate has gone right down and more people can be fitted into clinics. Some 'do not attend' rates are horrendous, run at about twenty-five per cent. Such a waste.

I'm on the team from the patient's point of view, so I look at specimen letters and draft letters, think whether I'd like to get a letter like that. Would I understand it? Is it confusing? How best to contact the patient? Then other people from Outpatients look at it from their point of view. And people from the Records department from their point of view – how awkward is it going to be to send out letters, make appointments, etc. There are some consultants there who have their own lists and who might say, 'I don't like the fact that they can make appointments. What do we do with urgent cases? If we have routines how do we fit those in?' So everybody brings how it will affect them and we can look at where there are hiccups. The manager co-ordinates and chairs the meetings and draws it all together. So no-one has a real lead, more of a co-ordinator with everyone having a strong voice.

Example 4.20 suggests that not only is local change best made by those in the particular area of work, but also that helpful change can often be made without additional resources if people share the existing resources more effectively.

Example 4.20

Encouraging teamworking to manage local change

They might not co-operate as a team. It's a threat. They'll have to share offices. Each consultant wants a named personal assistant – you have almost a cultural thing about one doctor, one secretary. No-one wants to share. This is silly. We're producing review after review after review, which isn't getting anywhere. Writing lengthy documents and doing desk workload exercises – how many people have long letters to write, how many have short letters to write, how many are filing . . . it ain't working. You can have piles of work one week, different others.

If there is a limited resource, left to themselves people will help each other out and get it done. I'm not going to tell them how I think it should operate. Part of the change process is not to help them necessarily in the way they want to be helped. We're going to start changing teams but not because we've had a review or produced a document for consultation. We'll work on changing things naturally. I delegated and got them to set up groups to look at their work. They'll look at their working practices and things and they'll come out with the best system that will be sharing what they do and sharing resources.

In an area where staff turnover is slow, with frequent changes in the ways in which services are organised, people often move from one role to another. In Example 4.21 this is presented as an advantage because staff gain wider experience of taking different perspectives in different roles. This may enable people to have better understanding of the variety of views about an issue and to be more flexible about negotiating solutions.

Example 4.21

Same people, new roles

In a place like this, the players stay the same but the structures change. You have the same faces but they're in slightly different roles. You see people with different hats on. In many ways it is an advantage because they can understand from someone else's point of view, might say, I used to feel like that too – how can we get round it?

PERSPECTIVES ON LEADERSHIP

Example 4.22 discusses how leadership in health and care in the political environment is setting helpful frameworks and direction for local service improvement.

Example 4.22
Political leadership and clinical needs

Leadership and the political environment are tied together. If you have your heart attack here today, the standard of care you will receive from the local hospital is actually relatively rather good. It would stand up to the standard of care you would receive anywhere else. The National Service Frameworks are excellent in that they set down a standard of care that should be uniform across the country. In other words you try as a national political leader to say to the clinicians, and I think it's a rather brave thing to do, you tell me what the standards should be and we'll try to reach the standards uniformly across the country. Which is brave. Which is good.

At local level, the issues for leaders are more about balancing service development within available resources. Example 4.23 describes some of the tensions involved when making choices about service development when there are competing priorities.

Example 4.23
Managing resources and expectations

I think the two leaders, the chief executive of the Trust and the chief executive of the Local Health Board, had an understanding. I think they said, we could do this now, and then in a couple of months when more money comes on stream perhaps we can do that. We can't do it all now. This is the understanding we'll work on. Everybody will be happy and calm, all the politicians. The newspapers will be cool.

But then you get a clinician firing off in a meeting, wanting it all on day one, for all the right reasons, but politically naive. Either more money will come or it will backfire and you'll have people wandering around wondering what is the future of that hospital. It's a very dangerous ploy. Leadership is a balancing act, between clinical need and the realisation that rationing really does exist. A balanced distribution of resource is necessary for the benefit of all the patients. It's no good having a clinician firing off in his own particular area when the outcome might cripple several other very important areas.

Example 4.24 comments on the need for an overview of service provision and commitment to provision of a complete local service from all those that contribute.

Example 4.24
Need for overarching vision

When you have crossover you've got to have some form of leadership otherwise things fall between two stools – that's their responsibility . . . no that's their responsibility. I think you have to have overarching vision, perhaps even more than leadership if people are coming from two different perspectives and don't want to lose power. Overarching and with some sort of commitment to taking one service forward coming from both sides.

Example 4.25 describes a leadership role in structuring meetings to enable wider participation in discussion about change.

Example 4.25
Developing a structured process

This is a partnership process, so everyone has a right to have their view, everyone has a right to be heard, but everyone has the right to have their views listened to, discussed and debated. Just because you want your thing to go ahead doesn't mean that it will be accepted and implemented. So it's how you manage that process.

That's a particular challenge we have. If you're involving people in meetings in ways they haven't been involved before, asking them to make a contribution, particularly when it's something that they're impassioned about, there has to be a way of educating them, showing them, demonstrating, how best to participate in the process. You could ask whether the group is the right mix, right people. You have to have structure and order.

Example 4.26 describes leadership as encouraging and shaping developments in ways that support the agendas of influential participants.

Example 4.26
Pulling the strands

With leadership you've got to have charisma so that you draw people along with you. I don't think it would work at all if I made decisions and said we're going to go this way or that way. I like to think I pull all the strands, the important ideas other people have got, and try and translate them to some sort of positive action. I can decide this is a good idea or yes, we should be doing that. It's very intuitive in many ways. You have to be quite well read as you get tomes and tomes of reports from everywhere. You need to know what the current thinking is because thinking goes in trends – what's flavour of the month one month might not be another month. What's attractive to the politicians, especially when there's an election in May. Anything that gets them in the headlines will be good. So you have to know in a sort of underhand way how to fit in your messages to best effect.

Another example of leading through influence rather than by having power is given in Example 4.27.

Example 4.27 ▬▬▬▬▬▬▬▬▬▬▬▬▬▬▬▬▬▬▬
Leading by influence

I try to analyse. Dealing with members and politicians, they obviously have a vision, but say, 'We want that.' When they want something to happen and can only see the pros, I try to see the cons, see the bigger picture, to steer a way through it. Otherwise, we'd be caught out. Often we know far more about what's going on than people who come from one service area, particularly if they don't get on. Sometimes I could bang their heads together. Like you do with kids when they're quarrelling, try to make them see each other's point of view. Sometimes someone from outside can take the heat out of a situation. Sometimes I just say, 'Can I just clarify? You say your problems are so and so, you say your problems are so and so.' Just articulating it for them. Move away from the confrontation. Then I might say, 'What if?' Make some suggestions. Some might be completely silly and they'll say, 'That won't work', but then things evolve and they become less antagonistic towards each other.

Leadership in a public forum can bring personal conflict. Example 4.28 describes having to act on a decision that seemed wrong.

Example 4.28 ▬▬▬▬▬▬▬▬▬▬▬▬▬▬▬▬▬▬▬
The power of the people

Once a decision was made that I totally disagreed with. In hindsight I think it was made for a political end. Nobody could see where this decision had come from. In the end, we had to take the decision through because so many people wanted it, but it hadn't been carefully thought through.

I had to do a radio interview following the decision and I'd written it out for the other decision that I'd expected. I had to cancel the interview because I didn't have any idea what to say. No idea how to say 'support this decision', why they voted in this way, what were the reasons. I had to do a lot of thinking about this afterwards and it took a lot of smoothing over. We were among many making this decision and although I think that it would actually have gone this way in the end, I still don't support the decision.

It taught me a salutary lesson. I learnt that it's not just leadership, there are so many other things at play. Politically where votes are and who's trying to support who for what reason. What seems eminently sensible to me might for some other reason just not get through. I hold the cards but there still might be a joker in the pack that I'm not seeing. So I know now that I do have to be careful. To be aware that until the decision is actually taken, it's not taken. Until we know, I've learnt not to sound confident, to hedge my bets, not go around assuming it. It completely turned pear shaped on me and I realised that this is what democracy really is. That actually you can't say, 'This is how we're going to go', even as a leader. It is the power of the people.

Example 4.29 describes leadership in public service more as a type of 'servant leadership'.

Example 4.29
Servant leadership

In many ways, one would query whether I am a leader – really I serve the members. It's the members and the chair who actually should lead – ask the members and they'd say, 'She's the dogsbody, she does what we tell her.' But I suppose I lead by perhaps suggestions, by ways of bringing knowledge too. I help the members and guide them.

Example 4.30 comments on some of the skills that a leader needs in such a public environment.

Example 4.30
Some necessary leadership skills

Personality is very important, people skills, in this type of job. You've got to be able to get on with members of the public. You've got to have empathy, compassion with people who have complaints. You've got to be able to speak in a public meeting, when you're saying something that perhaps people don't like, so you've got to be able to take the flak, to be able to take quite a bit of stress. You've got to be confident enough to deal with people at Board level, with Chief Execs and to be able to say your piece. Be able to speak articulately and sensibly. So a good education is quite useful as well. People skills are the most important, and intuition.

Another member of this team explains in Example 4.31 how agreement is obtained to progress a plan. This person also commented on a lack of project management skills within the service.

Example 4.31
Agree the plan

My role is to lead the process and also to do it, which is an incredibly time-consuming role. You get the guidance, you get the information, you think of the changes. The one thing that it's worth getting people's approval for is a plan. That's certainly where you need partnership working. You say, here's a plan, comments please, let me know what's right, what's wrong, agree the plan, from that point get an action plan. Fine. Settle on that plan. That's the point at which everyone's happy to buy into the vision.

LEARNING FROM THIS CASE STUDY

The case study says much about leadership as a political process, one that involves influence, relationships and knowledge of the most effective channels to work through. Leadership takes place within a democratic political environment that is inherently 'messy'. It is unpredictable, changeable, and characterised by tension, conflict and competition for scarce resources. The price of democracy and winning votes means that change is sometimes conflated with service improvement, where shifting funding patterns can be an advantage, but sustainability of established services can suffer.

Team members talk about leadership as a political process at both a macro or large-scale level, and at a micro or teamworking level. The large-scale, political environment is one where clinical and political/management drivers for change can and do clash. Reconciliation requires an overriding vision. Political leaders provide that vision by articulating the needs and wants of an increasingly well-informed public. One of the difficulties is the degree to which the political players ought to determine the way in which services are delivered.

At a more local level, the team gives many examples of how any change influences the complex patterns of interrelationships. Change in one department inevitably requires change in others. Making a referral decision has implications for the individual patient, the local provider in the near environment and the specialist centre in the far environment. Leadership at a local level involves effective teamworking and a meeting 'etiquette' to facilitate participation. Leadership requires building alliances with those who have power and influence.

Example 4.23 talks about leadership as a balancing act between clinical need and the realisation that rationing really does exist. A balanced distribution of resource is necessary for the benefit of all the patients. Do you agree that this is a key focus of leadership? Where would you place this view in the management/leadership continuum? This seems to be a statement that respects the status quo. Where might challenging the status quo come in? What alternative views of leadership might you consider?

In reading through the case study and examples consider the following questions:

- How might various and alternative views of leadership such as those discussed in Part 3 make a difference to the examples in the case study?
- What role does leadership have in considering the ripple effects of change?

What leadership approaches are used in your own current team or organisation? What could you do differently given that you have the power and influence to make a difference? What can you do now?

CHAPTER 5

CANCER COLLABORATIVE NETWORK

INTRODUCTION

This Cancer Services Collaborative Network is supported by the National Health Service Modernisation Agency and was set up specifically to bring about practical improvements in cancer services. Cancer services in the UK have lagged behind North America and Europe particularly around survival rates for people who have had cancer. This appears to be not because the treatment or specific services were poor but because people have accessed services much later in cancer, making curative treatment more difficult. Once this became apparent, it was clear that more emphasis had to be placed on providing early access to services and providing better integration of services.

There are many similar local networks in the UK supported by this modernisation programme. The scheme uses an American approach called Health Improvement Methodology. This focuses on introducing continuous incremental change as opposed to large-scale planning and implementation. Both local government and Strategic Health Authorities provide strategic co-ordination but many other public, private and voluntary organisations have become involved.

How the team works

This local collaboration involves several teams. There is a small team of facilitators who work with teams from health organisations, Social Services and social care voluntary agencies to improve access to services and the patient's journey through sequential services. Areas of improvement that the teams are working on include waiting times, appointments, communication between primary and secondary care, patient information pathways and meeting targets for urgent treatment. They are also beginning to address palliative care services.

Improvement of services is part of everyday work although this often runs alongside maintaining the existing services until they can be replaced by more integrated ones. The improvements are designed and developed by staff already involved in service delivery. This is core to the philosophy underlying the approach, which places importance on application of local knowledge and skills to address local problems. The locally employed facilitators are trained and supported by the Modernisation Agency and are also supplied with a range of tools and techniques that they can use and share to support staff making local developments.

PERSPECTIVES FROM THE TEAM

Network service improvement lead

This network is made up of two acute Trusts and six Primary Care Trusts. My role is to lead service improvement for cancer patients, to enhance their experiences and to enable them to have a better outcome at the end. It's not about the clinical aspects, it's about the processes that go along the patient pathway. I lead a team of service improvement facilitators and I am talking about facilitating and not doing. So they go into a clinical team when invited in and they use their tools and techniques to enable that team to move that work along.

We learn specific tools and techniques for modernisation methodology, which is mapping a patient journey, capacity and demand, and out of that comes an action plan for the team. The team take ownership of that plan and take it away, but we are there with the skills to help if a facilitation day is needed or some input. For example, how do we do this, what sort of numbers do we collect here, how do we collect the numbers? It's about supporting and facilitating rather than doing. The initiative has been going three years but has gone through some changes of identity and role. This facilitation phase has only been going a few months and we changed the title and looked at the role of facilitators.

Within your mandate you are working with different organisations. That's where you have the different challenges and the human dimensions. The Network Board is made up of membership from the acute Trusts and the Primary Care Trusts. So if we say service improvement is on the agenda this year, this is how we are going to do it, there is a process. It is up to the lead to work out which is the best way of working to gain the most. I have one of the smallest networks in the country but the issues and challenges are exactly the same.

Our team changed from being project managers to facilitators. I was told to do it, but now my thought processes have changed. I have had to think about facilitation and support compared to project management. I also had to get my team to think that way. Before they got an action plan and implemented it. Their job now is to go in and facilitate to get an action plan, but the action plan has other names on it, not theirs, because it has to have the ownership of the clinical team. That team has to take the work forward but they can ring us anytime to say, 'We are stuck here, what are we doing and where do we go? We need some help on this or we need training on this.' So it's a different way of working.

It wasn't difficult to bring the team on board. I started gently saying things about how we'll have to change the way we work. So the team worked out how we would take this forward. We modelled in our own team what we hoped we would do in the settings. There are five on the team from a range of backgrounds. They can be anything. A radiographer, a nurse, etc. It's about learning the skills. It's good to have insider knowledge, but it's also good for the dynamics of the team to have outsider knowledge. The current team have all worked in health but one of the members comes from Australia. Another person works two jobs, one in the public health sector. One worked in information and audit.

I feel my team are together. If any of us have a problem it comes to the team and we try to work it through. As a leader, I can bring some things to the team, but there are other things I need to sort out outside of the team. It can be very difficult but I have made sure there is a system in place for my team and I did that in the very beginning. You have to take all the old processes, put them to one side and think in a different way.

My resources come down from a national pot and I have another pot for new service improvement. That pot of money is about a service improvement where we've identified what we have to put in place but haven't got resources. For example, this will let us fund a nurse for twelve months, see what the outcome is and evaluate. If we find that's what's needed, then it's up to the Trust to pay for it in future because my pot of money runs out. Often they want it, but they don't want to fund it next year. One guy was very sceptical about the team's work but he's gone outside and seen what value he has here and has changed his mind. I'm glad that I will be able to relay that to my team, because he gave them problems. I am proud of all of us.

Lead facilitator

I'm a service improvement facilitator with the Cancer Services Collaborative that was established to bring about practical changes. It has made some great inroads into breast cancer. One in three people will get cancer at some time in their lives and one in four will die from cancer. It is very much a disease of the elderly. Not exclusively, but as the population grows older more people will get cancer. The NHS Cancer Plan aimed to reduce the risk of cancer, to improve cancer services in the community, to improve and give faster access to treatment, improve the lives of cancer sufferers and also to improve research.

Cancer Collaborative people are employed by local health organisations to assist with these improvements. We have a team leader who is the service improvement lead. I am employed by a Primary Care Trust and work across the five in this region that form the Cancer Network. Cancer Networks are loose organisations that bring good practice together.

I helped to facilitate a baseline assessment of General Practitioners' cancer services in the community. There was a questionnaire that asked things like, 'What information do you have in the surgery on cancer? Do you keep a list of cancer patients? Do you keep a list of palliative care patients? Do you use the fax referral system for the hospital?' At the moment I'm following that baseline assessment up. I might go to a Primary Care Trust Executive Committee and give a presentation on the results of the assessment, which says things like only one in five practices keep a list of palliative care patients. The question is, if they don't know who they are looking after how can they develop a service? Last week I presented a 'Time to learn' session, which was when all the general practitioners come together.

My frustrations are about having influence but no power. The baseline assessment had been sitting in the doldrums, so I spurred it into action. Now, I am trying to spur the Primary Care Trusts to do something about the results. But, the report sits on people's desks, among the priorities. To push the cancer corner is an uphill struggle because the new contract does not emphasise cancer as a primary care issue. It is seen as an acute issue. People want to move in the same direction but their own agendas can get in the way.

Social service lead

I've been involved since phase three of the Collaborative. Before this I was managing the community Macmillan nurses. So it was all palliative care. Getting to grips with what's going on in the acute Trusts has been quite a steep learning curve.

I've had to learn about using the Modernisation Agency's redesign methodology – process mapping, capacity and demand. It was something I hadn't come across before – the techniques and things. Cancer Collaborative is changing in the third phase, becoming more about sustainability. People who were programme managers have become facilitators, so staff are changing their own service. Being the lead means working with them, making sure that it's fitting in with national and local priorities, feeding that information back to the national team and also taking a strategic view.

We meet up very regularly and have a service improvement steering group. We get together with the cancer services managers in the acute Trusts and the network team. We also have a clinical lead for service improvement who works one day a week with us. I take a linking role and get the overall view and try to move it forward in a strategic direction, making sure that we are actually achieving what we set out to do. It's basically about improving the patient's journey through various methods. We are looking at things like waiting times, patients being seen, urgent referrals from their general practitioners to the target of first (definitive) treatment within sixty-two days. Also improving communication between primary and secondary care and looking at patient information pathways. Palliative care is a big issue for us as well.

One of my biggest challenges is engaging with clinical teams and getting them on board, because a lot of them have worked very hard on their services and have already done a lot to improve things. What works well is getting together with them and talking it through. Getting them to come up with some of the areas they can improve, working with them on those ideas. To be a good lead you have to be able to communicate well and listen to some of the problems they have. Have a strategic view. Have a vision of where you want them to be and be able to demonstrate it. Trying to get people out of some kind of silo.

My personal strategic view is keeping the patient at the heart of the journey on whichever pathway their care is taking, be it acute, primary or palliative. How you improve that patient experience. We get lots of information back from clinical teams about what the patient experience is. Also from mixing with the national team and the other networks and what's going on in their area. Now we have a reporting system where we put everything on to a database and look at what other teams are doing. A lot of work is available on line. We also get an update on key implemented changes. This gives us something to discuss with clinical teams about whether there is anything they think can be done here. That is the idea of the team going in to help the clinical team look at their service and any redesign needs so that if there is an improvement it can be sustained.

The service improvement leads meet up together and with our associate director from the national team, who is very supportive. The clinical lead is a palliative care consultant. She helps us to engage with the clinicians. It's about credibility. Even in this day and age sometimes peer to peer is more effective. If we are trying to engage general practitioners we would write joint letters. People are doing joint training now. When I trained it wasn't like that. You were very much doing a nursing course.

Service manager for Older People's Services

My role is multifaceted. I'm employed by the local authority in a joint-funded post with the Primary Care Trust. I have management responsibility for all Older People's Services in the locality provided through the county council but I also now have responsibility for instigating and overseeing partnership schemes. It's a fairly new concept. We were asked to move into a locality base for social work for provider services as well as external commissioning. It aligns far more with health colleagues and it really went in the right direction with regard to the NHS Plan and as a way forward for partnership schemes.

My background is in social work though mainly in health. This new approach is key to the merging of services in the locality. I am working so closely with primary care colleagues and acute Trust colleagues that it gives a much more partnership approach. It doesn't contradict or conflict with your own professional identity. It's about seeing how together you can work to provide a service.

I am very fortunate that in this part of the county there is a very open communication. In that people have been very willing to talk and explore different options. Primarily I am here to manage county council services and to move forward with commissioning that affects local authority money. But I also have a direct link through to the director of Integrated Care Services within the Primary Care Trust. My line manager is within the county council but I also have an indirect route through to the director and the chief executive within the Primary Care Trust. If there is any confusion, the way forward is to talk it through to find a solution to the problem. We deal with each situation as it comes up. We have to value people's professional identity and their interest base that has brought them into a particular role.

The palliative care pilot that we are looking at initially started with conversations and individuals just networking. The facilitators came in a little bit later but have been extremely helpful and bring a different perspective. The initial group was a 'hospice at home' service, including myself and my social work staff within the hospital who have a particular interest in palliative care, my home care staff and our Primary Care Trust colleagues.

What we wanted to achieve is a seamless service so that patients and their families could come in one door and they didn't have to open six others. Our prime action was about a more integrated way of working. Not everybody being based together but a far more integrated way of working and knowing who to network with if somebody needs to pull in another service. As part of that, it was about a certain number of home care workers developing their skills to work alongside the 'hospice at home' service so that they could do the same job. At times you want to run before you can walk and you make mistakes that way. You must plan it and work with people on what needs to happen. We have to be clear on what needs to be offered before we take it out to general practitioners because they will want to grab it and run with it.

I've asked the home care manager to work with the manager of the hospice and the Macmillan nurses and with other colleagues to talk through what the roles are and what we need to achieve because that has implications for costs. For them to have ownership of what's going on they need to identify what it is that's required. If they're not involved from the word 'go' they can't see where this is going and they can't own what's going on. There are some quite painful changes to be made to the way things work across both health and social care and they have supported us in doing that. But that has to come from them owning the service that they're involved in and wanting to see it achieve. So they are prepared to work with us even if we have to make difficult changes.

We will eventually end up with groups of people who are offering a common service. Not a 'one-stop shop', but a streamlined service. So that someone might go out and see a patient but say that a bit more involvement is needed. So we might offer respite care for the carer, or something like that. The hospital home service had been the initial port of call but they'd found it very difficult to access other services along the way because it wasn't being seen as a high priority. This way we're hoping that they will be able to access services because we'll have put in the network to do that. You need to identify what the issue is and what the gap is, then look at how that can be remedied. Sometimes you can put in place what other people have done. But sometimes it is a case of having to look at it and saying, 'What do we have to do to achieve this?'

I think it has been right for my post to be based here because people have been able to get to know me. They've also got to know social care a lot, lot better. For health colleagues understanding the local authority system has been a steep learning curve. At times social care is seen to drag its feet, but there is a political process that has to be followed because we are led by elected members of the county council who are responsive to the public. So there is a clear route that things have to take. Because I've been based here people can see it working day by day – the constraints that I have to work to as well as the advantages.

There are formal and informal structures. My colleague is community nursing manager for adults and we're directly opposite, office to office, so we spend quite a lot of our time working things through together. Up until two weeks ago we shared the same office but because of the noise have been given our own offices, so now we're next to each other. It has been a real relief but you do lose some of that daily contact. You'd take a phone call and they'd hear what it was, I'd take a call, ask their advice, whatever. A two-way street really.

I think what motivates it here is the strong staff base, an extremely committed force of people. They are quite practical people and so am I, sometimes too practical and not strategic thinking, but we can talk things through and that's what makes it work. I have an optimistic view but not unrealistic. If I can get district nurses and social workers talking better together they'll have a better understanding and feel more at ease and comfortable with each other. Then the next time a district nurse phones up and says, 'I've just been to see Mrs

Smith and she really isn't that well and doesn't look too comfortable. She could probably do with a bit more care packaging, more than twice daily calls for a couple of weeks just to get her through this.' If the social worker accepts that without going out to see for herself, it is a big step forward. I think we're getting there and it isn't a pie in the sky dream.

PERSPECTIVES ON CHANGE IN HEALTH AND SOCIAL CARE

The issues raised in this case study have focused on continuous improvement in the context of cancer services. Everyone we interviewed gave a range of examples, many of which we have drawn out of their individual stories to discuss below.

This team are unusual in sharing an approach to their work that has been developed through a national initiative by the NHS Modernisation Agency. This is explained in Example 5.1.

Example 5.1
Health Improvement Methodology

Health Improvement Methodology aims to take a good idea, try it out to see how it goes and study it. If it works out well, do it again, and do it more, and keep doing that. Look for constant little change and build up evidence that these changes are good. If things don't work out you've done small changes and you haven't done a lot of damage.

So you might work with one patient, or one practice, or one consultant and their list of patients. It might include something like introducing a new form with a space to put a mobile telephone number on. It's only a small change, but part of the problem in making an appointment is that you only have a home phone number. Try it out, see if it works. If it does, you might put it on all of the forms.

Although that example is of an improvement that could be easily introduced, most of the change discussed by this team involves working across organisational boundaries. Services that have been provided for many years have particular characteristics. The policy drive to modernise service provision usually requires closer integration of these services in order to provide a quicker and smoother journey for service users. Some of the issues are outlined in Example 5.2.

Example 5.2
Reconfiguring local services

We're trying to work across different systems, different management styles, different organisations. We're working across a Primary Care Trust then a county council. Some of the work in this local sub-economy around our acute Trust is with a different unitary authority. It does at times prove extremely complicated and frustrating because you can't always move things on in the way you want or as quickly as you want. But because we work closely together we can usually find a way through without it becoming too bureaucratic.

The formalities of different funding systems and different areas of responsibility represent boundaries that have to be overcome in joint working. Another set of issues arise from the nature of the work and the attitudes and experience of staff. In Example 5.3 some of the problems of working differently are outlined.

Example 5.3
Changing people's mind sets

The issues and challenges are about change management, human dimensions of change, vision. Sometimes we think people have the same vision but they don't. We are trying to bring a national programme to fit into local priorities and it's how you do that. Also there is the historical aspect of how people have always done things and you are trying to get them to think and work in a different way. It's about changing people's mind sets. The Modernisation Agency have given us the tools, the techniques, the technology, to do this, but what they had not concentrated on was the human dimension within it so not done enough work on that.

So provision of techniques and tools is not enough – time must be spent on working with staff to ensure that everyone understands how the new approach will work. Service users can't wait until new services are tried and tested, therefore existing services have to be continued until improvements can be introduced without too much disruption. This team has developed an approach to incremental change that accommodates the necessity of keeping existing services running while introducing improvements. This process is discussed in Example 5.4 where an interagency collaboration is proposed.

Example 5.4
Incremental change

We've had to take it very, very slowly because we are asking people who have been established in roles for a very long time to make some quite fundamental changes. The team has been running for eighteen months but there are still changes that need to happen, so you have to take it at a steady pace. At a pace that the service can be provided, because that's why we're there – to provide the service. But it's also about bringing your staff along and not making them feel displaced or unsafe with what's going on around them.

We try to target certain areas at certain times. What we're beginning to do came out of some initial discussion with the independent sector. Service users are used to having a home care worker from Social Services going in, but at a certain point, because of the deterioration of their condition, they may feel that that a nurse or somebody else needs to come in. It often leads to a disjointed approach with the best intentions in the world. So that's where the discussions first started.

From there we've been able to highlight that there are a small group of people within the home care sector who would be really interested in extending their skills to work alongside other agencies, both in the independent sector and health. To develop their skills so that we could have a more streamlined service. And that's where it started. The group are looking at an operational policy – how could this work and what do we need to do. They're also looking at the training needs of individual staff. So it's been a fairly slow process but we need to put those bits in place before we start asking staff to make changes or take this development on board.

One of the reasons for the emphasis on incremental change rather than large-scale change is the opportunity it gives to try new approaches without the risk of damage if the new ideas do not work satisfactorily. Example 5.5 explains a little more about the potential benefits of incremental change.

Example 5.5
Small steps to significant results

I'm not sure how the initiative will work out. The initial aim is purely and simply to hone the skills of home care workers within social care to become able to work alongside colleagues in health and the voluntary sector. To provide a more seamless route through for patients at an extremely difficult time in their lives. The pilot is really just to tease out how that might work. We're building it with a facilitator's help against the 'gold standard' framework and trying to look at how that models out in this particular field and how it could fit in and enhance that. A pilot to me is a really good way of just teasing something out, to see if it's viable, how it will work, what are the teething problems and what do we need to consider for the future. They are often quite small changes but can produce big changes.

Many professionals fear loss of identity if they work in multiple skills areas. The training, experience and commitment to a Code of Practice that denotes professional status represents a considerable investment to the individual. There is often a fear that interprofessional working will demand significant blurring of professional boundaries, to the point where the expertise that a professional has developed may seem not to be valued. Example 5.6 presents joint working as a potential advantage, providing a way of working in which different expertises can be complementary and enhance the experience of the service user. It is clear, however, that for this approach to succeed, professionals from different backgrounds would have to both respect and trust each other.

Example 5.6
Benefits of integrated services

A couple of years ago we were a bit panicky about all having to integrate. But integrating doesn't mean that you're going to lose your identity. For me, it's meant that I can still bring my social work identity to what I'm doing and I can enhance what they're doing and they can enhance what I'm doing. What it primarily does is cut down bureaucracy. Achievement will be the day when no matter who goes in to make an assessment, we will all be able to look at their information and respect their professional credibility in making a judgement of what's required. We won't then expect to go in and make our own assessment, do it all over again. That would be a real achievement.

Perhaps we can do it with the palliative care pilot. We're looking at using the single assessment process. It means that the services can be provided quicker and can be more appropriate for the person who requires it. It doesn't matter whether it is a nurse, social worker or who is going in, the service user will be confident in knowing that the information will be passed on and the right person will come to see them.

We're starting to see changes coming into place that are beginning to make a difference to delays in hospital and to the types of care that are given in the community. If you can do that you've still got job satisfaction.

If real benefits from change can be demonstrated it can help staff to overcome some of the more trivial issues that hinder improvement. In Example 5.7 we hear how attitudes can change once staff see improvement and understand how it can be achieved.

Example 5.7
Motivation from service improvement

It's important to develop followership for the vision so that they start to want the vision as much as I want it. No one wants to work in a rubbish organisation. The staff know what's needed. But there isn't necessarily someone there to point out a possible solution. A lot of my work is about linking and saying why don't we bring those two things together because that might help what you want to achieve.

Everybody gets bogged down by the day-to-day routines and their own badges and stuff. They don't realise that all the badges are interlinked somehow and if you start to make those links work for you, you can make the job and the service better. And that's what most people are in it for. They want to see an improvement in the service for the people they are working for.

If most staff want to improve services for the benefit of service users we might expect that collaboration to identify and implement improvements would be easy to secure. This is not necessarily so. In Example 5.8 we are given an outline of how improvements can be identified collaboratively.

Example 5.8
Identifying opportunities for improvement

Recently we did a networkwide processing session. We mapped the patient's journey, right from primary care through being referred to the hospital, being discussed in the multidisciplinary team, having treatment and then the follow up. We got all the team together from both sites and we tracked the patient's journey. We had booking people there, clerks, so that everyone could have a say. We looked to see if there were any areas of duplication or any areas where the patient had to come up to the hospital and it wasn't actually of benefit to them. Sometimes you can cut it right down in terms of days. Also sometimes visits to hospital can be cut down if they can come up and have more than one test done in one go.

Other mechanisms are needed to ensure that service developments are planned and co-ordinated. Example 5.9 comments on some mechanisms that are being introduced to enable better planning so that the service can be proactive rather than always reactive. It also mentions the impact of using different ways of measuring performance.

Example 5.9
From reactive to proactive

When the patient is dying everyone pulls the stops out to achieve a reasonable service. What I am trying to do is to turn a reactive service into a proactive service so that people are planning and co-ordinating and thinking ahead. For example, so that a palliative care patient can die in their own home if they would like to. A survey in 2002 suggested that of 65,000 people three-quarters would like to die at home. Yet three-quarters die in hospital. My biggest satisfaction is knowing that the local team of general practitioners and district nurses are working to achieve that choice. It's satisfying personally for me, when I am talking about the 'gold standards' framework, when general practitioners say, 'Yes, we are interested in that.' Because it means I've presented it in a way which answers 'What's in it for me?'.

General practitioners are having a new contract next year and for the first time they will be measured on quality. There's still some number-counting. It's made up of 1,000 points and for every point they get money. They will get six points for listing their cancer patients. If they see them within six months of diagnosis they will get points. A firefighting reactive service will be turned into a well-planned, well-co-ordinated and well-communicated service. There are quality points for organisation, and for having proper summary information on patients. So with the 'gold stan-dards' framework I am able to introduce it and say, 'What's in it for you is a tool to help you achieve not only what's good for your patients but also points for your quality pot.'

There are, however, reasons why some people are not immediately ready to co-operate. In Example 5.10 the General Practitioner con-tracts are mentioned again as mechanisms that do not always encourage participation in innovative projects.

Example 5.10
Will they co-operate?

How open are practices to the kind of work we are doing? They are not. It comes down to the leadership thing. In terms of actually getting people to buy into any of these things one's got to find out what interests them. General Practitioners are self-employed business people who happen to be doctors. They are paid for what they do. They are interested in what's in it for them in terms of money. So, for instance, when we did the baseline assessment, the Primary Care Trusts paid them to return the completed forms. Which ensured they were completed. It's as basic as that. People become very cynical about this. For example, people say General Practitioners won't do anything unless you pay them. The basic facts are that that's how they earn their money.

There are also reasons why individuals do not co-operate as we see in Example 5.11, even if they seem to have agreed to be involved. In some cases the team might be able to overcome resistance but the key people have to be committed if they are part of achieving change.

Example 5.11
You must have the key people on board

We wanted to change the direction of a clinic because when people come in they need certain diagnostic tests. What the clinician was trying to do was change the actual dynamics of the clinic, so that the patient wasn't waiting every step of the way. We co-ordinated the clinic so that they would go in and have a test at a certain time and they would come out and know where they were going next, whether it was to see the surgeon or whatever. Before they would sit and wait until they were called and then would go back and wait. So it was to try to manoeuvre that so they knew more or less exactly where they were going.

Everyone was on board with it. It was a small 'plan–do–study–act' cycle. But on the day that we trialled it, put it into action, it didn't work. The rea-son it didn't work, unbeknownst to us, was that the clinician involved decided on that day that her patients needed a lot more tests than would normally have been needed. So that threw the whole thing out.

When we got talking afterwards, nobody challenged that. But was there something else going on? Something about thinking that everybody was on board although there was scepticism. So next time we did it, we worked very closely with that person. We got all her issues and challenges out and asked her what she thought should happen. In the regular meetings, she hadn't said anything, but maybe she felt the environment wasn't right.

We run the 'plan–do–study–act' cycle. Although it seems simplistic, it isn't easy and it isn't easy to say we failed. But it's alright to fail, because a failure is a learning now. In a lot of organisations, including the National Health Service, we are not allowed to make mistakes, but what they are trying to be now is a learning organisation.

When people feel that they are likely to be blamed and penalised for failure it is very difficult to innovate. Innovation always involves some degree of risk of failure. There is risk in doing anything differently. There are ways of overcoming this type of 'blame culture'. As mentioned in Example 5.11, one way is to see failure as an opportunity to learn. In health and care services people are often risk averse because so many service users are vulnerable and staff would not want to put them at risk. The incremental approach to change used by this team (and many other similar teams) makes small, sequential changes that can be evaluated quickly and developed further only if they are successful. There are techniques that can help to assess potential risks and contingency plans can be made to limit any potential damage.

Another approach that can build confidence in change is the use of standard-setting, so that standards are identified as targets for good practice that can provide direction for those planning improvement. Example 5.12 discusses the use of a new framework of standards for palliative care.

Example 5.12
A framework for change

A major part of my work is around palliative care and the introduction of the 'gold standards' framework for community palliative care. It's a framework which has been developed by a General Practitioner working with the Macmillan cancer relief organisation, a charity that has been established for 100 years and works very closely with the government around cancer services. The Macmillan sponsors General Practitioners to spend some of their time focusing on cancer and educating other General Practitioners on cancer. The one who developed the framework is a General Practitioner Macmillan facilitator. She spent some time looking at palliative care in the community and came up with this framework of best practice. Basically there are seven steps in the framework. The first one is listing your palliative care patients and the seventh one is around care of the dying in the community. So the framework aims to co-ordinate good practice in the community.

It's been tried out the past two or three years in dozens of practices in the community, and it has been firmly established as a good way to go, so I am rolling it out in my area. I send out leaflets to practices, saying, 'Here is the "gold standards" framework. Let me come and give you a presentation on it and encourage you to adopt the framework.' Already several practices are adopting it and I meet up with them every three weeks.

These new initiatives are focused on improving the patient's journey through whatever services they need, but if they are to be successful in the long term they will need to be resourced. The incremental approach to change takes place alongside existing provision and often has to compete for funding with the current well-established and familiar services. In Example 5.13 this conflict is illustrated in a discussion about how new initiatives might influence the commissioning process.

Example 5.13
Commissioning to meet needs

In the commissioning process it is up to the Primary Care Trust to decide how money is being spent. It isn't always specific pots for this and specific pots for that but a decision about where you want to spend for your patients. So that decision-making process is part of the commissioning process.

That has been a hodge-podge in the past. Everybody has done it differently. How do you get to this decision? What makes you do this and leave that out? How do we commission and what makes us consider that is right? Should we be looking at this in a different way and turning it on its head? Have we looked closely at what we need? How did we do that? What were the processes we went through and what were the outcomes of that process to get us there?

That is about service improvement. That's about what we look at in mapping the patient pathway. Where the gaps are. What it is that we have to influence to make it better. If there is anything we can make better that doesn't cost more but is about doing something differently. And then looking at the demand for this particular thing and whether the capacity meets that demand and if it doesn't, in what ways it doesn't. Then taking that whole equation to the commissioning process and saying what we've done and that this is here to inform commissioning. It's a new way of informing commissioning. It's a very reflective process and time consuming. It might not happen next year but the next year.

Commissioning processes can only be informed by these new initiatives if information about the impact of the service improvements is produced and understood. Incremental change produces gradual improvements rather than dramatic ones that might gain greater publicity, but where there are networks of groups able to share experience and information there is a potential to develop an evidence base to inform future investment in improvement. Example 5.14 discusses the extent to which learning in other groups can inform planning and development elsewhere.

Example 5.14 ▬▬▬▬▬▬▬▬▬▬▬▬▬▬▬▬▬▬▬▬
Learning from other initiatives

Quite a bit can be learnt from other groups. With collaborative care we did look at other schemes. We went to visit other schemes in the country, just to look at how things could be developed. For example, I was asked to visit, with two county councillors, a home care scheme in another county. This was about three years ago and we were just at the beginning of looking at ours. One of the things that came out was that they hadn't been able to involve the home care aspect from Social Services, as much as they would have liked to.

So from that visit I was able to come back and think to myself, well, if we are going to do this, we really do need to bring social care and health in together. Although I took from them some really good ideas I also think that we've sorted some things in a different way. It helps you to balance out what you're doing yourself and also to get other ideas. So we try to look at other schemes when appropriate, as and when we can. To look at other examples.

Leaders who are developing new initiatives often want and need personal support. Example 5.15 comments on the possible need to look wider than one's own organisation to find appropriate mentorship.

Example 5.15 ▬▬▬▬▬▬▬▬▬▬▬▬▬▬▬▬▬▬▬▬
The need for development skills at all levels

I am looking for mentorship now with the Strategic Health Authority. My line manager is a clinician. And they are not the best to be your line manager as far as a personal development path. The director of modernisation is the person I should be looking to. But the way things are in the NHS the people with that hat on in the acute and Primary Care Trusts are not necessarily skilled in the skills that I have. If I went to them, they would not necessarily understand what I am doing and what I need.

There is a need not only for senior staff who can mentor change agents but also for staff who have appropriate experience of change and understanding of the complexity of interprofessional and interagency working. In Example 5.16 we hear more about the issues that arise in developing staff in more flexible collaborative services.

Example 5.16
Developing staff in collaborative services

We are going to be doing some work with the General Practitioner about a proper referral route. So that if they have a patient requiring a certain service there is a single access point. Refer them through and then from there it would be looked at from a multidisiciplinary perspective – who can best meet the needs of that person, rather than, 'Oh this is social care. We can only deal with this bit'. It's to try to take some of those barriers down that often stop the service getting to the person in time when they actually require it. It's about an understanding of everybody's role. The pilot has shown that from an auxiliary nurse to a social care point of view they didn't really understand what each other did. It's about breaking down some of that.

In addition to providing standards and frameworks to support change and appropriate staff development, Example 5.17 demonstrates that the structural and physical arrangements within organisations can be significant in enabling change.

Example 5.17
Physical signals

My role was welcomed within the Primary Care Trust, whereas in some other areas there was a little bit of suspicion of what the job was about and why this social care person needs to be here. But this Primary Care Trust have actively made me part of their management structure. I am based with them. I am in their office space, not in Social Services. Therefore it was automatically seen that I was part of their structure as much as within the local authority.

PERSPECTIVES ON TEAMWORKING

In this case study, one of the issues was difficulty in bringing people together to form teams, as discussed in Example 5.18.

Example 5.18
Taking the first step

I just can't get people together to talk and meet, can't do it by phone, we have to get people physically together to spend a few minutes to actually make a decision. This idea of a multidisciplinary team meeting is a fundamental aspect of the cancer plan. That you get together in the same room. It's about making quality decisions. In the past, you had individuals making decisions because they worked on their own. These days the aim is to get them to be part of a team and for the team to produce a good-quality decision. This can happen in smaller ways and bigger ways, though. With teleconferencing and showing slides on TV screens they can have joint decision-making without being in the same room.

Trying to make change is the first step. What are the first three things you are going to do when you leave this room? What tiny thing can you do to start this process moving? This thing about getting people together is a stumbling block. The rest won't happen if this doesn't happen. I see it as the handle to grab hold of the whole thing, because sometimes you don't know where to start, you don't know how to get people moving. If there is a clear, almost physical aspect, you can almost physically grab hold of it.

So if I can find some tick to put on some little step it will have consequences all the way down. Systemic management. You can't get change in one area without impact in another. It's difficult to know where to start but they can see things differently when you get people together.

Once the potential participants have been identified, it often needs the intervention of senior managers to enable a team to work together across organisational boundaries, as in Example 5.19.

Example 5.19
Starting a collaborative team

It's a bringing together of home care staff, auxiliary nursing staff, qualified nursing, social workers and therapists. All together in one team that provides rehabilitation and a focus to facilitate people coming out of the hospital but also preventing them from having to go in the first place.

It's not an easy process because you are trying to work with people who have come from very different persuasions. Yes, they have a common theme but they have a very different outlook and focus because of their training and where they come from. Asking them to work together and to start to take down the professional boundaries and some of the preciousness around the job.

That needed to happen first of all at my level. They needed to see that people like myself and my counterparts at the Primary Care Trust could put that aside and say, how is the best way to move this service forward? So we've worked it very, very much together. Even if there have been some specific issues for staff that are employed by the county council and staff that have been employed by the Trust, we've still worked it together. So that as far as the staff are concerned it's a joint focus and a joint voice that is speaking.

When a team are brought together from different backgrounds, they need to learn to work together. Example 5.20 explains how a common concern with the patient's pathway can provide a focus.

Example 5.20
How does this team work together?

Maybe that's about the team working differently. A team is made up of people with different skills. It's the skills that you bring together and the intuition and the vision that makes a whole team. The strength is within that team. Now when we do something we move it forward as a team. If we were mapping a patient pathway, which is the first thing you do to look at what's happening in the system, you can get people into different groups to bring key themes back, and the themes with the map end up as the work plan or the action plan.

The role of a facilitator is to help teams to work together, particularly in planning how they can identify and address service improvement. Example 5.21 explains how a facilitator can help a team to find solutions for themselves whereas bringing in a new manager to make improvements is less likely to work.

Example 5.21
The facilitator's role with the team

The facilitator's role is to help them. To lead them on thinking where the gaps are, what objectives to make and how we can move that forward.

When we brought the services together, the rotas were completely different. The nursing service kept their rotas in a completely different way to home care. But it took several months with a facilitator to work with their managers and the team to look at having one rota and one way of working for the whole team.

If we'd had a new manager to come in to take over from everybody else it would have put everybody's backs up. The facilitator came in to work with the team rather than to manage the team. To work with them to find a solution. It's not to say that we mightn't need a manager in the future, but if we'd tried that at the beginning it would have set us up to fail.

In Example 5.22 another member of the team commented on the way in which the facilitators had changed their roles from being the project manager responsible for carrying out a change to facilitating teams to make their own changes.

Example 5.22
Changing roles in teams

Project management to me is doing. It's a different role. A couple of years ago the team started out as project managers. They actually did the work. Now it's about using our skills to facilitate and also to train the people to do it themselves, to take ownership of it rather than giving it to us to do. The ownership is when they do it and we support and facilitate them doing it.

The facilitator is an outsider as far as the service delivery work of the team is concerned and Example 5.23 explains why the presence of an outsider can be helpful.

Example 5.23
Acting as a link

Although I felt completely involved in the hospice I was always slightly on the outside, which itself has an advantage. Although I was a social worker to that hospice we discussed everything and I could go to any of them. They always knew that I was just that little bit apart so I could give an objective overview. I feel the same here really. Although I'm very much part of it, my professional credibility is still within social care. So I can help them if they want to talk to anyone in Social Services. I can act as a link for them. So it acts on a formal and informal way.

The facilitators are not the only ones who have faced considerable change in roles. As the interprofessional service development teams are formed, all the team members need to develop new skills. Some of the practical issues are discussed in Example 5.24.

Example 5.24
Developing new roles

It's a question of working with them and their needs. If they want to extend their skills and looking at how to do that. It's trying to understand where people are coming from in the first place. We've had social care staff that have been employed by Social Services and we've had auxiliary nurses that have been employed by the Primary Care Trust. What we've said is that the ideal, eventually, would be to have a role that was generically across the two. So you didn't have this barrier of 'I am a home carer so I can't do this', or 'I am an auxiliary nurse so I am not supposed to do that'.

We looked at the job descriptions of both the home carers and the auxiliary nurses and we have produced a generic care worker. New people that have been taken on have come into that role so they are not one or the other. But they are working with the established staff. You need to give people time to make the adjustments.

Not only time is needed to create change across organisational boundaries. Staff also need the ability to reconfigure systems. This needs an understanding of the complexity of budgets and policies. In Example 5.25 some of these systems issues are discussed.

Example 5.25
Issues in reconfiguration of services

The auxiliary nursing staff and the generic care workers were on different contracts to the home carers that were employed by the county council. We agreed to look at pooled budgets or integrated services, whatever we wanted to call them, to get everybody on the same contract. We had consultation meetings with unions, human resources, finance colleagues to advise us on how that could happen. It was not as straightforward as we thought. But what we could do is to work with the staff who were on social care contracts and actually offer them the opportunity to move across onto a health contract in a generic care role, working on the same team. This then placed them on exactly the same contract as other people. We put that option to five people and four opted for it. So they moved across, feeling much safer than they would have a year ago. This allowed me to extend their hours. I could give them more stabilised hours to work, which is what they wanted. It freed up other money to work with and we could extend staffing numbers. We had to do it stage by stage. They needed to see that we'd followed it through, consulted on it, and put suggestions to them.

Once teams have formed and are working to deliver local improvements, they can develop very close working relationships. Example 5.26 describes some of the changes in team dynamics when one strong member of the team was away from work for a period of time.

Example 5.26
Managing loss in the team

One very strong personality who was absolutely fantastic and very driven has left the team recently. That person would see something and do it whereas other members of the team think differently. They will not necessarily do the job in the same way as that person either, but they relied a lot on them to move things forward quickly. So when the person left, there was a very down side to this team. I got them together then, and said, 'What is missing out of the team, what has gone away, what do we need to understand about that and how will that make a difference? Will it make a difference? What do we need to put into place so that it doesn't cause a great void that prevents us from moving forward.'

So we had that discussion. They decided we will have to do it ourselves. They were so delighted with themselves. They've organised this and that and found it was not so difficult. When the person comes back, the team will be different. They have taken on some challenges they were a bit worried about because somebody else had done them but they're not so difficult. The team will change again when the person comes back. They won't rely on one person so much and that may be good but may also be a challenge.

We faced it squarely and openly, confronted the anxiety, and helped people to take ownership of their own strengths. They had to accept that you are as good as the person who has gone away for a bit, and you can also do what that person does with a bit of support and help from everybody else.

Ultimately, respect is central to teamworking. Example 5.27 shows how mutual respect can help to overcome the different approaches that people bring in a team with such diverse backgrounds. The common focus on the patient experience is the key for their joint work.

Example 5.27
Respecting others

It's about respecting people's professional identity and professional judgement. We both know the objective, but we might have slightly different ways of getting there. You have to respect that. You can't cut it off and say you're not going to be that way. I know what my skills as a social worker and as a social work manager are, just the same as my colleagues do with nursing. That doesn't mean to say that you haven't got a partnership approach, because you have. You're both able to bring a philosophy to it that can enhance what's happening to the individual you're working with.

PERSPECTIVES ON LEADERSHIP

Leaders of teams in this case study have had to be able to take an overview of service delivery in a locality, linking closely with other organisations and agencies that contribute to service provision. In Example 5.28 some of these links are mentioned, along with the need for leaders to set a broad direction for change in the area.

Example 5.28
Linking with local and national developments

She provides leadership in terms of change management. She directs me and my hospital colleagues to focus on particular areas of change. The agenda gets developed partly by national initiatives and partly by local discussion with various clinical groups.

In such a complex environment, leaders have to be able to operate with people from different backgrounds and with different views about practice in health and care. Example 5.29 gives a description of this multifaceted role.

Example 5.29
A multifaceted role

What we now have is an intermediate care interprofessional lead who works across social care and the Primary Care Trust. She doesn't manage the service but she leads the service and therefore, she acts as the consultant for all the different facets. That has proven its weight in gold because she was able to give the time to it that neither I nor my colleagues could do. Our role is more about strategic planning and management rather than the day to day of how the team needs to work. She doesn't manage. She leads. If we had brought in a health person to purely manage the whole service it would have put some barriers up. Social care people might feel that a health person might not understand their role.

One of the key concerns for everyone in this context is how to work effectively across organisational and agency boundaries. In Example 5.30 the importance of respecting different views is emphasised again.

Example 5.30
Working across boundaries

Leading is about being able to see across the boundaries. I think that's what's held people back in the past really, the more traditional type of boundaries. See the other point of view and a bit of give and take.

Working across traditional boundaries raises problems in other ways for members of the team. Example 5.31 discusses the issues that were raised when staff were asked to change from their traditional uniforms to one that identified them as members of the new team.

Example 5.31
Working with change in identity

We were asking people to make some changes to what they've been wearing, been identifying with, for a very long time. To get them to work as one team we needed them to wear the same. They agreed that it needed to be a uniform. But then we had to make it a separate uniform from one you would normally wear as an auxiliary nurse in Health and what you wear as a home care worker within Social Services. So that was quite a major thing to ask them to do. It's such a visible identifier of who you are.

We talked to them about the reasons behind having this new uniform. We let them choose it once we had a decision about everybody doing the same. One afternoon we had all the swatches of material for dresses and tabards and we let them choose the colour, the pattern and the style. People still went away and had some misgivings about giving up their identity – there are probably still some people feeling like that. But they are wearing the uniform today. They were from the day that collaborative care started. So they have taken that on board and have done it. Some of the things they were saying were things like, 'How are we going to identify between us?' How are people going to know the difference between auxiliary nurses and those who are home care trained? Our argument back was that you don't need to because you're one team and you're going in there to work with a person on specific aspects of their rehab programme that you have been asked to do. So it doesn't matter what background you come from.

Even when the physical issue of uniform has been agreed, it is not easy for people to think from a more generic perspective. One team member explained in Example 5.32 that from time to time it is as though people temporarily put their original badges back on.

Example 5.32
Changing badges

Modernisation is doing things in a different way. It means having to get people to take off their own badges for a few minutes and become part of this virtual group or this virtual organisation that is in place. But when there is a crunch or a difficulty and when the discussions dry up and when the vision on the flip chart comes close to being the reality, people start putting their badges back on.

My role, and part of leadership, is not to fight that, but to appreciate it. To say, 'Let's look at some things we can handle in reality, let's look at some small thing we can do.' It's me trying to convince you that if we can get some little change there, maybe we can do other little changes and we can get an overall improvement.

I am in a position where I am required to push the vision, but I constantly turn to reality when people put their badges back on and I've got to find out where they are sitting, where they are thinking from and bring them back to the vision again. So there is this constant to-ing and fro-ing.

Other leaders in this team mention vision. In Example 5.33 the importance of sharing vision is stated.

Example 5.33
Leading to make the team effective

I think leadership makes it effective. I am not sure if they were left on their own that would have happened. So it was a bit about my vision and trying to see where their vision was and meeting in the middle somehow. They hadn't had a full-time leader before. When I came I explained how I see a team working together. Valuing the differences within the team so that the team always remains strong.

Development is also highly valued as noted in Example 5.34.

Example 5.34
Growth and development

I have put my time into my team, because if I don't have a strong team and they don't get their development, I am going to lose my team. They are the life blood of what we need to do. If you don't give them an approach that can be developed they will walk. They need a pathway. It's about growth and development and that is eternal.

In Example 5.35 some frustration is expressed about the ability of senior budget holders to consider alternative ways of delivering services.

Example 5.35 ▬▬▬▬▬▬▬▬▬▬▬▬▬▬▬▬▬▬▬▬▬▬▬
Thinking differently

They say we won't have the money. And that's about thinking differently. If we thought differently, maybe we wouldn't need that money somewhere else. It is about a massive thought process. I get very frustrated about the leadership gap at that level and above.

Frustrations can, however, turn into achievements as explained in Example 5.36.

Example 5.36 ▬▬▬▬▬▬▬▬▬▬▬▬▬▬▬▬▬▬▬▬▬▬▬
Highs and lows

Last week, I was going home and never coming back again. Then somebody says something to you and it makes it all worthwhile. One consultant was very sceptical but he's rung me today and asked if I can come and help him. He will become champion for what he needs to do. I don't think he knows that yet but I know. He will become a champion of change.

Frustration can lead to motivation once the obstacles are overcome, but leaders have to find motivation for themselves if they are to inspire others. In Example 5.37 this motivation is described as passion, a very emotional experience and one that might be considered to be a failing as well as a strength. In this example we are also offered an insight into how such passion can inspire a career pathway.

Example 5.37 ▬▬▬▬▬▬▬▬▬▬▬▬▬▬▬▬▬▬▬▬▬▬▬
Driven by passion

My failing is my passion. But it's my strength. It gets me up in the morning. I strongly want to make it right for the team and ultimately for the patients.

I came into health as an auxiliary nurse. No qualifications. Now in my fifties I have a Master's. It's all from passion. I started my career because people wouldn't let me do the next step because they didn't think I could do it. I have fought all the way.

Reflection on a role model can also help to motivate leaders as described in Example 5.38. In this case, the role model was also able to offer encouragement and an opportunity to gain experience in a leading role.

Example 5.38
Learning from a role model

Leadership is about oneself having a leader, a role model. I had a role model. A director of nursing came into post, and she became my line manager and she saw something in me that I didn't see. She said, 'I have a vision that other people don't and sometimes they have to catch up with you. That's why I know you'll do this job well because before you start in the morning you know what it should look like at the end of the day.' I know what I am supposed to be doing and why I am doing it. I have a vision and a sense of direction. She set me on my path. She saw something else in me.

They wanted to have a surgical unit and they wanted it commissioned and opened in three months. She gave me a file with letters and costings and she said get on with it and I did it. I did it for the first month alongside my bed management job. The bed management job is operational. So I knew what was happening in the whole hospital at any one time. I used my bed management skills, my skills and background as a nurse and my co-ordination skills. She allowed me to do what I needed to.

A significant aspect of leadership in this case study is the ability of those in leading roles to provide conditions in which staff can learn and work together. In Example 5.39 a leader explains how a team was identified and developed.

Example 5.39
Providing conditions for team-building

I identified a particular home care manager in this area who is interested in developing this side of work and a small number of home care assistants and co-ordinators to work with her on developing this pilot. They have identified that there are training needs and linked in to the hospice and other training via the acute Trust to build their skills and understanding so that they feel safer in what we are asking them to do. The Macmillan service and the occupational therapy service are interested to work collaboratively with the pilot to see how it could be developed in the future.

Facilitators also play a leading role in developing vision, direction and motivation for change as described in Example 5.40. This is linked with an ability to develop ideas by tracking, summarising and synthesising.

Example 5.40
Leading by facilitating

My job is about facilitating, about bringing change, about making things happen, but I have no power to do that. I have influence. I have got to get in there and make it happen because that's what I am paid to do. And there is a leadership quality needed. I have to present myself as upbeat, someone with vision, someone who can turn concerns into opportunities, someone who can pick up on contributions which others have overlooked. I often use a flip chart to bring things together which people have lost in the discussion and don't realise they've said. It's also a leadership job to draw people out from their own agendas.

LEARNING FROM THIS CASE STUDY

Members of the Cancer Collaborative Network discuss a number of stakeholders with multiple agendas in an environment where roles, structures and processes are changing rapidly. The broad vision focuses on improving access for cancer patients and the patient's journey and this requires cross-agency, cross-boundary working. Members of the Cancer Collaborative Network talk about the need to be proactive rather than reactive in bringing about small incremental change. Everyone is working with situations of considerable complexity and Example 5.2 gives a snapshot of some of these complexities. There are costs and benefits to integrated working and Example 5.5 highlights the benefits of a single assessment process. However, several examples identify potential 'trouble spots' in the change process.

To bring some coherence and understanding to the change process it can be helpful to ask questions such as why, who, what and how.

- What is changing? There are a number of comments about change on many fronts. What kinds of changes are happening?
- Who is implementing change? Who is receiving the impact of change and what are the consequences? Who is leading change?
- How is change being handled? How are individuals leading change? How is teamworking supporting change?
- Where does learning come in and how does it occur?
- Why are certain areas targeted for change?

What insights have you gained from considering the case study and how might you apply them to your own situation?

CHAPTER 6

REABLEMENT FOR HOMECARE TEAM

INTRODUCTION

The Reablement for Homecare Team was created by a locality manager and funded as a joint Health and Social Services project. The remit was to put together a joint rehabilitation team in the community, an area of a city. The purpose of the team is to assist people to be able to live in their own homes after disabling health incidents. For example, if someone had a stroke the team would help them to be able to function at home afterwards.

It was originally made up of an occupational therapist, a physiotherapist, a nurse and a social worker, all as twenty-hour posts, and an administration post. After the first year a full-time manager's post was funded by Social Services. Some additional jointly funded professional posts were added together with a number of care assistants. Most of the funding came from Social Services because the team were able to provide evidence of financial savings in avoiding frequent referrals to other services and, in terms of users' and carers' quality of life, could show year-on-year continued independence. The team work with approximately 2,000 clients.

How the team works

Referrals are made to the team from hospitals, social workers and General Practitioners. Occasionally a client refers themselves, usually because they've been a client before and wants a little more help, in which case funding is arranged through the appropriate social worker or general practitioner. A reviewer goes to visit the client in their home to discuss what the client wants to achieve and what they may be physically capable of. The team then plan a programme of tasks and/or exercises and the reablement assistants go out and supervise the tasks and work with the clients to try and achieve their goals. It could be a very simple task like being able to get up and go to the kitchen to make a cup of tea, being able to go to the toilet, or preparing a meal. Anything that the client feels that they need help with to enable them to gain similar independence to that which they had before they became unable to do these things.

Reviews are held with each client to make sure that the care package is working well and to arrange any necessary increase or decrease to the care package. Sometimes people need to be rehoused or need to have social worker input. The reviewer can put referrals into the reablement team to ask them to work with someone's mobility in the house or outdoors, or their social tasks, for example, cooking and meal preparation. The reviewer monitors, makes sure records are up to date and after about twelve weeks, checks if the package is still needed.

Team meetings are held every six to eight weeks, staggered to avoid always falling at the same times in shift patterns. People often come in for meetings even if it is their day off. Two team members work on each patch with one peripatetic worker. Handovers are carried out at the end of each shift to discuss any changes or problems.

PERSPECTIVES FROM THE TEAM

Team leader

When I am being the leader, I think about getting the best from the people that work with me. I say 'with' me, as opposed to 'for' me, because it really is about being with me. It's about giving them the space to think creatively and the encouragement to take calculated risks. For me, what's really important is to support those people and make them feel secure. What helps is like-minded people and without a doubt if I hadn't had people with the same beliefs as me, I doubt if we could have made it work.

I manage occupational therapists, physiotherapists and social care staff and getting them to think outside the box takes quite a lot of time. Often, if one person manages to get the service user's confidence, gets somebody believing in them, I don't feel it's necessary to bring another person in. For example, to look at finances or at how the carers or relatives are managing the situation. Physiotherapists and occupational therapists have come to me in the past to look at somebody's mobility. What I encourage them to do is to look at what motivates that user, what is it that is important to them. We have spent time taking people to the bookies, because that actually is what they want to do. They want to be able to walk or get the bus to go and do that – that's important to them.

I took on this job because I was a social worker in an acute care setting and so often I would hear consultants and nurses make a decision about somebody that would write off their life. A classic example, the turning point for me, was an elderly lady who had a stroke. She had been the main carer for her sister who had had polio as a child and had quite profound disabilities. Her stroke meant that she couldn't transfer from hospital to her home independently, and that was enough to stop her from going home. That she couldn't transfer independently meant that she had to go to the toilet without a home care assistant coming in three times a day. But the doctors in the hospitals wouldn't even consider catheterisation or other methods to manage that because it might mean then that she couldn't control her bladder. I have to say that in talking to clients, they would rather lose the control of their bladders and be catheretised but go home than have to go into a nursing home.

At that time there were no alternatives. It was a risk to open your mouth. Even today there is still a lot of pressure. It's about people not being prepared to take risks, going for the safe option and what they think is kind to users – although in reality it will often shorten their lifespan.

I was told, just put together a team. I had the freedom to go outside the box. In the whole of the six or seven months (and you still get it today) our in-house home care provider would say the right things but actually never really provide the service that was asked for because their carers would not stop 'doing for'. That makes a huge, huge difference. I took the money out of two nursing home beds. We took a risk. I went to a private agency and said, this is what I want, these are the hours I want. There was too much inflexibility with an in house. There were lots of risks. It was scary because the project only had two years' funding.

Certainly in the last six to nine months frustrations are beginning to get to me but I am hoping the tide will turn again. I put my staff first and try to keep them motivated. Structurally there is obviously a hierarchy. But all the reablement assistants are told from day one, and I reinforce it in front of the therapists, that when they come in and have a discussion they are all equals. Their input is of more importance than the therapists because they are the people seeing the clients seven days a week. Their ideas, their thoughts, their opinions are valued and will be taken on board because, they may be paid slightly less per hour, but the knowledge that they give us allows us to do a good job. I would hope that everybody is treated and valued as an individual regardless of the level, regardless of what their pay or title is.

The one thing I am probably most proud of is that if you look at sickness levels in home care staff, in residential care or in social work staff, the team as a whole have an incredibly low sickness level, because they feel responsible to each other. In particular, I'm thinking of the reablement assistants because they have a partner but are a group of seven, they come together very frequently to train and have workshops and away days. They have loyalty to each other. So they know if I go sick today, my partner's probably going to pick that up.

I will always put what I believe is the right of the service user first and if that means standing up to my staff I will do that. I will always put my staff next. I will always protect them against the outside world. I think that's why my staff will take risks and I hope why they respect me, because they know I will always support them.

Team administrator

Staff meetings are an update on anything that's happening. Our leader goes to team management meetings and updates us on what's happening, any information that might affect us or our work. Staff changes, procedural changes, anything really, any changes. She's very upfront. I think the idea is that if she tells us, we won't hear the gossip and start scaremongering between ourselves. For example, there was a rumour some time ago that one of the departments that we work with was going into the private sector, which might mean that our jobs would change or stop. She went to the team managers' meeting and was able to tell us the truth and what is probably going to happen. She started the team. Fought many a battle to maintain it. If Reablement hadn't been started, I think there'd be a lot more people in care, not in their own homes. This area is densely populated with elderly people so there's always someone who needs this. It's what service users want.

It can be tricky working with other agencies. It was difficult two or three years ago to get referrals from people. Social workers weren't making them because, well, perhaps it's a mental thing. You've got a client that you really, really care about and you want the best possible for them. It's like looking after a child, I think, you want to do everything for them.

If you've got a client who's just got out of hospital you'd probably see them several times a day. Then you'd report to the physio and very, very gradually cut down and concentrate on the programme of exercises and tasks rather than oversee the simple things. Once they can do the basic things we can say, alright, we've done this, let's do something on mobility now, like how about getting on a bus and doing some shopping? It's staged, according to what reports we give back. The physios will amend the programme according to what state the client is in. If it's running normally, we see the client contact sheet every week and send it back to the therapists unless it's a bit more pressing, or not clear, or we don't understand. When we start with a client they give us a pen picture; what caused their problem, what they'd like to be able to do, what their current restrictions are and, as a result of that, what work we need to be doing with them. So if any of that changes we need to tell the therapists and we report back.

In April we had an away day where we talked about the business plan for the team, for what Reablement were doing and where we thought we were going. The team leader outlined what sort of thing needed to go into a business plan and we brainstormed strengths and weaknesses of our team. Then we broke up into groups where we talked under the headings of the business plan about what it meant for us and came up with a series of statements. We needed to have training and support, to know where we are and what we're doing. We need to be able to satisfy our clients. We're all committed to restoring people to as much independence as they would like.

We have an emergency mobile phone to whoever is on duty, so if we need direct action we can phone. If there's a problem we would probably ask the person we work most closely with or the most experienced one here. We're not allowed to administer medicine – we're allowed to give them the packet and tell them what it says, but one gentleman got really confused with his medication. The chemist hadn't done what he should have done. So the reablement assistant phoned the OT who was on duty to come and sort it out. He was on a drug which changes, and he had his day's medicine in his box. On Friday the chemist turned up on his doorstep with another box of medication and said, your dose changed. He was taking fours but the chemist said, 'Now you take threes one day and fours the next and these are the threes.' In my opinion, he should have taken the current dose out and changed the dose in the box. He added to the confusion. The gentleman not only had the doses he had been taking in the box, he had part of the dose he should now take in another box. But there's always someone you can call in a case like that.

The same gentleman, I went one night and he wasn't there. Should I break the door down? Basically, I walked around the property to ascertain that no-one was there, then checked with the neighbours and nobody knew where he was. I rang the emergency line and they gave me advice. I went home and found the pen picture and found his daughter's phone number and it turned out he was at the pub – she knew exactly where he was. But it was my responsibility to make sure that wherever he was he was safe.

The manager is the leader. Even though we don't see her very much, she makes sure that we're alright, she's where the buck stops. She gets herself very much involved – if the therapists can't man the phone line, she does. Her door is always open.

Social care assistant

I mainly deal with people who've been discharged from the hospital. They may need some help from the reablement team when they go home, so they have a slow discharge and the reablement team link in. If I see something and think they would benefit from reablement, then I will put the referral in. One of us would then go out and assess them and they may feel there isn't anything more we can do for that person, then I would look at the picture as a whole.

The leader is the manager of the whole team. She's the one that supervises all the staff. Because they're jointly funded, obviously they have their manager that they go to, but she oversees the whole team.

I value my own supervision sessions because it's a time and a place where I can air my views and my feelings to somebody, and they can do the same to you, and it's all done above board, professionally. You feel comfortable about that. I feel comfortable talking about anything to do with work, or personal. If you've got that type of relationship that's good. It's all about confidentiality, you've got to be able to trust your manager. Others will say they can only talk about work, but that's fine, that's up to the individual. A good manager listens, is good at hearing what you say.

We have meetings on a regular basis. The therapist has regular meetings with our team leader about the clients and we meet every fortnight. The team leader always feeds back the information she's been given. The admin staff type up the notes so everyone has a copy. Supervision as well, it's relevant to your post and to you. If I ask her a question she'll find out for me, give me the information. She might give me some graphs about my work and I'll do the same for her, it's a two-way thing.

In the end, you're all working towards one thing, to make sure the client stays at home and that they've got the support that they need. We probably need to employ more people. You look at the whole system and think, are you wasting money in one area, could it be saved in another? But they're looking at it from a high point of view, not from our point of view. We're mixing with people, going to see them in their own homes. People do shout and say what about this and that, but I don't think it's being heard.

Occupational therapist

As occupational therapists we're ideally placed to influence policy, but nobody at a high enough level asks us. I keep saying we must get together and talk it through and if we come up with a plan we can say this is how we think this little area should work. But everybody's got different agendas and we're all at the same level so there's not somebody to say, you might think that but this is what we're going to do.

The structure is very piecemeal. It's very flat, across clinical abilities and everybody owns different little bits. Within this whole structural change we sit here in the Reablement team and it's difficult to see where it would go. We get on well and there's not a lot of point in changing something that works quite well unless it's going to make something else work better. There's no point in us breaking ourselves up if it's just going to add a bit to other teams – it does work quite well.

PERSPECTIVES ON CHANGE IN HEALTH AND SOCIAL CARE

One of the most important policy directions in public services is bringing the focus on the experience and involvement of the service user rather than on the convenient organisation of service provision. There is always a balance to be sought between efficient and effective use of resources, but the emphasis is now on providing what service users need, where and when they need it. Often, a range of different services are needed and this can cause difficulties when they have traditionally been provided by different organisations and agencies. There are many similarities in how services are organised that should facilitate closer working, but Example 6.1 demonstrates that it is not easy to bring services together.

Example 6.1
Issues in merging services

I think health and social care merging is a good idea because we're all aiming for the same results. We all have to do health and safety checks. They only do certain moving and handling, we only do certain moving and handling. Why can't they amalgamate the two? We're all working side by side at the moment and we need to get working together. It needs the hierarchy to realise that and to do something about it. It has to come from the top. We do it this way, they do it that way. Maybe culture needs to be changed slightly. It might be 'My way's best' kind of scenario. It may be that it's people like us that need to bring them together, say why don't you try this, this and this? We're the ones actually doing it, seeing it every day, hands on.

One barrier to collaboration between service areas is the difficulty organisations often encounter when they attempt to engage in interagency working, particularly when changes in practice are perceived to have implications for jobs and contracts. These issues are described in Example 6.2.

Example 6.2
Barriers to interagency working

It's been a tough battle because it's a threat to some departments. People's perception of the Reablement and Reviewing team is that 'They're going to go in, make people totally independent and then they're not going to need my service any more'. This happens if you've got an agency that's being paid to go in and get someone out of bed, put their breakfast in front of them, wash them. Then, all of a sudden, we go in and teach people how to do this with aids, so we seem a threat. We're not a threat. If we're working with someone who won't be able to be totally independent we'll involve other agencies. It works both ways, we can help them find clients too.

Even when things are working well and a team is able to demonstrate that it has developed good practice, it is not easy to share these ideas in ways that make it possible to reproduce this success elsewhere. As one of the team pointed out, 'They might say this works well in this county, maybe we should do exactly the same in this county. But people's cultures might be very different, staffwise. Their views, knowledge and experiences may be very different to the staff in that county. So the system that works very well in one place might not work here.' She went on to suggest that more standardised or national approaches to training might be helpful in enabling the spread of good practice (Example 6.3).

Example 6.3

Modernising services through staff development

Could everybody have the same kind of input everywhere, have the same training, same knowledge base? I'm a social care assistant and I've been one for twelve months. There are others that have been social care assistants for twenty years and they may not have had any training for ten of those twenty years. Whereas I've been having training for this twelve months and new systems have been coming in, so I'm quite fresh. They might not have had the training because they don't want to do it – it's not all mandatory, so they may stay at the level they were at ten years ago whereas maybe we should all be moving.

If you're in that position, no matter how old you are, you should be having the same training as everybody else at the same level. You may have had training twenty years ago but standards have changed, the world's changed. People's attitudes towards things have changed. You may think you don't want to know anything else and there are people out there who don't want to train, they just want to do their job. You do need to have some sort of training, though, and you should be made to do it to keep up with legislation and modern times.

This team had strong feelings about the potential for service users to be damaged by some of the approaches taken in traditional health care. This perception is potentially a very strong barrier to collaboration between health and care and is not one that is often openly discussed. The issues are complex because they involve challenges to behaviour and attitudes that people have often thought are humane. At the heart of this issue is the potential conflict between the focus on social empowerment, which is typically one that would be prevalent in social care, and a focus on treating illness, which is typical of traditional health care. For one of this team, the issue was illustrated starkly in different approaches in services for older people (Example 6.4).

Example 6.4 ▬▬▬▬▬▬▬▬▬▬▬▬▬▬▬▬▬▬
Writing off older people

I continually talk about integration with health, although I am not sure I believe in it because of the culture. I saw injustice, selling out, particularly with older people. I felt like we were selling them short. As we do so often, we fit our users into the service, rather than fit the service around our users. I would say that most people would rather go home and take the risk of having a fall, and maybe of dying in six months, than go into a nursing home for six years. It will take away dignity, kill them with kindness. And the user doesn't realise, doesn't make the connection that as long as they sit in the chair and have the nice lady make the tea, soon they won't be able to do it.

I can't bear bullying. I can't bear individuals being so trusting in the professional when the professional really doesn't lay open all the options. Older people are so vulnerable, so believing that what they are told is gospel. I saw the pattern of bullying over time. Watched how their lives can just become nothing. Even those who started off being resistant would often accept eventually that their children want them to be safe. So it was the easy route, the doctors saying there's nothing more for you. But I was able to prove, over a period of time of doing the job, that people who had been written off, sometimes two or three years before, still had something to come back.

Uncomfortable assertions are made in this example. The suggestion that it is commonplace to fit service users into inflexible services rather than ensuring that services are designed to meet the needs of service users. The suggestion that professionals do not always either offer a full range of options to service users or ensure that the users are fully involved in making decisions about their own care. The suggestion that older people may be deprived of quality of life.

Particular issues arise for older people when it appears that they will not be able to be fully independent. The potential for people to learn how to live with less than their former capability is not always fully considered and there is often a tendency to seek the apparent safety of care that provides for physical needs but removes meaningful day-to-day activity. In Example 6.5 members of this team talk about taking risks as something that is part of their practice but not easy to do in services that are publicly accountable.

Example 6.5 ▬▬▬▬▬▬▬▬▬▬▬▬▬▬▬▬▬▬
Looking after people

Although there are now government guidelines saying that we must try to keep people at home, the culture has not changed within many health and care organisations. You still have the culture of 'caring for' within home care context, and you have a huge proportion of social workers and care assessors who still want to 'look after' and not take risks. I think our county has one of the highest admission rates to residential care. So you have staff saying they are doing the right thing, and maybe believing they are doing the right thing.

One practical way to determine the best option is to involve service users in considering the options open to them and the potential consequences of choices. Not all service users expect to be involved in decisions about their care. Many have confidence that professionals know best. If service users are feeling worried about how they will be able to continue to live at home with less ability than before, there may be a tendency to opt for the 'safe' option.

There are obligations on professionals to ensure that service users are helped to understand the implications of decisions about treatment and care. In Example 6.6 these ideas are demonstrated in the team's practice.

Example 6.6
Training service users

Periodically the therapists will drop in on a client to see how things are going. We need to communicate with them, not just by looking at them, but if they think they're making progress. We have training sessions with them. They might discuss the effects of a stroke, different ways in which people might be affected, their reception might change, organisational skills might go. There are different ways in which they might use the equipment, of course.

There is a wider issue in society about how better understanding of the implications of choices about care can be developed. Service users are increasingly involved in developing services that are responsive to their needs.

PERSPECTIVES ON TEAMWORKING

Team members felt that there were some things about how they worked as a team that helped them to be successful. The processes and procedures that they had developed helped each member to work independently but also kept coherence in the team's approach. Their reporting and record-keeping, with use of client contact sheets, helped them to contribute to provision of individual programmes for each client. Several team members also mentioned the importance of good communications. The day-to-day work was reviewed through regular team meetings, arranged so that people who worked different shifts had opportunities to attend within their working hours. Away days were used for developing longer-term plans, with the whole team involved in considering the team's strengths and weaknesses and what they might do to improve. There were also arrangements for supervision within the team and for consultation between team members. One team member describes in Example 6.7 how much more quickly individual needs could be met within the team's resources through their good communications and approach to joint working.

Example 6.7
A team approach to improving service

I think it's good working in this environment because you've got physiotherapists, you've got the occupational therapist and you've got the care staff. You've got reviewing officers that go out and see people every day and you can ask them for advice, what they've seen, etc. You've got the admin staff there to support you and to find out information if you can't find it for yourself.

So you can pick people's brains. For example, you can say, 'So and so's got a bath board but doesn't know how to use it', and they can go out and help. It saves time. If you're working in different organisations it might take six weeks to get someone to go and show someone how to use a bath board. A lady doesn't want to wait six weeks to learn to use a bath board and it only takes ten minutes to go and show them, but because everyone has their workloads you can't always do it.

Staff in this team each have a specialist role but they also all take responsibility for considering the impact of the team's contribution to the care of an individual. This holistic approach to care can cause tensions for professionals whose training and experience has focused on developing expertise within a particular discipline. The team leader describes in Example 6.8 how she develops her team to be able to take this broader view.

Example 6.8
Holistic teamworking

It's about not just looking at their own discipline, but often taking risks with what might be somebody else's discipline. For example, when the occupational therapists or physiotherapists go out to visit somebody, what I expect of their assessment and work is not just about the physical and the practical things specific to their job. It's about not just looking at your specialism. It's leading on your specialism, but it's also about looking at the family dynamics, and how that might impact on what you are doing.

The team leader also felt that one of the most energy-draining aspects of her job was keeping the team's confidence in this interdisciplinary approach, particularly when there were disagreements about ways of working. As she points out in Example 6.9, if these disagreements are not addressed and resolved as interdisciplinary issues, the team would be working collaboratively, to some extent, but not in a fully interdisciplinary way.

Example 6.9

Keeping an interdisciplinary focus

That's the bit that takes the most emotional energy, trying to keep them up there believing in what they do while all the politics around them are going on. Keeping them a coherent team. It would be very easy to walk away from a team member who wants to do things differently and say, 'You just get on with it your way and I'll get on with it in mine.' Then, immediately, what you've got is a multidisciplinary team sitting together but working independently. And I would say there's certainly a lot of examples of that around.

Although much of the work went well, there were frustrations in the team. Low staffing levels were perceived to be a problem: 'If you've got low staffing levels, things get missed. Not with the clients, I don't think any of us would do anything with a client if we didn't feel safe doing it. When t's don't get crossed and i's don't get dotted, there's a very grey area.' There is always a risk that controlling and regulating practice will stifle innovation, but in health and care some degree of regulation is important to ensure that service provision conforms to safety guidelines. This team were aware of the need for staff to have back up when they were faced with a situation that they did not feel equipped to deal with adequately. The use of mobile phones and duty staff often provided the necessary cover. There was also mention of working with other community agencies, including pharmacists.

As this team became better established and more experienced Example 6.10 describes how policies and procedures increasingly provided a framework for decision-making and reduced the need for staff to call on the team leader for decisions.

Example 6.10

Routines and exceptions

The team leader's split into a million pieces. We all need pieces of her, various bits and bobs – she works very, very hard. She has an open-door policy – we don't have to wait for our meeting with her to raise anything that we're worried about or concerned about. But most of the time now, because we're well established, we can get on with it. Most things have happened before and we have procedures and can just get on with them.

The hard work of the team leader is also seen as an example for other staff to follow. The routine work is shared but she also encourages team members to take responsibility for areas of development. As she explains in Example 6.11, it is important to ensure that training, information and possibly other resources are provided to enable individuals to develop new projects.

Example 6.11
Individual development responsibilities

In their review and development I try and give each team member a responsibility and an ownership of something that they want. When they come to me with an idea I will try and encourage them to expand on it and, if appropriate, to actually be responsible for it. It's the same as I hope we do for our users. I try to motivate and enable people to take responsibility and do it themselves. I will give them whatever tools they need, be it formal training, be it time, be it information.

Information-sharing is one of the concerns in the team. Team members mention that the team leader shares information about the wider environment in which the team operate. In Example 6.12, however, a team member expresses frustration at not having easy access to updating in professional issues. In an interdisciplinary team individuals may feel that they have less access through shared practice to knowledge development in their own area of expertise. Some team members mentioned that there is a danger of feeling deskilled. Perhaps this is one of the issues to consider in developing staff within an interdisciplinary environment, particularly once an understanding of holistic ways of working has been established. There is, of course, also a personal responsibility in maintaining an up-to-date knowledge about one's area of practice. In a multidisciplinary team environment it is unlikely that specialist journals would be bought for each disciplinary area but different arrangements might be made for access to libraries and personal subscriptions where appropriate.

Example 6.12
Updating professional knowledge

I once had a manager who would go and find out about things. She was busy getting all the information. We had all the journals, British and American occupational therapy journals. She was always well up with what worked, the outcomes. It's about having your finger on the pulse, having the interest and the drive and the information you need because you can't change anything unless you have the information.

Performance management in interdisciplinary teams can also be an issue if staff are used to being supervised by someone with a similar professional background. In Example 6.13 the focus of performance reviews seems to be on the role of the individual and their contribution to teamworking. There appears also to be an opportunity for individuals to identify areas of personal development.

Example 6.13
Performance reviews

We have our performance reviews, she's always very supportive, very positive. I would imagine that unless we were really awful at our jobs she would emphasise the good. Then focus on the weak bits and look at what to work on. She asks what do we find negative and how do we want to work on it. Then at the next performance review will ask how we're getting on with so and so.

The team leader's view of how she supports the team puts emphasis on how she reduces the pressures on them. But there is a danger, which she acknowledges in Example 6.14, that this approach has the potential to increase pressure on herself.

Example 6.14
Who carries the baggage?

I am not sure whether it would be seen as a good management tool, but I actually make time for everybody, both to do with their profession but also to do with them as individuals and their personal issues. I listen to them. I listen to them when they want to come in and offload, because by offloading they can then go on and do a good job, because they are not carrying baggage around. That often doesn't bode well for me, but that's how I think they've kept together for seven years.

PERSPECTIVES ON LEADERSHIP

Several of the team associated leadership with appointment to a post, but commented that there was more involved. Several mentioned the importance of interpersonal skills and showing respect for others. There were comments about how differences in the team were addressed and how a leader might get the best out of the team. In Example 6.15 there is a description of a leadership approach that maintains a warm atmosphere but does not avoid confronting problem areas when improvement is needed.

Example 6.15
The best example of leadership I've seen

My last boss had very good leadership skills, very professional. She's very down to earth, doesn't think that she's something that she isn't. She is very warming. You could say that people might take advantage of that, but she has spoken to people and asks, 'Why are you doing it like this?' She looks at all aspects, doesn't just take on board what one person says, looks at it as a whole. I think that probably comes from her social work training. As a social worker you have to look at everything as a whole picture.

One of the team described these skills as 'personal skills rather than about the professional ones we learn or gain'.

Another important issue for this team was that a leader should give protection. Support was frequently mentioned and this team leader was noted as being approachable and having an open door. One said that 'the buck stops' with the team leader, who said herself, 'What's really important is to support those people and make them feel secure.' The need for a sense of security is often most necessary in times of change. In health and care services frequent change can be very disruptive. Example 6.16 outlines some of the dangers and how this leader created conditions that enabled staff to make a positive contribution.

Example 6.16
Leading culture change

She has put things in place. At one time she felt there was a lack of communication – she said she didn't want people to be talking about something that, if she knew about it too, she could help to put right. So the two longest-serving assistants started coming to the weekly team meetings and drew up a list of what needed looking at. It was very responsive. It was a time of upheaval and everyone was feeling a bit funny. We'd had a major change and people don't like change. It could have very easily have descended into a sniping session. She said that she realised that people are apprehensive but if you have anything personal to say about anyone or anything, say it to me. She was firm that she wouldn't allow any negative input, not voiced in a public meeting. It made a safe framework to work in. She's quite emphatic that if someone asks someone else a question it should be honoured and answered properly.

A good leader was seen as being able to involve staff in thinking creatively about the ways in which the team worked. This involved both making time to meet and discuss work together but also the 'safe framework' that enabled individuals to take decisions themselves and sometimes to take calculated risks.

If staff are to feel confident in making decisions that might contain an element of risk, the way in which these staff are supervised and given feedback has to contribute to their development. In Example 6.17 one of the team explains how she felt in performance reviews carried out by two different supervisors with very different styles.

Example 6.17
Leading performance improvement

We have our performance reviews, she's always very supportive, very positive. I would imagine that unless we were really awful at our jobs she would emphasise the good. Then focus on the weak bits and look at what to work on. She asks what do we find negative and how do we want to work on it. Then at the next performance review will ask how we're getting on with so and so.

I have worked in an environment in a residential setting where the manager wasn't a very good leader. Not very professional. Confidence in that leader was zilch. When you had a supervision session you knew that the supervision would be talked about to other members of staff, which obviously caused animosity between staff groups. You don't feel confidence in managing your own workload or leadership of staff groups because that leader might not be giving you the right vibes or encouragement because they can't lead other people. Even if you've done something yourself and think, 'Gosh, I shouldn't have done that', a good leader points out all of the positive things that you did do if you're in that situation and then says, 'Well let's have a look at where you felt you did go wrong.' Whereas a bad leader says, 'You shouldn't have done it like that and now I'm going to have to put it right.'

Another aspect of leadership is to make sure that people are given the opportunity to learn skills to carry out new aspects of work, as in Example 6.18.

Example 6.18
A good leader

It was somebody I worked with when I was younger. We were setting up a new department and they got this whizz kid from outside and he was excellent. He was dynamic, he set us up but at the same time he wasn't heavy handed. He set the system up then let us do the job ourselves. When you consider that none of us had ever done that, used these computers, he was there but he wasn't standing over your shoulder. He had a sense of humour, invaluable.

When considering what makes a good leader, one of the team said that 'it's about what they do, what they stand for'. In this team, the team leader explained why she took the lead in establishing the service. She spoke with passion about decisions and actions that she felt not only ignored the views of elderly people but which brought pressure on them to comply with choices that were not in their best interests. This team face complex options that involve making choices between risk and safety all the time. The emphasis that they place on having the support of the team leader reflects the context of this type of work. There are, however, dangers for the leader who invests so much in supporting others if this drains their own personal resources. These dangers are magnified when the leader's emotional commitment to the area of work encourages them to overwork. Someone who was leading professionals in an innovative service that worked with vulnerable people explained what happened to him in Example 6.19.

Example 6.19
Emotional drain: management and leadership conflict

Three years ago I reached the point of working to live rather than living to work. I did have a breakdown. The management recognised its role in that and I have had really good therapy support since that time. I think it's because they've forgotten. They said take the time it needs. I have the most superb therapist. It's one of the best things that happened because it stopped me dead in my tracks.

I found I could not control what emotion I was in at any one time. I was starting to show inappropriate emotion. Not anger, but I found it difficult to sit in a meeting. From having been a fairly outgoing person I started finding it hard standing in front of people. And that's about management not protecting us.

When I broke, I said enough's enough. There was restructure. I'm not sure you will ever get support from management because management has a different agenda. Yet I straddle that myself, the role between leader and manager. It's such a tough act. You still have to come up with whatever management want, and the price is high sometimes. The crucial thing is having support. Being able to pick the phone up and offload so you can go home and have a normal life.

This team raises issues about what professionalism means in health and care. One of the team said of a health professional, 'she would probably have difficulty in respect, because I suspect she would see it as a threat allowing people to be equal.' These services need expertise and professionalism but the modernisation agenda challenges professional attitudes that might claim to know best because of their expertise and insists on involvement of service users in making decisions. The emphasis on interprofessional and interdisciplinary working also challenges the notion that any one profession has a sufficiently complete view of a situation to be able to make well enough informed recommendations. In services that are intended to promote social inclusion, leaders must be able to embrace inclusiveness and equality of people, whatever their roles in health and care settings.

Motivation was another common theme in this team. Most spoke enthusiastically about their work and one commented that staff turnover was very low. Public services and, in particular, health and care services, attract staff who have a 'service ethic'. Example 6.20 explains what that meant to some staff who worked in an environment that they had joined thinking it to be a service but which became driven by productivity targets.

Example 6.20
Motivation for working in a service

I worked once in a bank and the girl who managed there had read all the books, believed it all, but it was gobbledegook. She couldn't understand that we didn't want pay rises and promotion, we just wanted to go in and do the business. But they had targets, you've got to serve so many people per hour, you've got to sell so many products per number of hours in the week. None of us did any of that, because we just couldn't be bothered. Our age group thought that banking should be a service but they saw it as selling products.

There were some features of this team that encouraged people to take a lead. One person commented that leaders needed personal confidence and skills and a sufficient knowledge base and experience. She considered this to be a mix of personal make up and things that could be learnt. Another considered that having appropriate knowledge was a duty: 'I think knowledge is very important. You've got to know what you're talking about and if you're not sure you need to find out. It's your role to find out and to support staff accordingly.' Training and development was seen as having a role in leadership development.

There were also features that facilitated shared leadership and enabled those not in an appointed leading role to take the lead over some areas of work. Everyone in the team was seen as needing to have an equal input into the decision-making arrangements. Individuals took the lead frequently because of the way that the team worked within predetermined agreements and frameworks for decision-making. Example 6.21 describes how different people took the lead for different things.

Example 6.21
Shared leadership

I think we're all leaders in our own departments. One is the leader of the rotas, the cover for the week for reablement staff. Another is a physiotherapist, a locum. The reviewing officers have their own workload on appointments and organising the work. I have my own workload, make appointments and go out and do visits. The team leader is aware that people are out and about but she expects us to take on our own workload and manage that, but if there is an issue or there are problems or concerns, or if we need advice, then she's there for that. So we have to take leadership. But we talk to each other if there are any concerns, ask each other about progress, how it's going – everyone interlinks.

In this team, the barriers that were experienced in taking a lead were closely related to the nature of the work. Several mentioned the strength of belief in the work of the team as being both motivating and, potentially, problematic if there were different views about either what should be done or how it should be done. Much of the work involved negotiation and sharing of information to ensure that service users and carers were well enough informed to make choices and engage fully in decision-making. In some cases, the focus that members of the team had on working with the service users could raise difficulties at the organisational level if it challenged the ways in which partner service providers contributed to the same area of work.

In discussing what was expected of leaders, members of this team were very aware of the political and interagency dynamics in which this service operates. Although government policies encourage increasing provision of care in the community, the practices of many of the collaborating agencies, including voluntary or private sector bodies, has not necessarily changed to reflect what is currently regarded as good practice in public services. In a team with this diversity it would be difficult for a leader to develop a sense of community of practice in which processes and practices could be openly reviewed and revised. The contracting processes that are required to operate in multiagency environments tend to set out agreements about levels and processes of service provision that are difficult to change. The most difficult issues, however, would usually arise if individuals felt that their practice was being criticised or challenged.

Example 6.22 suggests that a leader needs to have vision and give direction for developments and to be able to explain clearly why the team works in ways that may be unfamiliar or unconventional.

Example 6.22
Leading vision and direction

She has to be all-sighted. To see that this team is working alright now, in the confines of what is happening everywhere else in England. In general, looking at where this team is going to be in twelve months' time. She is actively seeking to promote us. We've always been slightly experimental and she is deeply committed to what we do. She's also deeply committed to the people she works with and wants to move us forward into what social services and healthcare will be doing in future. She gets herself actively involved in that in order for people to see what we do.

In a team in which individuals have so much autonomy we might expect there to be difficulties over balancing personal responsibility with sharing and mutuality. The team leader said that she always supports and protects staff. For members of her staff, the frameworks within which they operate usually provide guidance. For another, the social life of the team played an important part as described in Example 6.23.

Example 6.23
Making shared leadership work

How do we manage all leading? You need a good sense of humour, patience, a good knowledge of everybody's role – you've got to understand what an admin assistant needs to do, what a care assistant is supposed to do, what a reviewing officer does. You need to have a good understanding of people's positions, a good understanding of people's experiences. I might have weaknesses in one area and others might pick that up, but we need good humour and support. We gain that understanding through communication, through supervision, general chit-chat and spending time with each other in various ways.

Leadership is the person responsible for co-ordinating. Leadership is about the personal skills rather than about the professional ones we learn or gain. It's about the individual. We are so reliant on good will, on nurturing creativity, so that if you stunt somebody by being overpowering, dictatorial, you just stunt their creativity.

LEARNING FROM THIS CASE STUDY

Members of the Reablement team share a philosophy of holistic care and service user involvement. These approaches are aligned with legislation and policy developments. The team, however, describe a range of barriers involved to more integrated ways of working with other agencies and organisations. They see themselves as trail blazers and describe the difficulties of sustaining and promoting their views and ways of working across these.

Implementing a more shared approach to service provision relies on effective interprofessional working The team works at maintaining an interdisciplinary focus amongst themselves. Balancing mutuality and individual responsibility, shared leadership and individual leadership is key to this kind of working. Examples 6.8 and 6.9 discuss some issues related to keeping this balance.

Read the descriptions by each team member about how the team works and discuss with examples:

- Who took the lead, when, why, and over which issues?
- How did the team do it and how did this link to their 'expert' background and role in the team?
- How did leadership work in this teamworking context?
- Can you apply any of the comments in these accounts to your own situation?

What are the strengths of this team? How do they differ from those in your own team? Are there any in this team that you might develop in your own team? What are the weaknesses of this team?

How could they overcome them? How might these ways of improving effectiveness work in your own team?

In considering your responses to these questions, you may find it helpful to refer to Part 3, especially the sections on new forms of leadership and maintaining a team.

PART 3
THEORY AND PRACTICE

You have heard multiple voices giving perspectives on leadership, teamworking and change in the context of interprofessional teams. In applying a range of theoretical models to the case studies, this section draws together themes, key learning points, and potential applications that have emerged from practice.

The current climate is one that challenges each person involved in health and social care to develop a more inclusive and sustainable culture in which service users have ready access to seamless service and a coherent package of care. This challenge involves change, both large and small scale, in asking each person to take increased leadership responsibility and to work more effectively interprofessionally. Change is, in many ways, both the backdrop to and a focus of current practice.

CHAPTER 7

THEORY AND PRACTICE IN EXPERIENCE OF CHANGE

Studies of change initiatives in organisations have resulted in a number of models that attempt to answer the following questions:

- How can we understand complexity, interdependence and fragmentation?
- Why do we need to change?
- Who and what can change?
- How can we make change happen?

(Adapted from Iles and Sutherland, 2001, p. 22)

These questions can help practitioners to organise their thinking and action. We will follow them through in this chapter, focusing on complexity, interdependence and fragmentation.

The teams we interviewed were both producers and products of change. Many teams were created in response to top-down change, their formation directed by legislation and policy. At the same time, the teams also initiated change from the bottom up, change that had impact on their internal functioning and the external environment of colleagues and service users. Whether change comes from the bottom up or from the top down will have implications on how it is accepted. Team members operated on several levels at the same time. Reminiscent of Russian stacking dolls, they were members of teams within teams. They identified with their professional groups, and they had allegiances to their teams. There were time and resource constraints, tensions and controversy about models of care. Change efforts often spotlight traditional organisational dilemmas such as autonomy versus control, innovation versus 'no surprises', participation and ownership versus timely delivery and job security versus role changes. Juggling these complexities can be exhausting, frustrating and problematic. Some teams described the use of process-mapping techniques to help them to identify potential improvements in services. These techniques can demonstrate where tensions or limited capacity cause blockages in the flow of activities and can help teams to sort out dilemmas and find a way through the dynamic relationships. (If you would like to find out more about these mapping processes, consult Martin, 2003, pp. 112–119.)

WHY CHANGE?

The impetus for change often comes because the people involved have a vision. They can see how things could be improved and are committed to making things happen. Change is a process and involves:

- becoming aware;
- developing a vision;
- developing direction;
- inspiring action;
- reviewing, revising and reflection.

Handling change takes thought, emotional energy and practical action. Change often requires people to think about things in a different way as well as to do things in a different way. Learning is at the heart of change.

While all of us have experiences of learning, not everyone thinks or feels about learning in the same way. Learning involves letting go of the familiar and stepping into the unknown. For some, the journey into the unknown is an opportunity, an invitation to an exciting journey of discovery. In some of the case studies change was seen as opportunity, a reflective learning approach, which in many ways mirrors the change process itself and seemed to offer an important key to effective functioning. It was apparent that individuals and teams were using a process resembling Kolb and Fry's (1975) experiential learning cycle. Figure 7.1 demonstrates how learning moves through five stages.

The Assertive Outreach Team leader described how the team used just such a process in the early stages of developing their service when they were faced with situations of considerable risk and the need to develop new procedures. The Virtual Multidisciplinary Team had to consider a new 'etiquette' of meetings for video conferencing. Many staff in the case studies treated change as opportunity by:

- *Becoming aware of experience.* For example, when a nurse describes becoming aware that they 'were supposed to be humble' and their dissatisfaction with that realisation. This awareness in itself was a different way of seeing, a learning that opened the doors to new ways of doing.
- *Finding out more* by gaining experience, talking, reading and observing role models. Nurses talked about how they gained in confidence as a result of gaining experience and that experience

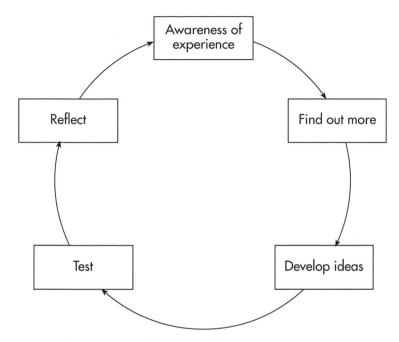

Figure 7.1. An experiential learning cycle.

often included discussion with peers, widening their circle of contacts and information.
- *Developing ideas* about the need for innovation in services and facilities, as well as new ideas about how they could participate and, indeed, catalyse innovation, as the Macmillan nurse on the Virtual Team described.
- *Testing*. In the Macmillan nurse's account, testing included drawing up a business plan and seeking resources to implement ideas.
- *Reflecting* on what went well and what they might have done differently as the members of the Assertive Outreach team describe.

The reflective learning process is not only an important tool in moving through a change process, but it also signifies a fundamental mind set, one of experimentation and hope. One Trust chief executive encouraged this experimentation and learning mindset when he said, 'Don't come to me for permission. Come to me for forgiveness.' The learning cycle approach encouraged team members to be on the look out for why change might be needed, while, at the same time, providing a framework for how change can happen.

WHO AND WHAT IS CHANGING?

The variety and the extent of change facing interprofessional teams magnifies the complexity of an already complex environment.

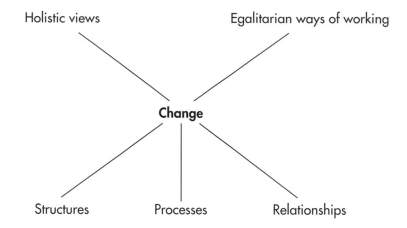

Figure 7.2. What is changing?

Clustering these changes, forming patterns, can bring an increased sense of control and meaning as the diagram in Figure 7.2 illustrates.

Two philosophical changes seem to be taking hold. The first of these is a move toward an increasingly holistic view of the service user and the need to adapt services to accommodate this view. The second change, which is separate but inevitably related, is the move from traditional, hierarchical ways of working to more egalitarian approaches. These philosophical 'shifts' have implications for structures, processes and relationships.

The formalising of interprofessional teamworking is a response to a servicewide commitment to a more holistic view of the service user. More egalitarian ways of working require that all voices be heard. These shifts have implications for decision-making processes, chains of accountability, access to and use of resources, roles and tasks expected from team members. Team leaders manage budgets as in the Assertive Outreach Team, consultants share decision-making as in the Virtual Multidisciplinary Team, and project managers become facilitators as in the Cancer Collaborative Network.

A systems model of change (see Figure 7.3) helps in understanding the dynamics of continuous and wide-ranging service change. Services are essentially processes that involve some sort of transformation. Once people have received a service they are, in some way, different. The systems model helps us to consider what resources and conditions contribute to enabling the transformation to take place, what activities and processes actually take place to cause the transformation and what outputs result. (For further reading, consult Martin, 2003, pp. 106–109.)

With so much change, it can be difficult to recognise the terrain. But many features of the terrain remain the same, serving as points of orientation. They are markers for taking stock of what remains

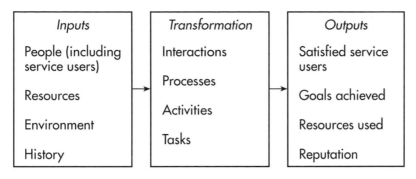

Figure 7.3. A systems model of service change.

the same and what is in the process of changing. In many of these case studies there are examples of change being introduced alongside existing services rather than as an immediate replacement for these services. Peter Senge *et al.* (1999) used the term 'balancing processes' and pointed out that these can sometimes look like resistance to change. Balancing processes play a role in conservation and it is important to pay attention to what is being conserved. Processes that conserve financial cash balances, adequate service capacity or technological know how are good examples. He suggests that many change strategies for developing learning organisations also rely on conservation of personal purpose, honesty and quality of relationships.

The Virtual Multidisciplinary Team offers an example not only of who and what is changing but *how change happens*. In Figure 7.4 this is set out as a systems model.

Systems, processes, tasks, roles and responsibilities are all subject to change. People, however, and the people involved in the change process, remain the pivot around which change efforts will succeed or fail. Not everyone will be fully committed to change, but a critical mass should be enough for a change to succeed (Senge, 1990). Some people will be more significant than others in influencing attitudes. It may be important to determine what level of support is actually needed from individuals and groups to develop a critical mass. Making connections between key people often creates a contagious excitement which can also increase commitment to innovation and change (Smale, 1996). Those who are fully committed or who readily comply with what is asked will take action whereas those who are not prepared to comply will actively oppose change. There may also be people who are apathetic about the proposed change but will comply sufficiently to retain their position in the setting.

Gleicher (1986) developed a pseudo-mathematical equation that sets out the conditions for successful change. The model begins to address the importance of considering the individual costs and

INPUTS

■ People – includes service users and various staff involved in service provision with varying attitudes, needs and abilities.

■ Resources – includes access to various new technologies such as video conferencing with tertiary centres. Other resources include grants to support the development of technology, space and time.

■ Environment – includes the particular features of the local community such as its rural nature, its isolation and its prominence as the only acute care provider in the region. Consideration of the wider environment includes the technical, economic and political climate.

■ History – many of the team members have worked together for several years. This is a small community and providers are also service users.

TRANSFORMATION

Interactions
Processes
Activities
Tasks

At the simplest level, the formalised process insists that all team members meet every two weeks to consider treatment of every patient. While views vary about the meetings, most agree that it is a time-consuming process, requiring preparation and development of a new etiquette. The process has encouraged shared decision-making, challenged practice and increased visibility of team members to each other.

OUTPUTS

Satisfied service users
Goals achieved
Resources used
Reputation

The transformation that has taken place has created a new way of working.
A somewhat simplified view is that treatment of the individual patient is more widely informed.
A greater range of treatment options may be considered. The outcome is increased quality of life for service users.

Figure 7.4 A systems model of the service provided by the Virtual Multidisciplinary Team

benefits in any change that are key to understanding the levels of enrolment, commitment and compliance to the first step of any change effort:

if A = the individual's or group's level of dissatisfaction with things as they are now;
and B = the individual's or group's shared vision of a better future;
and C = the existence of an acceptable first step;
and D = the costs to the individual or group;
then change is unlikely unless A+B+C is greater than D.

This proposal signals again the importance of ensuring that enough of the people involved see how they might achieve an improvement.

THE EMOTIONAL SIDE OF CHANGE

People in the case studies gave a range of responses to change. The leaders in both the Assertive Outreach team and the Reablement team talked about the dissatisfaction they had experienced personally with the way services had been provided prior to the formation of their teams. Taking advantage of changes 'in the air', including new policies and new funding arrangements, they created and led their teams, motivated by their dissatisfaction with the status quo and in accordance with a vision for a better future. Significantly, they recruited like-minded people to these teams, making a shared vision and collective action more likely. These teams deal with change in a coherent, cohesive manner.

In contrast, the Virtual team appears less cohesive, possibly because there has been less emphasis on developing a shared vision. Most significantly, membership on the team and the costs to some members of the team in status, power, command of resources and decision-making is greater than for others.

Bridges (1988) makes a helpful distinction between change and transition. Change is situational and external such as in a restructuring or a merge of services. Transition is an internal, psychological process that people go through to come to terms with a new situation. He developed a three-staged model that accounts for the often surprising, difficult and paradoxical emotions that many people experience while going through change. Transition always begins with the first stage, 'endings', a time of loss as well as opportunity. No matter how welcome a change might be, it will be necessary to let go of important aspects of the past. Transitions do not leap from endings to new beginnings but move through a 'neutral zone', an in-between time of confusion and disorientation, a disconnection from both the past and the present, sometimes without a clear and concrete vision or plan for the future. An example is moving house to a new neighbourhood. There may be a lot of excitement about being in a new place, closer to work perhaps or family. But a visit to the new supermarket may suddenly bring about a sense of disorientation, confusion, possibly sadness and a few tears. There is a sudden desire to 'go back'. The final phase brings new beginnings and means establishing new priorities, new activities, new ways of doing things.

Because of the links between change and loss, change involves bereavement. People involved in transition and change can feel overwhelmed. They may be mourning loss of belonging, loss of power, loss of familiar service models and loss of long-lived philosophies of care. We often identify with the circumstances of our lives, roles and responsibilities, those we like and those we do not. In the work of health and social care, many bring a profound sense of vocation, investing a lifelong passion and commitment. Change can threaten a sense of meaning and purpose and the very core of identity. Interprofessional teams are caught in a vortex of change and some members suffer in the face of paradox – there is both loss and gain to most change. Helping people to articulate their sense of loss and confusion, and to make explicit their personal and organisational gains, can encourage a movement toward exploration and commitment.

In practice, there are a number of actions that can assist the transition process.

Effective endings

Expressing open appreciation, celebrating past accomplishments, bringing people together to acknowledge loss, fear and anticipation of the future can help negotiate effective endings.

Handling the neutral zone

The visibility of leaders and managers, who provide empathy and reassurance is especially important during this time. Providing updated information gathering views from multiple sources can decrease the sense of disconnection characteristic of this stage.

Supporting new beginnings

New beginnings can be fragile and champions who provide encouragement, resources, support and linkages to information, networks and the wider context will help strengthen and consolidate new beginnings. In exploring perspectives on leadership with the teams in the case studies, leaders were reported to have nurtured the change process in the following ways:

- Attended to staff needs and the philosophy of the service early in the process. Consulted with staff involved to ensure that goals were shared and targets realistic.
- Placed staff support and supervision high on the agenda. Set priorities and stuck to them.

- Created ongoing mechanisms, such as formal and informal monitoring systems, to ensure continuous dialogue.
- Continually clarified roles and responsibilities and offered suitable rewards and a range of options.
- Provided clear information about new career structures, future career prospects and access to training and development.
- Took time during change to acknowledge personal reactions.
- Focused on progress that had been made and celebrated achievements.

Many of the leaders also commented on the need for personal support themselves.

LEADERSHIP, MANAGEMENT AND CHANGE

Leadership and change exist in a dynamic relationship with each other. Change is one of the cornerstones of leadership, and often it is the role of achieving change that distinguishes management from leadership. A number of people in the case studies describe the differences between management and leadership. While some preferred to see themselves as leaders rather than managers, they acknowledged the need to do both. Zaleznik (1993) suggested that managers and leaders are fundamentally different in personality. He proposed that leaders tolerate, indeed create, chaos, foster disruption, can live with a lack of structure and closure, and are actually on the look out for change. In his view, managers seek order and control through established processes, procedures and routines. They are interested in achieving closure on problems as quickly as possible. Leadership is characterised by change, while management is characterised by stability.

How leaders handle change will determine its success or failure. In the day-to-day reality of work in health and social care, it is important to discern when to lead and when to manage and to be able to balance the two. In the Assertive Outreach team and the Virtual Multidisciplinary team we saw leaders facing pressure from team members to 'take decisions', to act as a manager in attending to the process and procedural details. This suggests that balancing leadership and management is an important challenge.

The commitment to improving services requires large- and smaller-scale change, and a distribution of leadership to all levels. Systemwide change requires a strategic view of leadership, while change at a team level might require more operational leadership, with small, incremental clinical and service changes. The need to develop awareness of the context seems to be common to all forms and levels of leadership. Many external factors will drive service change, include policy and legislation, social and technological change. An important aspect of leadership is the ability to look ahead, 'scan' the environment and forecast issues and influences your team will face.

The Outpatient Referral team offered keen perspectives on the context of their particular service change. A STEEP analysis is a useful tool for organising the complex information that this team presented about external influences driving change. STEEP stands for the different types of influence:

S   Sociological
T   Technological
E   Economic
E   Environmental
P   Political

To carry out a STEEP analysis, you consider the current and anticipated influences in each of these categories and note the potential impact on your organisation or service. Figure 7.5 sets out how a STEEP analysis might look for the Outpatient Referral team.

Figure 7.5 STEEP analysis of the context of the Outpatient Referral team.

Sociological factors

Demographic, lifestyle factors, changes in patterns of work and consumption, have a profound influence upon the needs of the community and the expectations of individuals for service provision. With increased availability of medical information and an emphasis on patient choice, the outpatient referral group identified changing expectations, particularly in higher socio-economic levels of the population about access to referrals and levels of care. The area has a rapidly increasing population of older people and an exodus of younger people.

Technological factors

Technology is transforming referral patterns. With greater access to information, patients can participate knowledgeably in selecting their care. In addition, technology is enabling GPs to access wait lists directly and in some cases to refer directly. This can streamline things for the patient, decrease the uncertainty, allowing more control over planning their lives. On the other hand, some consultants are unhappy with the move to central wait lists and the perceived loss of control.

contd . . .

Figure 7.5 contd
Greater access and skilful use of innovative technologies may mean alternative treatments to surgery are possible. This means that referrals may move from a local provider to one a considerable distance away.

Economic factors

Broad economic factors include prosperity of the country and the local area, levels of poverty, inflation, and relationships with other countries including exchange rates that influence import, export and travel possibilities.

This is a very poor region of the country, qualifying for European Union Objective One status. It is an agricultural region and there is little industry. Unemployment is low and so are salaries. The region has difficulty recruiting highly skilled service providers. This has an impact not only on direct service but on the infrastructures and the ability to work in partnership with other agencies. Although one of the group referred to the population as 'iconoclastic', willing to move where the service is located, it is most unlikely that members of this population could take advantage of hip replacement surgery in France or other parts of Europe.

Environmental factors

Remoteness and poor transportation is the most significant feature of this environment. While the population is one of the healthiest in the country, possibly due to a pristine natural environment, distances make access to services, when necessary, very problematic.

Political factors

Many of the changes occurring in health and social care are the result of legislation.

Legislation is translated into improved service quality through systems that set standards, regulate staff, professions, health and safety.

Government has introduced league tables, in terms of wait times and outcomes. Although the interpretation of outcomes is complicated, these league tables can influence patient expectations. Acute care centres have to meet standards regarding the scope and level of service offered and the proposed cardiology unit in the local acute care centre is response to the standard requirement.

The STEEP framework is a useful structure for building an awareness of context and the factors that may have an impact on your service. Leaders synthesise and make meaning of the information, sowing the seeds of a vision for the future.

CHAPTER 8

A FRAMEWORK FOR UNDERSTANDING LEADERSHIP

Leadership is also about developing an awareness of oneself in context and how one might actively participate in moving the vision forward. While the interprofessional teams in the case studies offered multiple perspectives on leadership, there are some common themes. The work of Hartley and Allison (2000), who looked at the role of leadership in modernisation and improvement of public service, helps to identify those themes or elements of leadership, persons, positions and processes. Studies and observations of leadership have often focused on the characteristics, behaviours, skills and styles of leaders as *persons*. Individuals play key roles in shaping circumstances. The *position* of the leader may be important in giving authority. Equally, a person without a formal position of authority may be a leader because others perceive them as influential. Leadership also involves a set of *processes* that occurs among and between individuals, groups and organisations. These processes provide vehicles for motivating and influencing others in partnership working, working across organisational boundaries to find solutions together. We add a fourth P to this set of themes – *purpose*. Purpose is the reason for doing things and involves underlying values. Setting a vision and determining a strategy contribute to actualising these values. Purpose is related to the primary task of individual organisations. However, when groups, teams or agencies collaborate, the purpose of the joint programme is more encompassing (adapted from Rogers and Reynolds, 2003, p. 58).

BEING AND DOING AND BECOMING A LEADER

The Leadership Qualities Framework developed by the NHS Leadership Centre and their various leadership development programmes place a great deal of emphasis on developing the person. However, they go much further. They seek to develop an awareness of the larger context and ways and means of working with transboundary processes. Leadership development involves developing the capacity to articulate important values and to align leadership with them. The increasing emphasis on teamwork requires flexibility as we expect people to play a variety of roles in a team including, from time to time, a leading role. Health and social care recruits well qualified, competent staff and it makes sense to enable staff to work to their full potential. This includes the opportunity to make judgements and participate in decision-making at local levels. Although many staff are well informed within their professional area of work, working on interprofessional teams and across boundaries requires a greater understanding of the larger context and the capacity to listen and learn from each other. Team members in the case studies talked about their experiences of good leaders and identified some of the characteristics and competencies they particularly value in leaders. These included qualities such as enthusiasm, availability, support and respect. This sort of emphasis fits into traditional models of leadership as outlined in Figure 8.1.

Figure 8.1 Traditional models of leadership.

Trait theories

Historical perspectives on leadership took the view that leaders were born into the role. This 'great man' theory assumed people to be leaders because of lineage, or heroic deeds. Early in the twentieth century, studies attempted to discover what 'traits' successful leaders had in common and although there was no consensus on a range of attributes, emphasis was placed on the selection of leaders rather than on development. Adair discussed trait theory as including a need to have a distinct personality and proposed that an important aspect of this would be integrity. He described integrity as 'wholeness', 'the type of person who adheres to some code of moral, artistic or other values' (Adair, 1983, p. 12). Studies found that the situation in which a leader was operating was also very important and that successful leaders often needed to balance one trait against another to accommodate the issues in the situation (van Maurik, 2001, pp. 4–6). Although people became sceptical about a pure trait approach, because of implications about innate superiority, the focus on characteristics and qualities remains a part of contemporary perceptions of leadership.

contd . . .

Figure 8.1 contd

Behavioural theories

Later in the twentieth century, behavioural theory, which includes some learning theory, influenced our approach to leadership. Studies attempted to identify the behaviours of successful leaders in order then to teach and develop these behaviours in potential leaders. Behavioural theories are based on the idea that leadership is largely a matter of learning to display appropriate behaviour. Tannenbaum and Schmidt (1958) suggested that a person could choose a leadership style from a continuum that ranged from 'manager-centred' leadership through to 'subordinate-centred' leadership. This continuum demonstrates the tension between use of authority by a manager and the freedom of action allowed to subordinates.

Contingency theories

Contingency theories are variations on behavioural theories and suggest that leaders can and should adjust their behaviours or 'style' to the circumstances. These were developed in response to the failure of behavioural theories to acknowledge important differences in situations.

Fiedler (1967) suggested that a leader's style, whether task oriented or people oriented, should be 'contingent' upon the situation. He found that a situation is very favourable to the leader if:

- The leader is liked and trusted by group members.
- The task is clearly defined and well structured.
- The leader has the power to reward and punish.

Furthermore, he suggested that it was easier for the leader to change the situation rather than to change his or her style. Blanchard *et al.* (1986) disagreed and proposed that effective leaders change their styles in accordance with situational demands. The Situational Approach developed by Blanchard *et al.* (1986) is still one of the most widely used approaches in training and development of leaders today.

Most of us are more comfortable with some styles than others. Figure 8.2 draws upon an application for organisational settings of the Myers-Briggs Type Indicator of personality preferences. The full version lists sixteen types of personality preferences. The list in

Figure 8.2 Raising awareness of different personal styles.

■ You are most comfortable **conforming** to established policies, rules and schedules and you take pride in your patient, thorough, reliable style.

■ You are most comfortable **responding** immediately to problems and you take pride in your open and flexible style.

■ You are most comfortable when **communicating** organisational norms, values and making decisions by participation and you take pride in your personal, insightful style.

■ You are most comfortable **building** new systems, frameworks and pilots, and you take pride in your ingenuity and logical, analytical style.

(*Source:* Adapted from Hirsch and Kummerow, 1987)

Figure 8.2 is therefore not a comprehensive summary, but one you can use as a tool to focus your awareness on the particular strengths you bring to your leadership roles.

The checklist in Figure 8.2 moves from a more 'managerial' style, through an adaptable and communicative style, to one that favours visionary, creative and analytical styles. While they are not mutually exclusive, you may find it useful to apply the checklist to your reading and analysis of the case studies to 'detect' various leadership styles team members described and to make your own decisions about how adaptable leadership style may be.

Often people achieve positions of 'formal' authority because they have developed competencies and capacities to lead and to manage. However, many people without formal position exercise 'informal' authority through these same qualities and competencies.

THE ROLE OF EMOTIONAL INTELLIGENCE

We have already heard described in the case studies the high emotion that often accompanies work in health and social care. Martin noted the need for leaders to be able to deal effectively with our own emotions and those of others:

. . . as leadership often involves being passionate and demonstrating both anger and frustration about making a difference, leaders are in particular need of this range of competencies.

(Martin, 2003, p. 64)

Goleman (1996) highlights the key role of emotion in all human interaction. His concept 'Emotional Intelligence' is a type of social intelligence that involves the ability to monitor one's own and others' emotions and to make use of the information to guide actions. Emotional Intelligence means developing competence in:

- Self-awareness – insight into our own thoughts and feelings, how they interact with our communication and behaviours and how these impact others.
- Self-management – involves the appropriate handling of our feelings and impact on others.
- Self-control – includes the capacity to channel emotions in the service of a goal.
- Empathy – means sensitivity to the feelings of others, the ability and the willingness to take their perspective and an appreciation of differences in how people feel about things.
- Handling relationships – includes listening, negotiation and conflict resolution.

In a more recent work, Goleman *et al.* (2002) discuss how at a basic, physiological level we are connected to others for emotional stability. We participate in 'emotional contagion'. Other people are significantly influenced by the emotions displayed by those in leadership positions. This makes the emotional task of leadership a primal, priority task. The more open leaders are with their enthusiasm, humour and passion, the more open team members are to each other and the more talent and potential is unleashed.

These insights open the door to an understanding of transformational leadership and leadership as a social process, where mutual influence, shared vision and collective action can transform all those involved in the process and the services to which they are dedicated.

LEADING TRANSFORMATION

Traditional models of leadership are all about actions and transactions. Rost (1991) went so far as to say they were really about management, and psychological approaches to get people to 'mind the shop'. Burns' (1978) seminal work introduced the notion of transformational leadership, currently receiving widespread attention in health and social care. Referring to Maslow's hierarchy of needs, Burns observed that some leaders are able to inspire, to raise the expectations and the performance of followers beyond everyday needs for survival, safety, security and companionship to expectations that are concerned with, and can lead to, the greater good.

Transformational leaders can often articulate the unspoken but important values and vision of followers. A member of one of the interprofessional teams commented that leadership is about being led towards something that we realise we should have been doing for ourselves. Charismatic leadership is a form of transformational leadership, and charismatic leaders often display qualities of inspiration, enthusiasm, intensity and willingness to risk. They often emerge in times of change or crisis, but equally they are capable of creating the conditions of change. It is based on a heightened emotional relationship between leaders and followers and relies on a mutual sensitivity. You may recall times when you have worked with someone charismatic and you felt a sense of excitement, hope and purpose. You may have had a clearer sense of where things were going and how you fitted in. You may have felt more intensely involved with your own work as it took on a sense of greater meaning and importance. This may also have led you to understand yourself more:

> You got to get inside of people. That's where it all is. You can't get inside them unless you open yourself to be got inside of. Follow what I am saying? The key to other people's hearts is finding the key to your own.
>
> (Jesse Jackson, in Frady, 1992, p. 51)

Team members in some of the case studies describe just this sort of experience.

Beverly Alimo-Metcalfe and Robert Alban Metcalfe (2002) carried out large-scale research in the NHS and other public service organisations to understand how people perceive leadership and what they value in leaders. They identified the following qualities which form a 'transformational construct' or composite of leadership qualities.

- *Genuine concern for others* – They have a genuine interest in their team members as individuals.
- *Inspirational communicator, networker and achiever* – This is about being able to communicate the vision with passion and commitment.
- *Empowering others to lead* – They trust staff to take decisions and initiatives in important matters.
- *Transparency* – This quality relates to honesty and openness.
- *Accessibility, approachability and flexibility* – They are accessible to all levels of staff.
- *Decisive determination and a readiness to take risks* – They are decisive when required and can clarify shared values.
- *Ability to draw people together with a shared vision* – The leader engages internal and external colleagues, departments, agencies to draw together a shared vision.

- *Charisma* – This involves the ability to be in close contact with people and to encourage their contribution.
- *Encouraging challenge to the status quo* – They encourage challenge to traditions and assumptions about how things are done.
- *Supporting a development culture* – They empower others to take risks.
- *Ability to analyse and think creatively* – This quality is about being able to understand complex issues and to solve problems creatively.
- *Managing change sensitively and skilfully* – This quality is about being sensitive to the impact and the effects of external and internal change and being able to balance change with some stability.

Many team leaders describe themselves and were described by team members in just such a way. Not every team leader possessed all of these qualities but there are notable examples of team members contributing many of these attributes to their teams.

Alimo-Metcalfe and Metcalfe emphasise co-creation of a vision. Leadership does not so much involve the vision of one charismatic person, but the vision comes from the exchange among people in an environment of innovation. Senge (1990) identifies 'shared vision' as one of five essential disciplines that people and organisations need to develop to transform themselves. Transformational leadership is driven by values, in that leadership is not just about getting things done, but getting the right things done in the right ways.

The emphasis on *social process* distinguishes transformational leadership and newer models such as learning leadership and servant leadership from the more traditional approaches:

> Leadership is an influence relationship among leaders and followers who intend real changes that reflect their mutual purposes.
>
> (Rost, 1991, p. 102)

The notion of leadership as a social process underpins the ideas of distributed leadership and leadership at all levels.

LEADING SOCIAL PROGRESS

Purpose holds together the social process of leadership. This view of leadership relies on a collective view of the need for change and the direction of change. New ideas of leadership move from individual leaders to mobilising others and challenging all team members to reflect upon their influence in the achievement of mutual purposes. New ideas about leadership emphasise *leadership as negotiation*.

Leadership is a process that different people engage with at different times. Groups and teams do not have straightforward common purposes. There are always multiple issues, interests and agendas.

Effective leadership in these complex situations requires negotiation to reconcile different interests in order to work towards common goals. Ferlie and Pettigrew (1996) have noted that broker roles may develop in *leadership across boundaries*. The case studies showed many of these emerging forms of leadership. Most dramatically, the case studies exemplified *leadership as learning and servant leadership*. The 'learning leader' unlocks human potential, and nurtures people's commitment to and capacity for learning at all levels. Greenleaf (1977) defined leaders as those who serve others, whose ethic is a responsibility to guide and support the work of others. Foster also emphasises the individual's role in contributing to community development:

> Leadership is and must be socially critical. It does not reside in an individual but in the relationship between individuals and is oriented toward social vision and change, not simply or only organisational goals.
>
> (Foster, 1989, p. 46)

Foster, in the above quotation, takes a critical social process view of leadership. This process has three key elements: shared vision, collective action and social change, as can be seen in Figure 8.3.

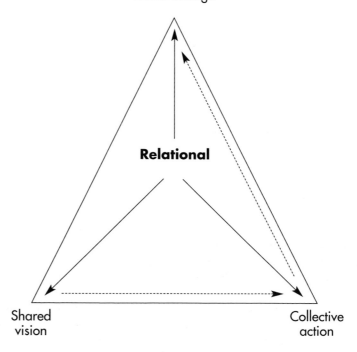

Figure 8.3 Leadership as a social process.

The shared vision that can be seen throughout the case studies, for example, is service improvement. Collective action means all of those committed to that vision working together to move closer to fulfilment of the vision. Social change, in this view, is the ultimate purpose, and it is hoped, the result, of collective action. Collective action brings changes in organisational and social structures and processes that result in a more fair, equitable service. Relationship is the pivot to this type of leadership, as it is to most forms of leadership. Relationship supports the development of the three elements identified above, hence the solid lines. The dotted lines show the direction of the process, from shared vision to social change, and represent the fluidity and flexibility needed in this process.

These newer, process views of leadership mirror the core value systems of health and social care that include an emphasis on:

- An egalitarian culture, one of openness and inclusiveness, where information, power and resources are shared;
- Individual and collective attitudes and behaviours such as empathy, respect, flexibility, accountability and good communication;
- Mechanisms and structures that both develop and support these, such as modernisation teams and efforts;
- Capacities that include both disciplinary expertise and the capacity to understand and change structures and processes.

This approach, however, is not easy to develop within strongly hierarchical structures and cultures.

The current Royal College of Nursing's Clinical Leadership programme draws upon the Kouzes and Posner (1987) approach, which sums up well key elements that characterise the newer models of leadership discussed here:

- Challenging the status quo
- Inspiring a shared vision
- Enabling others to act
- Modelling the way
- Encouraging the heart.

In these case studies we have seen the challenge and the inspiration of transformational leadership, the shared vision of leadership as a social process, the role modelling of learning leadership, the empowerment of servant leadership and the emotional engagement required by all.

Leaders influence how people think about issues but do not necessarily have formal power in the organisation. All members of a group or team can make leadership contributions. Different leadership capacities are required to develop strategy, develop team commitment and morale and progress detailed tasks. If everyone is committed to change, everyone needs to know something about the impact of forces in the wider environment and to understand why and how change is a response to these forces.

Team effectiveness is dependent upon the capacity of its members to draw from a whole range of leadership perspectives.

CHAPTER 9

THEORY AND PRACTICE IN TEAMWORKING

The belief that interprofessional teams, with multiple skills and expertise, will be able to deliver more effective, holistic and seamless patient care accounts for the growing emphasis on teams. Almost everyone will find themselves part of a team during their work in health and social care. Interprofessional teamworking is not new. But the context and expectations have changed. There is increasing formalisation of teams and accountability mechanisms and more distributed forms of leadership.

Interprofessional teamworking offers its own challenges and opportunities. The interaction of identity and diversity represents both a key challenge and opportunity. An interprofessional team is a type of multicultural environment, in which the unique cultures of professions, departments, agencies and disciplines come together for common purposes.

Our search for a range of interprofessional teams proved more complex than we had anticipated initially. As we heard more about current interprofessional teamworking we realised that teams and team members define themselves in a range of ways and identify with a variety of teams.

GROUPS AND TEAMS

All teams are groups and most organisations have formal and informal groups. Martin (2003) describes some important aspects of groups:

- Size – It is difficult to involve everyone if a group is larger than about ten people because participation becomes more difficult. But the more people, the greater the diversity.
- Work – Some groups exist for a long time working on fairly routine tasks and some are formed to work on a particular issue.

■ Status – A group that is recognised by the organisation will often have established channels of reporting to the organisation whereas informal groups may have to establish mechanisms in a more ad hoc way. Similarly, formal groups will probably have resources available whereas informal groups may have to negotiate these.

(Adapted from Martin, 2003, pp. 66–67)

The status of group or team has important implications for negotiating boundaries in multilayered, multifaceted contexts, and for the notion of leadership as 'networking' and 'brokering'.

Groups may rely less upon close collaboration and consensus than a team might. They can be useful when tasks are relatively simple and fast, innovative decisions are needed. Groups become teams when there is a joint product or goal upon which its members are focused. Katzenbach and Smith (1993) point out that in teams there is a shared understanding of the goals, and members of the team are mutually accountable for both their purpose and approaches. Teams are needed when tasks or problems are complex, consensus decisions are essential, there is a high level of choice and uncertainty and a mix of different competencies are needed.

DEFINING INTERPROFESSIONAL TEAMS AND THE CONTEXT

Interprofessional teams are a unique form of team which involves significant collaboration and the breaking down of boundaries, although these teams can be formed within the same department or organisation. The Virtual Multidisciplinary team, the Assertive Outreach team and the Reablement team are examples of teams working within the same organisation. Interprofessional team working can also involve cross-agency working, such as we saw in the Outpatient Referral team, whose membership included the head of a local agency, a General Practitioner and a hospital administrator. Teams can be *tight knit*, working in close tandem and sharing the same locale. The Assertive Outreach and the Reablement teams are good examples. Interprofessional teams do not have to involve everyone all the time, or be in the same location, but can be a *network* team, as in the Cancer Collaborative Network.

In many early stages of interprofessional teamwork it would be more accurate to use the term 'multiprofessional' to describe the degree of interaction. There is a distinction to be made between people who come together and, perhaps, agree to exchange some information or to collaborate over some issue of mutual interest, and a team that share vision and overcome boundaries to work collectively to achieve common goals. These terms tend to be used to indicate a difference between teams where individuals are defensive in protecting and preserving their professional boundaries and those where individuals agree to blur or to work across those boundaries, accepting some loss alongside the gains.

Hudson *et al.* (1998) suggested that collaborations move through different stages. Although he was referring especially to cross-organisation, cross-agency collaboration, these stages have some application to many interprofessional endeavours:

1. Isolation (no joint working);
2. Encounter (informal and ad hoc contact);
3. Communication (involving formal joint working, frequent interaction, sharing of information);
4. Collaboration (high level of trust, common interests, joint planning and service delivery);
5. Integration (organisations integrate teams or even merge with loss of individual identity).

(Adapted from Charlesworth, 2003, p. 145)

Interprofessional working involves joint working and joint working has three levels. Members of the Cancer Collaborative Network case study talk about the complexities and overlaps involved in working across these levels.

■ *Strategic planning:* Agencies need to plan jointly for the medium term and share information about how they intend to use their resources towards the achievement of common goals. In most of the case studies we heard about ways in which people had succeeded in working with other agencies and organisations within a local health economy to plan together and to initiate collaborative local improvements.
■ *Service commissioning:* When securing services for their local populations, agencies need to have a common understanding of the needs that they are jointly meeting and the kind of provision likely to be most effective. In the context of the Cancer Services Collaborative, a lead facilitator works for a Primary Care Trust. The money comes from government to the Primary Care Trusts, who decide what's needed for the patients and they then buy secondary services from the hospital. The Strategic Health Authority will ask pertinent questions about how the money is spent.
■ *Service provision:* Regardless of how services are purchased or funded, the key objective is that the user receives a coherent package of care, with the greatest of ease. We saw in the Cancer Collaborative Network that priorities included waiting times, appointments, urgent referrals, communication between primary and acute care and patient information pathways.

The context within which teams work is one of shifting structures, alliances and processes. Each context too has its own unique, idiosyncratic features. There are, however, some common themes with regard to what makes teams effective within an uncertain and ambiguous environment. Approaches to joint working:

■ Need clarity about roles, powers, accountability requirements and differing expectations of stakeholders at all levels.
■ Must be set in the context of the wider political agenda of modernisation.

(Adapted from Charlesworth, 2003)

The teams in the case studies are all very conscious of the extent to which their initiatives contribute to the modernisation agenda and there were many examples of role negotiation.

DEVELOPING EFFECTIVE TEAMS

Tuckman and Jensen (1977) identified five stages to team development which provide a useful framework for considering the factors that make a team effective in sharing responsibility during times of change. Although the original model implied that performance was delayed until several stages had been successfully negotiated, a more contemporary approach would suggest a dynamic relationship among the stages that would help account for the requirements on many teams to achieve early results.

Forming

This stage in the original model is one in which team membership is established, in which individual and team purposes are clarified and in which interpersonal relationships and processes begin to take shape. Michael West (2003) has identified how important it is to the team's future effectiveness to decide proactively on team membership and roles and the boundaries of the team with regard to the organisation and to other teams. The Assertive Outreach team and the Reablement team spoke explicitly about the power of recruiting 'like-minded' people to the team. West, using a needs-based approach, suggested that team members look to their membership of the team for belonging, growth and control.

Storming

Storming is the stage where conflict emerges and, if unresolved, can inhibit progress and derail the team. Interprofessional teams will inevitably have conflict and there were examples of overt and covert conflict in many of the teams. One team member spoke about shouting and 'getting the conflict out in the open'. A team leader spoke about how she encourages team members to resolve their interpersonal difficulties without her intervention. The Virtual Multidisciplinary team talked about 'breaches' of etiquette. A member of the Outpatient Referral team talked about conflicting priorities and processes for negotiating scarce resources.

There are psychological explanations that account for conflict and derailment too. Bion (1961) suggested that team development involved two parallel processes, a conscious one and an unconscious one. When teams have a clear 'primary task' and agree to work to the task at hand, their members will act constructively and consciously. However, there can be unconscious processes occurring at the same time, almost as if a parallel team is operating. This parallel 'unconscious' team makes sure that anxiety is handled by using a number of defensive manoeuvres to dispense with strong emotion. One defensive mechanism involves 'disowning' strong emotions and placing them in the team. The team comes to represent a mother figure, for example, that can contain or handle strong emotion. This kind of defence manoeuvre happens when the team task is especially anxiety provoking. Teams may use any one of the three following basic assumptions to avoid the primary task.

1 *Dependency:* Team members expect the leader to protect them from anxiety about the primary task. Members will rely on the leader to have all the answers. Individuals will not use their own capacity to make choices, but the leader will carry the eventual responsibility for the outcomes.
2 *Fight–Flight:* If the team becomes too intense emotionally, an individual might take flight or might fight. One form of flight might be the use of humour and jokes to diffuse the levels of anxiety or tension. This is not to suggest that all uses of humour are inappropriate, but the uses of humour that divert from attending to the primary task. Alternatively, an individual might not attend team meetings, or might not participate fully. Scapegoating is another manoeuvre of a fight or flight group. Management might be blamed for all that is wrong or other teams and departments may not understand the service the team is providing.
3 *Pairing:* The group believes that some future event will bring resolution to their anxiety. A 'selected pair' who are in conflict or who are allied in some way may carry the hope of the group for resolution either by resolving the group's problems in their alliance or acting them out in conflict.

It often helps a team to consider its basic values and principles. Reviewing difficulties is not a one-off event, but must be a continuous one. A robust process needs to be developed and maintained by the team to ensure continuing development of team awareness about their own interactions. In addition, if the team agree to value and respect diverse views, disagreement becomes a way of reviewing perspectives. In any change situation the views of all of those involved are important in determining whether progress will be made and to ensure that wide consultation accompanies its progress in parallel with achievement of the team's tasks.

Norming

At this stage the team settles into agreed routine ways of working. These routines must serve the needs of the team members as well as the task and purpose around which the team was initially formed. West (2003) has identified three needs that members bring to the team initially and the team must establish norms and processes to fulfil these needs for: belonging, growth and control.

- *Belonging:* Leaders and team members find ways to show interest in each other's well being. To fulfil the belonging need, the team should establish processes that build confidence, and ensure equality and consistent treatment.
- *Growth:* Personal development, planning, appraisals and objective-setting are most important. There needs to be follow through to ensure that these processes have helped the person to do his or her job better.
- *Control:* Norms and processes to keep motivation up and ensuring participation are some effective ways of giving all team members a greater sense of control.

There is a correlation between sophistication of appraisal and mortality after hip fracture. The more sophisticated the appraisal, the less mortality (West, 2003, Conference presentation).

In progressing change, however, the processes that have been agreed for the early stages of an initiative may not be the best as time moves on and situations change. It can be a constraint for a team to develop norms that inhibit change within the team and its ways of working. The balance of the team dynamics and progress towards achievement of the purpose may need to be revisited frequently to ensure that the team is not putting too much attention into maintaining itself at the cost of progressing the task.

The case studies provided many examples of 'norming in progress'. The members of the Assertive Outreach team, the Reablement team and the Virtual Multidisciplinary team talked about the various mechanisms, rituals and regular feedback processes that they had developed together to ensure their continuing effectiveness.

Performing

This is the stage at which the team is working efficiently towards its goals. As in the previous stages, nothing stands still and the situation constantly changes. The only way to be sure of effective performance is to monitor and review regularly against targets. The Assertive Outreach team described a constant process of review embedded in mechanisms that the team had developed together. The processes that are needed here are detailed management routines and these are not always the approaches that people oriented towards achieving change welcome. Everyone needs to be engaged in the routine monitoring activities if the reviews of progress are to be meaningful. The Reablement team described the value of having decision-making frameworks in place to handle routine situations and enable each member to make decisions autonomously.

Adjourning

One of the characteristics of a team is that it has a limited life that completes with the achievement of its purpose. If members of the team have enjoyed working together and found the work satisfying there is often some reluctance to break up the team. However, with people who are interested in change there will also be an attraction in moving on to the next challenge. It is helpful if some attention is paid to closure by ensuring that team members have all given each other feedback where appropriate. Achievements can be recorded in appraisals and other documentation. It is important that learning as a team and as individuals is discussed and noted, so that people are able to use the experience gained from this team when they move into new roles.

While the teams we interviewed were still teams very much in process, the Cancer Collaborative Network described quite major changes in roles and activities from project manager to facilitator that took place in the move from phase two to phase three. Collaborative team members talked about how these changes had emerged from systematic review of their interventions with collaborating agencies and about the importance of learning from small change efforts.

MAINTAINING THE TEAM

Each team member brings strengths and perspectives grounded in their discipline and experience. Coupled with personality and behaviour preferences, this combination of attributes has an impact on the sorts of roles team members will choose to play. Belbin's work (1981) identified a number of significant roles in teams. These roles each offer positive contributions to teamworking, but each also has what Belbin called 'allowable weaknesses'. Each role could be linked with taking a lead on an area of the team's work:

- *innovator*: original ideas, imagination, creativity (but may be weak in communication skills and reluctant to abandon or build on ideas);
- *implementer*: turns ideas and decisions into tasks and actions (but may be inflexible and reluctant to change plans);
- *completer*: sees tasks through to completion, good on detail (but can be inclined to worry and dislike casual attitudes in others);
- *evaluator*: offers critical analysis, takes a strategic view, considers options and makes judgements (but can lack drive, warmth and imagination and can dampen morale);

- *investigator*: explores opportunities and resources from many sources, enthusiastic communicator (but can jump from one task to another and lose interest);
- *shaper*: drives the team to address the task, dynamic and challenging (but can be impatient and intolerant);
- *team maintainer*: focuses on harmony, developing ideas, listening, reducing conflict (but can be indecisive and avoid confrontation);
- *co-ordinator*: clarifies goals, promotes decision-making, communicates effectively (but can be seen as manipulative and not fully contributing to the work of the team);
- *expert*: provides specialist skills or knowledge (but can be narrowly focused on their own area of work and fail to see the big picture).

Many people are strong in one or two of the roles and could also contribute in others. It can be helpful for a team to discuss who will take on each of the roles and whether they have sufficient resources or need to add members. The discussion might also consider how the team will accommodate the potential difficulties that can arise from the associated characteristics of each role. Belbin's research (1981) suggested that consistently successful teams contained a mix of these roles.

   Features of the current context introduce the need for some modification and expansion to these roles, and of the treatment of allowable weaknesses:

- *Change:* Teams that are engaged in change might need rather broader interpretations of some of these roles or other roles added in order to address some of the wider issues. Any change has the potential to affect people outside the team and often outside the area of work or organisation. The 'network' leader and the 'broker' leader are examples.
- *Joint working:* The team will need someone taking a lead on consultation and negotiation with all potential stakeholders. This might fall within the co-ordinator role or might be a more broadly ambassadorial role.
- *Technology:* Availability and expectations about the use of information technology have changed since Belbin identified these roles. There will be considerable information in the internal systems of many organisations and also information about benchmarking and best practice that can be important to consider before making significant changes. The person in the role of resource investigator now needs computer skills and ability to make appropriate and competent judgements about what information will be helpful for the team.
- *Distributed leadership:* We now expect team members to take a more holistic view of their work and their team involvement. We expect all team members to have a grasp on the context, the reasons for change, to lead some work and to share responsibili-

ty in work led by others. It is no longer enough for someone to confine themselves to their own area of expertise. You may find as you review the case studies and your own work that the 'allowable weaknesses' suggested by Belbin still have a place in the current context of interprofessional teamworking.

(Adapted from Martin, 2003, pp. 74–75)

Another way to consider team maintenance is to think about the kinds of behaviours the team needs to keep a balance between the task and relationships. An effective team requires a balance of *task* and *maintenance* behaviours. Task behaviours concern themselves with the primary tasks and purpose of the team, while maintenance behaviours are concerned with the team's interpersonal process and environment (see Figure 9.1).

Figure 9.1 Team task and maintenance behaviours.

Task progression	Maintenance
Proposing ideas to progress the task	Involving contributions to discussion
Building on ideas	Creating a friendly and welcoming atmosphere
Challenging ideas	Compromising and accommodating
Providing data, information, opinions	Emphasising positive feedback for individual
Summarising, noting action points	Recognising personal feelings

CHAPTER 10

REFLECTIONS AND CONCLUSIONS

We have referred to interprofessional teamworking as a multicultural experience. A study (Rogers, 1994) on effective multicultural working suggested an integrative framework that synthesises a number of attitudes, characteristics and behaviours that team members in the case studies revealed. Working across cultures requires:

- *Personal integration:* The capacity to self-reflect, to accept feedback, to develop self-awareness, leading to a real desire to change and grow.
- *Experiential agility:* Flexibility in thinking and action, leading to crossing boundaries, willingness to engage, asking questions, listening, trying to understand, working through conflict and toleration of uncertainties and ambiguities.
- *Power-sharing:* Inviting participation from others, encouraging growth and development in others, delegating, mentoring and creating systems and structures that support distributed forms of leadership.
- *Transcendence:* Having a sense of things beyond oneself to live for, a belief in service and inclusiveness, sharing commitment to an overriding purpose.

These elements exist in dynamic relationship to each other and reflect a holistic perspective that seems to be at the heart of change in health and social care today.

The case studies open the door to many different possibilities for future research. Areas we have identified include:

1 Ways of supporting small incremental change so that it contributes to significant organisational change.
2 Identification of processes that enable development of successful small change efforts into larger-scale initiatives.
3 Identification of features and processes that facilitate cross-boundary working.

4 Identification of features and processes that facilitate interprofessional working.
5 Gender and response to change.
6 Career trajectories and their contribution to innovation in health and care.
7 Service user involvement in co-development of services.

Service user involvement, not surprisingly, emerges as a significant theme in many of the case studies, and one which reflects broader legislation and policy development. Research might build on work already in the literature, continuing to explore the range and boundaries of service user input into shared ownership of individual health and well being and the co-creation of services. Investigation might explore more fully the effectiveness of education and training interventions in shifting attitudes and expectations for service users and for health and social care staff. The public service emphasis on inclusion and choice raises broader issues about the expectations and demands of citizenship and how these sit alongside capitalism and private sector provision. There is growing evidence that effective teamwork leads to significant increase in well being for team members, for the organisation and for service users. Many of the teams in the case studies are using a number of the tools, techniques, philosophies and theories explored here in an integrated, organic way.

Most importantly, effective interprofessional teams are driven by a collective passion, held together by deep and abiding commitment to service and to service users, consolidated by courage and a willingness to face down adversity, and sustained by a quest for learning and change.

RECOMMENDED READINGS

PERSPECTIVES ON CHANGE

Kotter, J.P. (1996) *Leading Change*. Boston, Harvard Business School Press.
(A contemporary exploration of leading change in organisations.)

Lewin, K. (1947) 'Frontiers in group dynamic: Concept, method and reality in social science; social equilibria and social change'. *Human Relations,* Vol. 1, pp. 5–41.
(A classic theory of the change process.)

Martin, V. (2002) *Managing Projects in Health and Social Care*. London, Routledge.
(Improving services by planning and implementing projects.)

Nadler, D.A. (1983) 'Concepts for the management of organizational change', in Hackman, J.R., Lawler III, E.E. and Porter, L.W. (eds) *Perspectives on Behaviour in Organizations*, pp. 551–61. New York, McGraw-Hill.
(A model and analysis of the different factors involved in organisational change.)

PERSPECTIVES ON LEADERSHIP

Adair, J. (1983) *Effective Leadership*. London, Pan Books.
(An influential, contemporary approach to leadership and leadership development.)

Grint, K. ed. (1997) *Leadership: Classical, Contemporary and Critical Approaches*. Oxford, Oxford University Press.
(A review of traditional and newer models of leadership.)

Martin, V. (2003) *Leading Change in Health and Social Care*. London, Routledge.
(Leading change as a process and with a focus on learning.)

Mintzberg, H. (1998) 'Covert leadership: notes on managing professionals'. *Harvard Business Review,* November–December, pp. 140–147.
(An innovative way of looking at leading professional teams.)

Rost, J.C. and Smith, A. (1992) 'Leadership: a postindustrial approach'. *European Management Journal*, Vol. 10, No. 2, June. (A political model of leadership.)

Starratt, R.J. (1993) *The Drama of Leadership*. London, Falmer Press. (A compelling exploration of charismatic leadership.)

PERSPECTIVES ON TEAMWORK

Menzies Lyth, I. (1988) *Containing Anxiety in Institutions: Selected Essays*, Vol. 1. London, Free Association Books. (Looks at unconscious strategies and interactions used to handle anxiety in health and social care.)

Morgan, G. (1997) *Imaginization: New Mindsets for Seeing, Organizing and Managing*. San Francisco, Berrett: Koehler. (Creative approaches to the use of metaphor in understanding and changing team performance.)

West, M. (2002) 'The HR factor'. *Health Management*, August 2002, London, Institute of Health Care Management. This research is reported more fully in 'A matter of life and death', *People Management*, 21 February, 2002, London, Chartered Institute of Personnel and Development.

REFERENCES

Adair, J. (1983) *Effective Leadership*. London, Pan Books.

Alimo-Metcalfe, B. and Alban-Metcalfe, R. (2002) 'Heaven can wait'. *Health Services Journal*, Vol. 12, Oct., pp. 26–29.

Barr, H. (2002) *Interprofessional Education Today, Yesterday and Tomorrow*. Commissioned and published by the Learning and Teaching Subject Network for Health Sciences and Practice, King's College, London.

Belbin, R.M. (1981) *Management Team*. Oxford, Heinemann.

Bion, W. (1961) *Experiences in Groups and Other Papers*. London, Tavistock Publications.

Blanchard, K., Zigarmi, P. and Zigarmi, D. (1986) *Leadership and the One Minute Manager*. London, Collins.

Bridges, W. (1988) *Transitions: Making the Most of Life's Change*. London, Nicholas Brealey Publishing.

Burns, J.M. (1978) *Leadership*. London, Harper & Row.

Charlesworth, J. (2003) 'Managing across professional and agency boundaries', in Seden, J. and Reynolds, J. (eds) *Managing Care in Practice*. London, Routledge.

Department of Health (1998) *Modernising Social Services*, www.doh.gov.uk

Department of Health (1999) The Health Act, www.doh.gov.uk

Department of Health (2000) The NHS Plan, www.doh.gov.uk

Department of Health (2001) *Working Together, Learning Together: a Framework for Lifelong Learning for the NHS*, www.doh.gov.uk/lifelonglearnng/index.htm

Department of Health (2002) *HR in the NHS plan – a document produced by the National Workforce Taskforce and HR Directorate for consultation*, www.doh.gov.uk/hrinthenhsplan/index.htm

Ferlie, E. and Pettigrew, A. (1996) 'Managing through networks: Some issues and implications for the NHS'. *British Journal of Management*, Vol. 7/ Special issue March, S81–S99.

Fiedler, F.E. (1967) *A Theory of Leadership Effectiveness*. New York, McGraw-Hill.

Foster, W. (1989) 'Toward a critical practice of leadership', in Smyth, J. (ed.), *Critical Perspectives on Educational Leadership*, pp. 39–62. London, Falmer.

Frady, M. (1992) 'Profiles (Jesse Jackson–Part 1)'. *The New Yorker*, 3, February, p. 57.

Gleicher, D. (1986) quoted in Turrill, T., *Change and Innovation: A Challenge for the NHS*. London, Institute of Healthcare Management.

Goleman, D. (1996) *Emotional Intelligence*. London, Bloomsbury.

Goleman, D., Boyatzis, R.E. and McKee, A. (2002) *The New Leaders: Transforming the Art of Leadership into the Science of Results*. London, Little, Brown.

Greenleaf, R. (1977) *Servant Leadership*. New York, Paulist Press.

Hartley, J. and Allison, M. (2000) 'The role of leadership in the modernisation and improvement of public services'. *Public Money and Management*, (April–June) Vol. 20, Issue 2, pp. 35–40.

Hirsch, S.K. and Kummerow, J.M. (1987) *Introduction to Type in Organizations*, (2nd edn). Palo Alto, CA, Consulting Psychologists Press.

Hudson, B., Exworthy, M. and Peckham, S. (1998) *The Integration of Localised and Collaborative Purchasing: A Review of the Literature and a Framework for Analysis*. Leeds, Nuffield Institute for Health.

Iles, V. and Sutherland, K. (2001) *A Review for Health Care Managers, Professionals and Researchers*. London, National Co-ordinating Centre for NHS Service Delivery and Organisation R&D.

Katzenbach, J.R. and Smith, D.K. (1993) *The Wisdom of Teams: Creating the High Performance Organization*. Boston, MA, Harvard Business School Press.

Kolb, D.A. and Fry, R. (1975) ' Towards an applied theory of experiential learning', in Cooper, C.L. (ed.) *Theories of Group Processes*, pp. 33–57. London, John Wiley.

Kouzes, J.M. and Posner, B.Z. (1987) *The Leadership Challenge: How to Get Extraordinary Things Done in Organizations*. San Francisco, Jossey-Bass.

Martin, V. (2003) *Leading Change in Health and Social Care*. London, Routledge.

Rogers, A. (1994) *Barriers To Community: Development of an Instrument to Assess Components of Prejudice*. University of San Diego, unpublished doctoral thesis.

Rogers, A. and Reynolds, J. (2003) 'Leadership and Vision', in Seden, J. and Reynolds, J. (eds) *Managing Care in Practice*. London, Routledge.

Rost, J.C. (1991) *Leadership for the 21st Century*. New York, Praeger.

Senge, P.M. (1990) *The Fifth Discipline: The Art and Practice of the Learning Organization*. London, Doubleday/Century Business.

Senge, P.M., Kleiner, A., Roberts, C., Ross, R., Roth, G. and Smith, B. (1999) *The Dance of Change: The Challenges of Sustaining Momentum in Learning Organizations*. London, Nicholas Brealey Publishing.

Smale, G.G. (1996) *Mapping Change and Innovation*. London, National Institute for Social Work.

Tannenbaum, R. and Schmidt, W.H. (1958) 'How to choose a leadership pattern'. *Harvard Business Review*, 36/2, pp. 95–101.

Tuckman, B. and Jensen M. (1977) 'Stages of small group development revisited'. *Groups and Organization Studies*, Vol. 2, pp. 419–427.

van Maurick, J. (2001) *Writers on Leadership*. London, Penguin Books.

West, M. (2003) *Connecting the Jigsaw*. NHS Confederation in Wales, Conference Proceedings, November.

Zalzenik, A. (1993) 'Managers and leaders: Are they different?', in Rosenback, W.E. and Taylor, R.L. (eds) *Contemporary Issues in Leadership* (3rd edn). Oxford, Westview Press.

INDEX

SAGE COURSE COMPANIONS

KNOWLEDGE AND SKILLS *for* SUCCESS

Social Research Methods

Nicholas Walliman

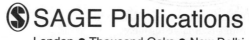
SAGE Publications

London • Thousand Oaks • New Delhi

SAGE Publications Ltd
1 Oliver's Yard
55 City Road
London EC1Y 1SP

SAGE Publications Inc.
2455 Teller Road
Thousand Oaks, California 91320

SAGE Publications India Pvt Ltd
B-42, Panchsheel Enclave
Post Box 4109
New Delhi 110 017

British Library Cataloguing in Publication data

A catalogue record for this book is available from
the British Library

ISBN10 1 4129 1061 7   ISBN13 978 1 4129 1061 3
ISBN10 1 4129 1062 5   ISBN13 978 1 4129 1062 0 (pbk)

Library of Congress Control Number: 2005930766

Typeset by C&M Digitals (P) Ltd., Chennai, India
Printed on paper from sustainable resources
Printed in Great Britain by The Cromwell Press

contents

part one
social research methods

1	
introduction to your companion	

Introduction to the series

This book is part of a series called Sage Course Companions. They are designed to be just that: 'companions' to your studies, books to take with you anywhere, that provide you with an easy-to-use reference and guide to your subject. They present you with enormously useful information and tips that will help you to be successful in your work.

Every course recommends textbooks that tend to be both long and complicated, providing great volume and detail of information but that can be overwhelming to the student. Sage Course Companions provide you with a simple guide to help you to steer a route through the detail by summarizing the main ingredients of the subject, their interrelationships and background. You will gain a clear overview of your course that will enable you to fill in detail as required, and support you in writing your essays and assignments and in passing your exams.

Navigation

This book is in three main parts. Part 1 is the Introduction to the Course Companion and gives guidance about how to use this book, how it relates to your subject, and how to think like a social science researcher. Part 2 covers the core areas of the social science research methods curriculum. This section presents a condensed summary and commentary on the subject, providing you with a useful revision guide to your course material plus suggestions for further reading. Part 3 offers guidance in study, writing and revision skills so that you can present your knowledge in the best possible way in your essays, assignments and exams. At the end, there is a glossary of the main terms used in the subject and a list of references. An index is provided to help you to locate subjects in the book.

How to use this book

This book is designed to help you to succeed in your undergraduate or postgraduate level course on social science research methods. This

> *It was only by the beginning of the 1960s that Popper (1902–92) formulated the idea of the hypothetico-deductive method, even though it must have been used in practice for decades before.*

There are certain assumptions that underlie scientific method, some of which are regarded by interpretivists as unacceptable when doing social research:

- **Order**
- **External reality**
- **Reliability**
- **Parsimony**
- **Generality**

The positivist/interpretivist divide

There is an important issue that confronts the study of the social sciences that is not so pertinent in the natural sciences. This is the question of the position of the human subject and researcher, and the status of social phenomena. Is human society subjected to laws that exist independent of the human actors that make up society, or do individuals and groups create their own versions of social forces? The two extremes of approach are termed **positivism** and **interpretivism**. Again, as in the case of ways of reasoning, a middle way has also been formulated that draws on the useful characteristics of both approaches.

Positivism

According to Hacking (1981, pp. 1–2), the positivist approach to scientific investigation is based on realism, an attempt to find out about one real world. There is a sharp distinction between scientific theories and other kinds of belief, and there is a unique best description of any chosen aspect of the world that is true regardless of what people think. Science is cumulative, despite the false starts that are common enough. Science by and large builds on what is already known. Even Einstein's theories are a development from Newton's.

There should be just one science about the one real world. Less measurable sciences are reducible to more measurable ones. Sociology is reducible to psychology, psychology to biology, biology to chemistry, and chemistry to physics.

Interpretivism

Although scientific method is widely used in many forms of research, it does not, and never has, enjoyed total hegemony in all subjects. Some of the world's greatest thinkers have disagreed with the tenets of positivism contained in scientific method. The alternative approach to research is based on the philosophical doctrines of idealism and humanism. It maintains that the view of the world that we see around us is the creation of the mind.

This does not mean that the world is not real, but rather that we can only experience it personally through our perceptions which are influenced by our preconceptions and beliefs; we are not neutral, disembodied observers. Unlike the natural sciences, the researcher is not observing phenomena from outside the system, but is inextricably bound into the human situation which he/she is studying. In addition, by concentrating on the search for constants in human behaviour, the researcher highlights the repetitive, predictable and invariant aspect of society and ignores what is subjective, individual and creative.

In order to compare the alternative bases for interpreting social reality, Cohen and Manion (1994, pp. 10–11) produced a useful table which they had adapted from Barr Greenfield (1975).

> ***Common pitfall****:* Just because the differences of perspective between positivist and interpretivist approaches are so radical, don't think that you need to espouse purely one or the other approach. Different aspects of life lend themselves to different methods of interpretation.

Critical realism

Critical reasoning can be seen as a reconciliatory approach, which recognizes, like the positivists, the existence of a natural order in social events and discourse, but claims that this order cannot be detected by merely observing a pattern of events. The underlying order must be discovered through the process of **interpretation** while doing theoretical and practical work in the social sciences. Unlike the positivists, critical realists do not claim that there is a direct link between the concepts they develop and the observable phenomena. Concepts and theories about social events are developed on the basis of their observable effects, and interpreted in such a way that they can be understood and acted upon, even if the interpretation is open to revision as understanding grows.

Table 2.1 Comparison between positivist and interpretivist approaches

Dimensions of comparisons	Positivist	Interpretivist
Philosophical basis	Realism: the world exists and is knowable as it really is. Organizations are real entities with a life of their own.	Idealism: the world exists but different people construe it in very different ways. Organizations are invented social reality.
The role of social science	Discovering the universal laws of society and human conduct within it.	Discovering how different people interpret the world in which they live.
Basic units of social reality	The collectivity: society or organizations.	Individuals acting singly or together.
Methods of understanding	Identifying conditions or relationships which permit the collectivity to exist. Conceiving what these conditions and relationships are.	Interpretation of the subjective meanings which individuals place upon their action. Discovering the subjective rules for such action.
Theory	A rational edifice built by scientists to explain human behaviour.	Sets of meanings which people use to make sense of their world and human behaviour within it.
Research	Experimental or quasi-experimental validation of theory.	The search for meaningful relationships and the discovery of their consequences for action.
Methodology	Abstraction of reality, especially through mathematical models and quantitative analysis.	The representation of reality for purposes of comparison. Analysis of language and meaning.
Society	Ordered. Governed by a uniform set of values and made possible only by these values.	Conflicted. Governed by the values of people with access to power.
Organizations	Goal-oriented. Independent of people. Instruments of order in society serving both the society and the individual.	Dependent upon people and their goals. Instruments of power which some people control and can use to attain ends which seem good to them.

(Continued)

Table 2.1 *(Continued)*

Dimensions of comparisons	Positivist	Interpretivist
Organizational pathologies	Organizations get out of kilter with social values and individual needs.	Given diverse human ends, there is always conflict among people acting to pursue them.
Prescriptions for change	Change the structure of the organization to meet social values and individual needs.	Find out what values are embodied in organizational action and whose they are. Change the people or change their values if you can.

Source: Cohen and Manion, 1994, pp. 10–11

The belief that there are underlying structures at work that generate social events, and which can be formulated in concepts and theory, distinguishes critical realists from interpretivists, who deny the existence of such general structures divorced from the specific event or situation and the context of the research and researcher.

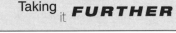
Taking it *FURTHER*

Social science, a brief theoretical history

As with any subject, some knowledge of its history provides a deeper perspective of why things are how they are at present, and how they come to be so. As you are not actually studying social science as such in this course, the history of the subject is not of central importance, but does show how research methods developed and were used in different contexts.

Social science, the study of human thought and behaviour in society, is a very large area of study that is divided into a range of interrelated disciplines. According to Bernard (2000, p. 6), the main branches are anthropology, economics, history, political science, psychology, social psychology, each with their own sub-fields. Other disciplines also involve social research, such as communications, criminology, demography, education, journalism, leisure studies, nursing, social work, architecture and design and many others.

A wide range of research methods have been developed and refined by the different disciplines, though these are not specific only to them.

Positivist beginnings

Social science, understood here as the study of human society in the widest sense, is a rich source of research problems. This important, and sometimes controversial, branch of science was first defined and named by Auguste Comte (1798–1857), the nineteenth-century French philosopher. Comte maintained that society could be analysed empirically, just like other subjects of scientific inquiry, and social laws and theories could be established on the basis of psychology and biology. He based his approach on the belief that all genuine knowledge is based on information gained by experience through the senses, and can only be developed through further observation and experiment.

The foundations of modern sociology were built during the end of the nineteenth century and beginning of the twentieth century. Prominent thinkers were Marx (1818–83), Durkheim (1858–1917), Dilthey (1833–1911) and Weber (1864–1920). Marx developed a theory that described the inevitable social progress from primitive communism, through feudalism and capitalism to a state of post-revolutionary communism. Durkheim is famous for his enquiries into the division of labour, suicide, religion and education, as well as for his philosophical discussions on the nature of sociology.

Unlike Marx, who tended to define the moral and social aspects of humanity in terms of material forces, Durkheim argued that society develops its own system of phenomena that produce collectively shared norms and beliefs. These 'social facts', as he called them, for example economic organizations, laws, customs, criminality etc., exist in their own right, are external to us and are resistant to our will and constrain our behaviour. Having 'discovered' and defined social facts using scientific observation techniques, the social scientist should seek their causes among other social facts rather than in other scientific domains such as biology or psychology. By thus maintaining sociology as an autonomous discipline, the social scientist may use the knowledge gained to understand the origins of, and possibly suggest the cures for, various forms of social ills.

In summary, this approach looks at society as the focus for research, and through understanding its internal laws and establishing relevant facts, we can in turn understand how and why individuals behave as they do. However, not all philosophers agreed that human society was amenable to such a disembodied analysis.

The rise of interpretivism

Another German philosopher, Wilhelm Dilthey, agreed that although in the physical world we can only study the appearance of a thing rather than the thing itself, we are, because of our own humanity, in a position to know about human consciousness and its roles in society. The purpose here is not to search for causal explanations, but to find understanding. As a method, this presupposes that to gain understanding there must be at least some common ground between the researcher and the people who are being studied. He went on to make a distinction between two kinds of sciences: *Geisteswissneschaften* (the human sciences) and *Naturwissenschaften* (the natural sciences).

Max Weber, developing and refining Dilthey's ideas, believed that empathy is not necessary or even possible in some cases, and that it was feasible to understand the intentionality of conduct and to pursue objectivity in terms of cause and effect. He wished to bridge the divide between the traditions of positivism and interpretivism by being concerned to investigate both the meanings and the material conditions of action.

Three main schools of thought can be seen to represent opposition to positivism in the social sciences: **phenomenology**, as developed by Husserl (1859–1938) and Schutz (1899–1959), **ethnography**, developed by Malinowski (1884–1942), Evans-Pritchard (1902–73), and Margaret Mead (1901–78), **ethnomethodology**, pioneered by Garfinkel (1917–87), and **symbolic interactionism**, practised by members of the Chicago School such as George Herbert Mead (1863–1931) and Blumer. They all rejected the assertion that human behaviour can be codified in laws by identifying underlying regularities, and that society can be studied from a detached, objective and impartial viewpoint by the researcher.

Husserl argued that consciousness is not determined by the natural processes of human neurophysiology, but that our understanding of the world is constructed by our human perceptions about our surroundings – we construct our own reality. In order to cope with this, Schutz believed that in social intercourse, each person needs to perceive the different perspectives that others have due to their unique biographies and experiences in order to transcend individual subjectivity. This constructed intersubjective world produces 'common sense'. He saw everyday language as a perfect example of socially derived preconstituted types and characteristics that enabled individuals to formulate their own subjectivity in terms understandable by others.

The work of anthropologists in the ethnic tribes of the Pacific (Malinowski, M. Mead) and Africa (Evans-Pritchard) developed the ethnographic techniques of studying society. By employing the method of participant observation, knowledge can be gained of the complexities of cultures and social groups within their settings. The central concern is to produce a description that faithfully reflects the world-view of the participants in their social context. Theories and explanations can then emerge from the growing understanding gained by the researcher thus immersed in the context of the society.

Garfinkel developed a method of studying individual subjectivity by observing interaction on a small scale, between individuals or in a small group. He maintained that people were not strictly regulated by the collective values and norms sanctioned by society, but that they made individual choices on the basis of their own experiences and understanding. It was they that produced the social institutions and everyday practices, developing society as a social construction. The analysis of conversation is used as the main method of investigation.

Language was seen by G.H. Mead to be central to human interaction. Human beings are able to understand each other's perspectives, gestures and responses due to the shared **symbols** contained in a common language. It is this symbolic interaction that not only defines the individual as the instigator of ideas and opinions, but also as a reflection of the reactions and perceptions of others. To be able to understand this constantly shifting situation, the researcher must comprehend the meanings which guide it, and this is only possible in the natural surroundings where it occurs. This approach was developed in the University of Chicago from the 1920s and was used in a large programme of field research focusing mostly on urban society in Chicago itself, using interviews, life histories and other ethnographical methods.

The reconciliatory approach

Weber disagreed with the pure interpretivists, maintaining that it is necessary to verify the results of subjective interpretative investigation by comparing them with the concrete course of events. He makes a distinction between what one can perceive as facts (i.e. those things that are) and what one can perceive as values (i.e. those things that may, or may not, be desirable). A differentiation must be maintained between facts and values because they are distinct kinds of phenomenon. However, in order to understand society, we have to take account of both of these elements.

Weber maintained that in order to describe social practices adequately we must understand what meanings the practices have for the participants themselves. This requires an understanding of the values involved, but without taking sides or making value judgements. This understanding (often referred to as *Verstehen*) is the subject matter of social science. It is then possible to investigate the social practices rationally through an assessment of the internal logic of the situation. In this way, one can make a meaningful formulation of the elements, causes and effects within complex social situations, taking into account the values inherent in it.

It is argued that it is impossible for the social scientist to take this detached view of values, as he/she is a member of society and culture, motivated by personal presuppositions and beliefs. Accordingly, any analysis of social phenomena is based on a 'view from somewhere'. This is inescapable and even to be desired.

The philosopher Roy Baskhar has provided an alternative to the dichotomous argument of positivism versus interpretivism by taking a more inclusive and systematic view of the relationships between the natural and social sciences. His approach, known as **critical realism**, sees nature as stratified, with each layer using the previous one as a foundation and a basis for greater complexity. Thus physics is more basic than chemistry, which in its turn is more basic than biology, which is more basic than the human sciences. The relationships between these domains, from the more basic to the more complex, are inclusive one-way relationships – the more complex emerging from the more basic. While a human being is not able to go against the chemical, physical and biological laws, he/she can do all sorts of things that the chemicals of which he/she is made cannot do if they are following only their specific chemical laws rather than those of biological laws that govern organisms, or social 'laws' which govern society.

Bhaskar also has a profoundly integrationist view of the relationship between the individual and society, called by him the transformation model of social activity. Rather than, on the one hand, studying society to understand individual actions or, on the other hand, studying individuals to understand the structures of society or, somewhere in between, checking the results of one study against that of the other, Baskhar argues that the reciprocal interaction between individuals and society effects a transformation in both.

Structuralism, post-structuralism and postmodernism
Based primarily on the view that all cultural phenomena are primarily linguistic in character, **structuralism** gained its label because of its assertion that subjectivity is formed by deep 'structures' that lie beneath the surface of social reality. Lévi-Strauss used a geological metaphor, stating that the overt aspects of cultural phenomena are formed by the complex layering and folding of underlying strata. These can be revealed by semiotic analysis. 'Cultural symbols and representations are the surface structure and acquire the appearance of "reality" (Seale, 1998, p. 34).

Post-structuralism was developed by French philosophers such as Derrida and Foucault in the latter part of the twentieth century. Through the method of 'deconstruction', the claims to authority made in texts and discourses were undermined. According to Seale (1998, p. 34), **postmodernism** subsequently developed and became more widely accepted through the appeal of its three basic principles:

1 **The decentered self** – the belief that there are no human universals that determine identity, but that the self is a creation of society.

2 **The rejection of claims to authority** – the idea of progress through scientific objectivity and value neutrality is a fallacy and has resulted in a moral vacuum. Discourse must be subjected to critical analysis and traditions and values should be constantly attacked.

3 **The commitment to instability in our practices of understanding** – as everything is put to question there can be no established way of thinking. Our understanding of the world is subject to constant flux, all voices within a culture have an equal right to be heard.

In view of the diverse range of theoretical perspectives, it is probably inappropriate to search for and impossible to find a single model of social and cultural life.

Questions to ponder

❝What role do epistemology and ontology play in understanding social research?❞

They form the theoretical basis of how the world can be experienced, what constitutes knowledge, and what can be done with that knowledge. Social research has been carried out subject to varied epistemological and ontological stances, so it is important to know what assumptions have been made at the outset of the research. You can explain this by outlining the main approaches and describing how these affect the outcomes of the research.

❝What is the difference between inductive and deductive thinking? Why is this distinction important in the practical aspects of doing a research project and in theory development?❞

Inductive thinking – going from the specific to the general. Deductive thinking – going from the general to the specific. You can explain this in greater detail. This distinction is important because it determines what data you collect and how you collect it. You can give examples of these. An inductive approach is used to *generate* theory whereas a deductive approach is used to *test* theory.

❝In what ways does the interpretivist approach particularly suit the study of human beings in their social settings?❞

Because humans are reflective beings, they are not simply determined by their surroundings. Cause-and-effect relationships are complex and difficult to determine, so a less deterministic approach can provide useful understanding about society, without the need for the kind of verifiable facts aimed for in the natural sciences. It is also impossible for a researcher to take a completely detached view of society, so investigation is necessarily dependent on interpretation.

References to more information

You can go into much greater detail about the philosophy of knowledge and the history of social research if you want to, but I suspect that you will not have enough time to delve too deeply.

For the theoretical background to social research, it might be worth having a look at these for more detail:

Hughes, J. (1990) *The Philosophy of Social Research* (2nd edn). Harlow: Longman.
Seale, C. (ed.) (2004) *Researching Society and Culture* (2nd edn). London: Sage.

For topics that are more into scientific method see:

Chalmers, A. (1982) *What Is This Thing Called Science?* (2nd edn). Milton Keynes: Open University Press.
Medawar, P. (1984) *The Limit of Science*. Oxford: Oxford University Press.

For a simple general introduction to philosophy, seek this one out. This approachable book explains the main terminology and outlines the principal streams of thought:

Thompson, M. (1995) *Philosophy*. Teach Yourself Books. London: Hodder and Stoughton.

And here are books that deal in more detail with some aspects of philosophy – for the real enthusiast!

Husserl, E. (1964) *The Idea of Phenomenology*. Trans. W. Alston and G. Nakhnikian. The Hague: Martinus Nijhoff.

Collier, A. (1994) *Critical Realism: An Introduction to Roy Baskhar's Philosophy*. London: Verso.

If you are doing a course in one of the disciplines associated with social research (e.g. healthcare, marketing etc), delve into the specific history that has led up to the present state-of-the art thinking. You will have to make a library search using key words to find what is easily available to you.

3	
research basics	

Research methods are the practical means to carry out research. In order to give them a meaning and purpose, you should be clear about the basics of research and the process of carrying out a project. The central generating point of a research project is the research problem. All the activities are developed for the purpose of solving or investigating this problem. Hence the need for total clarity in defining the problem and limiting its scope in order to enable a practical research project with defined outcomes to be devised.

Mostly, social science research methods courses at undergraduate level culminate not in an exam, but in a small research project or dissertation where you can demonstrate how you have understood the process of research and how various research methods are applied. Hence the need to be clear about the process as a whole so that the methods can be seen within the context of a project.

Overview of the research process

A research project, whatever its size and complexity, consists of defining some kind of a research problem, working out how this problem can be investigated, doing the investigation work, coming to conclusions on the basis of what one has found out, and then reporting the outcome in some form or other to inform others of the work done. The differences between research projects are due to their different scales of time, resources and extent, pioneering qualities, and rigour.

Whatever the research approach, it is worth considering generally what the research process consists of and what are the crucial decision stages and choices that need to be made. The answers to four important questions underpin the framework of any research project:

- What are you going to do?
- Why are you going to do it?
- How are you going to do it?
- When are you going to do it?

The actual doing of the research is subject to the nature of these answers and involve the most crucial decision making. Obviously the answers are not simple – this book has been written to help you formulate your own answers in relation to your own research project.

Figure 1.1 (see page 6) shows a rather linear sequence of tasks, far tidier than anything in reality, which is subject to constant reiteration as the knowledge and understanding increases. However, a diagram like this can be used as a basis for a programme of work in the form of a timetable, and the progress of the project can be gauged by comparing the current stage of work with the steps in the process.

> *Notice how, in the latter stages, the requirement for writing up the work becomes important. There is no point in doing research if the results are not recorded, even if only for your own use, though usually many more people will be interested to read about the outcomes, not least your examiner.*

The research problem

One of the first tasks on the way to deciding on the detailed topic of research is to find a question, an unresolved controversy, a gap in knowledge or an unrequited need within the chosen subject. This search requires an awareness of current issues in the subject and an inquisitive and questioning mind. Although you will find that the world is teeming with questions and unresolved problems, not every one of these is a suitable subject for research. So what features should you look for which could lead you to a suitable **research problem**? Here is a list of the most important.

Checklist: features of a suitable research problem

✓ You should be able to state the problem clearly and concisely.
✓ It should be of great interest to you.
✓ The problem should be significant (i.e. not trivial or a repeat of previous work).
✓ It should be delineated. You will not have much time, so restrict the aims of the research.
✓ You should be able to obtain the required information.
✓ You should be able to draw conclusions related to the problem. The point of research is to find some answers.

The problem can be generated either by an initiating idea, or by a perceived **problem area**. For example, investigation of 'rhythmic patterns in conflict settlement' is the product of an idea that there are such things as rhythmic patterns in conflict settlement, even if no one had detected them before. This kind of idea will then need to be formulated more precisely in order to develop it into a researchable problem. We are surrounded by problems connected with society, healthcare, education etc., many of which can readily be perceived. Take, for example, social problems such as poverty, crime, unsuitable housing, problematic labour relationships, and bureaucratic bungles. There are many subjects where there may be a lack of knowledge which prevents improvements being made, for example, the influence of parents on a child's progress at school or the relationship between designers and clients.

> *Obviously, it is not difficult to find problem areas. The difficulty lies in choosing an area which contains possible specific research problems suitable for the type and scope of your assignment.*

> *Common pitfalls:* when choosing a research problem:
> - Making the choice of a problem an excuse to fill in gaps in your own knowledge.
> - Formulating a problem which involves merely a comparison of two or more sets of data.
> - Setting a problem in terms of finding the degree of correlation between two sets of data.
> - Devising a problem to which the answer can be only yes or no.

Aids to locating and analysing problems

Booth et al. (1995, p. 36) suggest that the process for focusing on the formulation of your research problem looks like this:

How to focus on a research problem

- Find an interest in a broad subject area (problem area).
- Narrow the interest to a plausible topic.
- Question the topic from several points of view.
- Define a rationale for your project.

> *Initially, it is useful to define no more than a problem area, rather than a specific research problem, within the general body of knowledge.*

Research problem definition

From the interest in the wider issues of the chosen subject, and after the selection of a problem area, the next step is to define the research problem more closely so that it becomes a specific research problem, with all the characteristics already discussed. This stage requires an enquiring mind, an eye for inconsistencies and inadequacies in current theory and a measure of imagination. The research problem is often formulated in the form of a theoretical **research question** that indicates a clear direction and scope for the research project.

> *It is often useful in identifying a specific problem to pose a simple question. Such a question can provide a starting point for the formulation of a specific research problem, whose conclusion should aim to answer the question.*

The sub-problems

Most research problems are difficult, or even impossible, to solve without breaking them down into smaller problems. The short sentences devised during the problem formulation period can give a clue to the presence of sub-problems. **Sub-problems** should delineate the scope of the work and, taken together, should define the entire problem to be tackled as summarized in the main problem.

Questions used to define sub-problems include:

- Can the problem be split down into different aspects that can be investigated separately (e.g. political, economic, cultural, technical)?
- Are there different personal or group perspectives that need to be explored (e.g. employers, employees)?
- Are different concepts used that need to be separately investigated (e.g. health, fitness, well-being, confidence)?
- Does the problem need to be considered at different scales (e.g. the individual, group, organization)?

Second review of literature

A more focused review of literature follows the formulation of the research problem. The purpose of this review is to learn about research already carried out into one or more of the aspects of the research problem.

The purposes of a literature review are:

- to summarize the results of previous research to form a foundation on which to build your own research
- to collect ideas on how to gather data
- to investigate methods of data analysis
- to study instrumentation which has been used
- to assess the success of the various research designs of the studies already undertaken

For more detail on doing literature reviews, see Chapter 19.

Taking it **FURTHER**

Evaluation of social research

How can you tell whether a piece of research is any good? When doing your background reading, you should be able to assess the quality of the research projects you read about, as described by the research reports. Taking a critical look at completed research is a good preparation for doing some research yourself. You may later also have to defend the quality of some research that you have done.

It is not unusual that you will have to make comments on a particular research report as part of an assignment. If you can scrutinize it in a critical way, rather than just providing a description, you will impress your tutor with your expertise.

Below is one approach of how to do an evaluation of a social research study. It is only a short summary of the things to evaluate. You will have to refer to your textbooks for examples and a more detailed explanation of the process.

Consider these four major factors:

- Validity
- Reliability

- Replicability
- Generalizability

Validity of research is about the degree to which the research findings are true. Seale and Filmer (1998, p. 134) usefully list three different types of validity:

- **Measurement validity** The degree to which measures (e.g. questions on a questionnaire) successfully indicate concepts.
- **Internal validity** The extent to which causal statements are supported by the study.
- **External validity** The extent to which findings can be generalized to populations or to other settings.

Bryman (2004, p. 29) adds one more:

- **Ecological validity** The extent to which the findings are applicable to people's everyday, natural social settings.

Reliability is about the degree to which the results of the research are repeatable. Bryman (2004, p. 71) lists three prominent factors that are involved:

- **Stability** The degree to which a measure is stable over time.
- **Internal reliability** The degree to which the indicators that make up the scale or index are consistent.
- **Inter-observer consistency** The degree to which there is **consistency** in the decisions of several 'observers' in their recording of observations or translation of data into categories.

Replicability is about whether the research can be repeated and whether similar results are obtained. This is a check on the objectivity and lack of bias of the research findings. It requires a detailed account of the concepts used in the research, the measurements applied and methods employed.

Generalizability refers to the results of the research and how far they are applicable to locations and situations beyond the scope of the study. There is little point in doing research if it cannot be applied in a wider context. On the other hand, especially in qualitative research, there may well be limits to the generalizability of the findings, and these should be pointed out.

Read news reports about research projects (education, old age, criminality, etc.) critically. Look for 'spin', vested interests, choice of evidence and use/misuse of statistics.

Questions to ponder

❝ What are the desirable qualities of a research problem? ❞

You can provide a simple list. Here are some suggestions. It should be:

- Limited – to the scope of the research project.
- Significant – no point doing trivial research.
- Novel – ideally some new knowledge or greater understanding should be uncovered.
- Clearly defined – so that the purpose of the research is obvious.
- Interesting – in order to motivate you whlle doing the work.

❝ What relationship do sub-problems have to a research problem, and what function do they carry out? ❞

The sub-problems break the main problem down into researchable components. The main problem is usually couched in rather abstract concepts. The sub-problems help to make the concepts more concrete by suggesting several indicators and even variables that can be investigated and together may provide answers to the main problem. You could give examples to illustrate the points.

❝ Why review the literature again once you have decided on your research problem? ❞

Once you have decided on your research problem, you can narrow down your review of the literature to concentrate on the specific topics raised by it. It is always possible to go into greater depth when you are clear about the subject you are investigating. You will need to find out about similar research and the 'state of the art' in the subject, and you can check on the methods that were used in projects with similar aims.

References to more information

At an undergraduate level, most advice on locating and assessing research problems appear in books on how to write dissertations. Specific guidance on topics in a particular subject can be gained from books dedicated to one particular discipline. Explore your own **library catalogue** for both general and subject-related guides to dissertation writing. But do be careful not to get bogged down in technicalities – peck like a bird at the juicy pieces useful to you now and leave the rest. The list below is in order of detail and complexity – the simplest first. Here is a selection:

Ajuga, G. (2002) *The Student Assignment and Dissertation Survival Guide: Answering the Question Behind the Question!* Thornton Heath: GKA Publishing.
See pp. 46–55. Do you want to become the teacher's pet?

Mounsey, C. (2002) *Essays and Dissertations*. Oxford: Oxford University Press.
Chapter 2 looks at ways to develop research questions.

Swetnam, D. (2000) *Writing Your Dissertation: How to Plan, Prepare and Present Successful Work*. Oxford: How To Books.
See Chapter 1 for simple guidance on how to get started.

Naoum, S.G. (1998) *Dissertation Research and Writing for Construction Students*. Oxford: Butterworth-Heinemann.
Chapter 2 gives advice on choosing a topic (not just for construction students).

Blaxter, L. Hughes, C. and Tight, M. (1996) *How to Research*. Buckingham: Open University Press.
A much bigger book, but see Chapter 2 on how to get started.

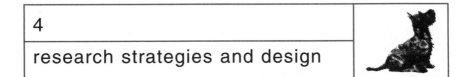

4	
research strategies and design	

Research strategies – quantitative and qualitative research

A common distinction is made between two different strategies in research, the one using quantitative methodology and the other using qualitative methodology. Apart from the simple distinction of the use of measurement or description as the main approach to collecting and analysing data, there is seen to be an underlying epistemological difference in the two approaches. Bryman (2004, pp. 19–20) lists three characteristics in each that make the point:

Quantitative research

- Orientation – uses a deductive approach to test theories.
- Epistemology – is based on a positivist approach inherent in the natural sciences.
- Ontology – objectivist in that social reality is regarded as objective fact.

Qualitative research

- Orientation – uses an inductive approach to generate theories.
- Epistemology – it rejects positivism by relying on individual interpretation of social reality.
- Ontology – constructionist, in that social reality is seen as a constantly shifting product of perception.

These distinctions are useful in describing and understanding social research, but are not to be seen as mutually exclusive, but rather as polarizations. There are many examples of social research that do not conform to all of the conditions listed above. There are also examples of research that combine the two approaches, usually to examine different aspects of the research problem.

The two different methodologies imply the use of different methods of data collection and analysis. Quantitative techniques rely on collecting data that is numerically based and amenable to such analytical methods as statistical correlations, often in relation to hypothesis testing. Qualitative techniques rely more on language and the interpretation of its meaning, so data collection methods tend to involve close human involvement and a creative process of theory development rather than testing.

However, Bryman (2004, pp. 437–450) warns against a too dogmatic distinction between the two types of methodology. He concludes that research methods are not determined by epistemology or ontology and that the contrast between natural and artificial settings for qualitative and quantitative research is frequently exaggerated. Furthermore, quantitative research can be carried out from an interpretivist perspective, as can qualitative research from one of natural science. Quantitative methods have been used in some qualitative research, and analyses of quantitative and qualitative studies can be carried out using the opposite approaches.

Research objectives

The objectives of a particular research project delineate the intentions of the researchers and the nature and purpose of the investigations. The range of possible objectives can be listed as:

- to describe
- to explain and evaluate

- to compare
- to correlate
- to act, intervene and change

Description

Descriptive research relies on observation as a means of collecting data. It attempts to examine situations in order to establish what is the norm, that is what can be predicted to happen again under the same circumstances.

'Observation' can take many forms. Depending on the type of information sought, people can be interviewed, questionnaires distributed, visual records made, even sounds and smells recorded. The important point is that the observations are written down or recorded in some way, in order that they can be subsequently analysed. It is important that the data so collected are organized and presented in a clear and systematic way, so that the analysis can result in valid and accurate conclusions.

The scale of the research is influenced by two major factors:

1 The level of complexity of the survey.

2 The scope of the survey.

For example, seeking relationships between specific events inevitably requires a more complex survey technique than aiming merely to describe the nature of existing conditions. Likewise, surveying a large number of cases over a wide area will require greater resources than a small, local survey.

> *As descriptive research depends on human observations and responses, there is a danger that distortion of the data can occur. This can be caused, among other ways, by inadvertently including biased questions in questionnaires or interviews, or through the selective observation of events. Although bias cannot be wholly eliminated, an awareness of its existence and likely extent is essential.*

Explanation and evaluation

This is a descriptive type of research specifically designed to deal with complex social issues. It aims to move beyond 'just getting the facts' in order to make sense of the myriad human, political, social, cultural and contextual elements involved. The latest form of this type of research, named by Guba and Lincoln as fourth-generation evaluation, has, according to them, six properties (Guba and Lincoln, 1989, pp. 8–11):

1 The evaluation outcomes are not intended to represent 'the way things really are, or how they work', but present the meaningful constructions which the individual actors or groups of actors create in order to make sense of the situations in which they find themselves.

2 In representing these constructions, it is recognized that they are shaped to a large extent by the values held by the constructors. This is a very important consideration in a value-pluralistic society, where groups rarely share a common value system.

3 These constructions are seen to be inextricably linked to the particular physical, psychological, social and cultural context within which they are formed and to which they refer. These surrounding conditions, however, are themselves dependent on the constructions of the actors which endow them with parameters, features and limits.

4 It is recognized that the evaluation of these constructions is highly dependent on the involvement and viewpoint of the evaluators in the situation studied.

5 This type of research stresses that evaluation should be action-oriented, define a course which can be practically followed, and stimulate the carrying out of its recommendations. This usually requires a stage of negotiation with all the interested parties.

6 Due regard should be given to the dignity, integrity and privacy of those involved at any level, and those who are drawn into the evaluation should be welcomed as equal partners in every aspect of design, implementation, interpretation, and resulting action.

A common purpose of **evaluation research** is to examine programmes or the working of projects from the point of view of levels of awareness, costs and benefits, cost-effectiveness, attainment of objectives and quality assurance. The results are generally used to prescribe changes to improve and develop the situation, but in some cases might be limited to descriptions giving a better understanding of the programme (Robson, 2002, pp. 201–15).

Comparison

The examination of two or more contrasting cases can be used to highlight differences and similarities between them, leading to a better understanding of social phenomena. Suitable for both qualitative and quantitative methodologies, **comparative research** is commonly applied in cross-cultural and cross-national contexts. It is also applicable to different organizations or contexts (e.g. firms, labour markets, etc.).

Problems in cross-cultural research stem from the difficulties in ensuring comparability in the data collected and the situations investigated. Different languages and cultural contexts can create problems of comparability. It is also criticized for neglecting the specific context of the case in the search for contrasts, and that this search implies the adoption of a specific focus at the expense of a more open-ended approach.

The strength of the comparative approach using multiple-case studies is that it may reveal concepts that can be used for theory building, and that theory building can be improved in that the research is more able to establish the extent to which the theory will or will not hold. Comparative design is akin to the simultaneous scrutiny of two or more cross-sectional studies, sharing the same issues of reliability, validity, replicability and generalizability.

Correlation

The information sought in **correlation research** is expressed not in the form of artefacts, words or observations, but in numbers. While historical and descriptive approaches are predominantly forms of qualitative research, analytical survey or correlation research is principally quantitative. 'Correlation' is another word to describe the measure of association or the relationships between two phenomena. In order to find meaning in the numerical data, the techniques of statistics are used. What kind of statistical tests are used to analyse the data depends very much on the nature of the data.

This form of quantitative research can be broadly classified into two types of study:

- Relational studies.
- Prediction studies.

Relational studies investigate possible relationships between phenomena to establish if a correlation exists and, if so, its extent. This exploratory form of research is carried out particularly where little or no previous work has been done, and its outcomes can form the basis for further investigations.

Prediction studies tend to be carried out in research areas where correlations are already known. This knowledge is used to predict possible future behaviour or events, on the basis that if there has been a strong relationship between two or more characteristics or events in the past, then these should exist in similar circumstances in the future, leading to predictable outcomes.

In order to produce statistically significant results, quantitative research demands data from a large number of cases. Greater numbers of cases tend to produce more reliable results; 20–30 is considered to be about the minimum, though this depends on the type of statistical test applied. The data, whatever their original character, must be converted into numbers.

One of the advantages of correlation research is that it allows for the measurement of a number of characteristics (technically called variables) and their relationships simultaneously. Particularly in social science, many variables contribute to a particular outcome (e.g. satisfaction with housing depends on many factors). Another advantage is that, unlike other research approaches, it produces a measure of the amount of relationship between the variables being studied. It also, when used in prediction studies, gives an estimation of the probable accuracy of the predictions made. One limitation to what can be learned from correlation research is that, while the association of variables can be established, the cause-and-effect relationships are not revealed.

Action, intervention and change

This is related to experimental research, although it is carried out in the real world rather than in the context of a closed experimental system. A basic definition of this type of research is: 'a small-scale intervention in the functioning of the real world and a close examination of the effects of such an intervention' (Cohen and Manion, 1994, p. 186).

Its main characteristic is that it is essentially an 'on the spot' procedure, principally designed to deal with a specific problem evident in a particular situation. No attempt is made to separate a particular feature of the problem from its context in order to study it in isolation. Constant monitoring and evaluation are carried out, and the conclusions from the findings are applied immediately, and monitored further.

Action research depends mainly on observation and behavioural data. As a practical form of research, aimed at a specific problem and situation, and with little or no control over independent variables, it cannot fulfil the scientific requirement for generalizability. In this sense, despite its exploratory nature, it is the antithesis of experimental research.

Research design

Once the objectives of a research project have been established, the issue of how these objectives can be met leads to a consideration of which research design will be appropriate. Research design provides a framework for the collection and analysis of data and subsequently indicates which research methods are appropriate.

Fixed and flexible design strategies

Robson (2002, pp. 83–90) makes a useful distinction between fixed and flexible design strategies.

- **Fixed designs** call for a tight pre-specification at the outset, and are commonly equated with a quantitative approach. The designs employ experimental and non-experimental research methods.
- **Flexible designs** evolve during data collection and are associated with a qualitative approach, although some quantitative data may be collected. The designs employ, among other things, case study, ethnographic and grounded theory methods.

Short descriptions of the main designs follow, starting with fixed designs.

Cross-sectional design

Cross-sectional design often uses survey methods, and surveys are often equated with cross-sectional studies. However, this kind of study can use other methods of data collection, such as observation, content analysis and official records. Bryman (2004, p. 41) summarizes the characteristics of this kind of design in the following way:

- It entails the collection of data on more than one case (usually many more than one), generally using a sampling method to select cases in order to be representative of a population. Random methods of sampling lead to good external validity.

- The data is collected at a single point in time, that is, it provides a snapshot of ideas, opinions, information etc. Because the data collection methods tend to be intrusive, ecological validity may be put at risk. When the methods and procedures of data collection and analysis are specified in detail, replicability is enhanced.
- Quantitative or quantifiable data is sought in order that variations in the variables can be systematically gauged according to specific and reliable standards. The variables are non-manipulable, that is, the researcher cannot change their values in order to gauge the effects of the change.
- Patterns of association between variables are examined in order to detect associations. Causal influences might be inferred, but this form of design cannot match experiments in this respect due to weak internal validity.

Longitudinal design

Longitudinal design consists of repeated cross-sectional surveys to ascertain how time influences the results. Because this design can trace what happens over time, it may be possible to establish causation among variables if the cases remain the same in successive surveys. Because of the repeated nature of this research design, it tends to be expensive and time consuming, unless it relies on information that has already been collected as a matter of course within an organization (e.g. initial interview assessments and final exam results of students in different years at a university). Some large national surveys are based on longitudinal design, such as the British Household Panel Survey, National Child Development Study, Millennium Cohort Study.

Two types of study are commonly identified:

- **Panel studies** – these consist of a sample of people, often randomly selected, who are questioned on two or more occasions.
- **Cohort studies** – these concentrate on a group that shares similar characteristics, such as students from a particular year of matriculation or people on strike at a certain time.

Experimental

Experimental research differs from the other research approaches noted above through its greater control over the objects of its study. The researcher strives to isolate and control every relevant condition which determines the events investigated, so as to observe the effects when the conditions are manipulated. Chemical experiments in a laboratory represent one of the purest forms of this type of research. The most important characteristic of the experimental approach is that it deals with the phenomenon of 'cause and effect'.

> *At its simplest, an experiment involves making a change in the value of one variable – called the independent variable – and observing the effect of that change on another variable – called the dependent variable.*

However, the actual experiment is only a part of the research process. There are several planned stages in experimental research. When the researcher has established that the study is amenable to experimental methods, a prediction (technically called a hypothesis) of the likely cause-and-effect patterns of the phenomenon has to be made. This allows decisions to be made as to what variables are to be tested and how they are to be controlled and measured. This stage, called the design of the experiment, must also include the choice of relevant types of test and methods of analysing the results of the experiments (usually by statistical analysis). Pre-tests are then usually carried out to detect any problems in the experimental procedure.

Only after this is the experiment proper carried out. The procedures decided upon must be rigorously adhered to and the observations meticulously recorded and checked. Following the successful completion of the experiment, the important task – the whole point of the research exercise – is to process and analyse the data and to formulate an interpretation of the experimental findings.

> **Common pitfall:** Do not believe that all experimental research has to, or even can, take place in a laboratory. What experimental methods do stress is how much it is possible to control the variables, in whatever setting.

Writers of textbooks on research have classified experimental designs in different ways. Campbell and Stanley (1966) make their categorization into four classes:

1 Pre-experimental

2 True experimental

3 Quasi-experimental

4 Correlation and ex post facto

Pre-experimental designs are unreliable and primitive experimental methods in which assumptions are made despite the lack of essential control of variables. An example of this is the supposition that, faced with the same stimulus, all samples will behave identically to the one tested, despite possible differences between the samples.

True experimental designs are those which rigorously check the identical nature of the groups before testing the influence of a variable on a sample of them in controlled circumstances. Parallel tests are made on identical samples (control samples) which are not subjected to the variable.

In **quasi-experimental designs**, not all the conditions of true experimental design can be fulfilled. However,the nature of the shortcomings is recognized, and steps are taken to minimize them or predict a level of reliability of the results. The most common case is when a group is tested for the influence of a variable and compared with a non-identical group with known differences (control group) which has not been subjected to the variable. Another, in the absence of a control group, is repeated testing over time of one group, with and without the variable (i.e. the same group acts as its own control at different times).

Correlation design looks for cause-and-effect relationships between two sets of data, while **ex post facto designs** turn experimentation into reverse, and attempt to interpret the nature of the cause of a phenomenon by the observed effects. Both of these forms of research result in conclusions which are difficult to prove and they rely heavily on logic and inference.

Case study design

Sometimes you may want to study a social group, community, system, organization, institution, event, or even a person or type of personality. It can be convenient to pick one example or a small number of examples from this list to study them in detail within their own context, and make assessments and comparisons. These are called case studies.

Commonly, in **case study design**, no claim is made for generalizability. It is rather about the quality of theoretical analysis that is allowed by intensive investigation into one or a few cases, and how well theory can be generated and tested, using both inductive and deductive reasoning.

However, if the research is based on the argument that the case studies investigated are a sample of some or many such systems, organizations, etc., and what you can find out in the particular cases could be applicable to all of them, you need to make the same kind of sampling choice as described above in order to reassure yourself, and the reader, that the cases are representative.

If there are large variations between such systems/organizations, etc., it may not be possible to find 'average' or representative cases. What you can do is to take a comparative approach by selecting several very different ones, for example those showing extreme characteristics, those at each end of the spectrum and perhaps one that is somewhere in the middle and compare their characteristics. Alternatively, choose an 'exemplifying' or 'critical' case, one that will provide a good setting for answering the research question.

Both quantitative and qualitative methods are appropriate for case study designs, and multiple methods of data collection are often applied.

Case study design tends to be a flexible design, especially if the research is exploratory. Despite this, it is desirable to devise an explicit plan before starting the research, even in the expectation that aspects of the plan may change during the course of the project.

Taking it **FURTHER**

Ethnographic and grounded theory approaches

There are other theoretical approaches that are not really a research design in the sense of the above, but do present a specific way of working that greatly influences the research efforts of the researcher. The two that are commonly mentioned in relation to social science research are ethnographic approach and the grounded theory approach. Look in your course description and lecture notes to see if these are included in your course. If they are, then what follows is necessary reading. If not, some knowledge about these will stand you in good stead when answering exam questions or writing an essay or dissertation. They are probably too sophisticated for you to use as a research method if you have to do a research project.

RESEARCH STRATEGIES AND DESIGN | *47*

Ethnographic approach

This approach is based on the techniques devised by anthropologists to study social life and cultural practices of communities by immersing themselves in the day-to-day life of their subjects. Robson (2002, p. 188) describes **ethnography** as follows:

- The purpose is to uncover the shared cultural meanings of the behaviour, actions, events and contexts of a group or people.
- This requires an insider's perspective.
- The group must be observed and studied in its natural setting.
- No method of data collection is ruled out, although participant observation in the field is usually considered essential.
- The focus of the research and detailed research questions will emerge and evolve in the course of the involvement. Theoretical orientations and preliminary research questions are subject to revision.
- Data collection is usually in phases over an extended time. Frequent behaviours, events, etc. tend to be focused on to permit the development of an understanding of their significance.

This is a difficult design for beginners as it requires specialist knowledge of socio-cultural concepts, and also tends to take a very long time. Writing up succinctly is problematic due to the complexity of the observations and it is easy to lose one's independent view because of the close involvement in the group.

Ethnographic studies concentrate on depth rather than breadth of inquiry.

Grounded theory

Glaser and Strauss (1967) developed **grounded theory** as a reaction to the then current stress on the need to base social research on pre-defined theory. Grounded theory takes the opposite approach – it does the research in order to evolve the theory. This gives rise to a specific style of procedure and use of research methods.

The main emphasis is on continuous data collection process interlaced with periodic pauses for analysis. The analysis is used to tease out categories in the data on which the subsequent data collection can be based. This process is called 'coding'. This reciprocal procedure continues until these categories are 'saturated', that is, the new data no longer provides new evidence. From these results, concepts and theoretical frameworks can be developed. This gradual emergence and refinement of theory based on observations is the basis for the 'grounded' label of this approach.

Although mostly associated with qualitative approaches, there is no reason why quantitative data is not relevant. A grounded theory design is particularly suitable for researching unfamiliar situations where there has been little previous research on which to base theory.

Because of its flexible design, grounded theory is not an easy option for novice researchers, despite a wide range of examples of this kind of research in many different settings.

Questions to ponder

❝ What are the distinctions between quantitative and qualitative research. How do these relate to epistemological and ontological considerations? ❞

Quantitative research tends to measure, qualitative research tends to describe. You can go into more detail than this by describing how. The nature of data is defined by different epistemological viewpoints and what you can do with it is defined by ontological considerations. You can go on to explain how. These raise the issue of the appropriateness of quantitative or qualitative approaches, and the type of information that can usefully be gained by the methods associated with each approach.

❝ Describe four possible objectives of research, and describe each using a simple example. ❞

Here are three examples:

To explain – e.g. the motives of disruptive teenagers on a housing estate. This may help to find a solution to vandalism in a particular area.

To predict – e.g. how different options in the introduction of a new claim scheme for pensioners will affect take-up.

To compare – e.g. how different climates tend to affect people's leisure activities.

You could be more expansive in describing the examples by elaborating on what you might do to reach the objectives.

❝You want to investigate the important factors that should be taken into account when designing a children's play area. What factors could you explore by using different research designs? Outline how you would do it?❞

First think of a range of possible factors that could influence the design of a play area. Do this by looking at technical issues (e.g. design of play equipment, maintenance), community issues (e.g. surrounding housing, siting, access, surveillance, meeting place), age-related issues (e.g. supervision, different areas and facilities for different ages), play and movement questions (e.g. what is 'play', exercise, safety), family matters (e.g. who would come, parent's requirements and activities, older children, picnics and refreshment).

Then take some or all of the issues and select a research design that would be used to investigate it. For example, you could do experiments to test the strength of the equipment, do a case study on play activities in an existing play area, do a cross-sectional study of parents' and children's wishes, etc.

References to more information

All standard textbooks on social science research methods will have a section on research design. I found the following books to be particularly useful. Look in the contents and index to track down the relevant sections. There is usually a summary of designs near the beginning of the book, and greater detail about each one later.

Bryman, A. (2004) *Social Research Methods* (2nd edn). Oxford: Oxford University Press.
See Chapter 2.

Bernard, H.R. (2000) *Social Research Methods: Qualitative and Quantitative Approaches*. Thousand Oaks, CA: Sage.
No short summary here. You will have to look up each design.

Seale, C. (ed.) (2004) *Researching Society and Culture* (2nd edn). London: Sage.
See Chapter 11.

Robson, C. (2002) *Real World Research: A Resource for Social Scientists and Practitioner-Researchers* (2nd edn). Oxford: Blackwell.
See Part II, Chapters 4–7 for great detail.

5	
the nature of data	

Data means information or, according to the *Oxford English Dictionary*, 'known facts or things used as basis for inference or reckoning'. Strictly speaking, data is the plural of datum, so is always treated as plural. When you do any sort of inquiry or research, you will collect data of different kinds. In fact, data can be seen as the essential raw material of any kind of research. They are the means by which we can understand events and conditions in the world around us.

Data, when seen as facts, acquire an air of solidity and permanence, representing the truth. This is, unfortunately, misleading. Data are not only elusive, but also ephemeral. They may be a true representation of a situation in one place, at a particular time, under specific circumstances, as seen by a particular observer. The next day, all might be different. For example, a daily survey of people's voting intentions in a forthcoming general election will produce different results daily, even if exactly the same people are asked, because some change their minds because of what they have heard or seen in the interim period. If the same number of people are asked in a similar sample, a different result can also be expected. Anyway, how can you tell whether they are even telling the truth about their intentions? Data can therefore only provide a fleeting and partial glimpse of events, opinions, beliefs or conditions.

Data are not only ephemeral, but also corruptible. Inappropriate claims are often made on the basis of data that are not sufficient or close enough to the event. Hearsay is stated to be fact, second-hand reports are regarded as being totally reliable, and biased views are seized on as evidence. The further away you get from the event the more likely it is that inconsistencies and inaccuracies creep in. Memory fades, details are lost, recording methods do not allow a full picture to be given, and distortions of interpretations occur.

> *It is a rash researcher who insists on the infallibility of his/her data, and of the findings derived from them.*

A measure of humility in the belief of the accuracy of knowledge, and also practical considerations which surround the research process, dictate that the outcomes of research tend to be couched in 'soft' statements, such as 'it seems that', 'it is likely that', 'one is led to believe that', etc. This does not mean, however, that progress towards useful 'truths' cannot be achieved.

Primary and secondary data

It is important to be able to distinguish between different kinds of data because their nature has important implications for their reliability and for the sort of analysis to which they can be subjected. Data that have been observed, experienced or recorded close to the event are the nearest one can get to the truth, and are called **primary data**. Written sources that interpret or record primary data are called **secondary data**. For example, you have a more approximate and less complete knowledge of a political demonstration if you read the newspaper report the following day than if you were at the demonstration and had seen it yourself. Not only is the information less abundant, but it is coloured by the commentator's interpretation of the facts.

Primary data

Primary data are present all around us. Our senses deal with them all our waking lives – sounds, visual stimuli, tastes, tactile stimuli, etc. Instruments also help us to keep a track of factors that we cannot so accurately judge through our senses – thermometers record the exact temperature, clocks tell us the exact time, and our bank statements tell us how much money we have. Primary data is as near to the truth that we can get about things and events. Seeing a football match with your own eyes will certainly get you nearer to what happened than reading a newspaper report about it later. Even so, the truth is still somewhat elusive – 'was the referee really right to award that penalty? It didn't look like a handball to me!'

There are many ways of collecting and recording primary data. Some are more reliable than others. It can be argued that as soon as data are recorded, they become secondary data due to the fact that someone or something had to observe and interpret the situation or event and set it down in a form of a record, that is the data have become second hand. But this is not the case. The primary data are not the actual situation or event, but a record of it, from as close to it as possible – that is, the first and most immediate recording. 'A researcher assumes a personal responsibility for the reliability and authenticity of his or her information and must be prepared to answer for it' (Preece, 1994, p. 80). Without this kind of recorded data it would be difficult to make sense of anything but the simplest phenomenon and be able to communicate the facts to others.

There are four basic types of primary data:

1 **Observation** – records, usually of events, situations or things, of what you have experienced with your own senses, perhaps with the help of an instrument (e.g. camera, tape recorder, microscope, etc.).

2 **Participation** – data gained by experiences that can perhaps be seen as an intensified form of observations (e.g. the experience of learning to drive a car tells you different things about cars and traffic than just watching).

3 **Measurement** – records of amounts or numbers (e.g. population statistics, instrumental measurements of distance, temperature, mass etc.).

4 **Interrogation** – data gained by asking and probing (e.g. information about people's beliefs, motivations, etc.).

These can be collected, singly or together, to provide information about virtually any facet of our life and surroundings. So, why do we not rely on primary data for all our research? After all, it gets as close as possible to the truth. There are several reasons, the main ones being time, cost and access. Collecting primary data is a time-consuming business. As more data usually means more reliability, the efforts of just one person will be of limited value. Organizing a huge survey undertaken by large teams would overcome this limitation, but at what cost?

> *It is not always possible to get direct access to the subject of research. For example, many historical events have left no direct evidence.*

Secondary data

Secondary data is data that has been interpreted and recorded. We could drown under the flood of secondary data that assails us every day. News broadcasts, magazines, newspapers, documentaries, advertising, the Internet, etc. all bombard us with information wrapped, packed and spun into digestible soundbites or pithy articles. We are so used to this that we have learned to swim, to float above it all and only really pay attention to the bits that interest us. This technique, learned through sheer necessity and quite automatically put into practice every day, is a useful skill that can be applied to speed up your data collection for your research.

Books, journal papers, magazine articles and newspapers present information in published, written form. The quality of the data depends on the source and the methods of presentation. For detailed and authoritative information on almost any subject, go to refereed journals – all the papers will have been vetted by leading experts in the subject. Other serious journals, such as some professional and trade journals, will also have authoritative articles by leading figures, despite the tendency of some to emphasize one side of the issue. For example, a steel federation journal will support arguments for the use of steel rather than other building materials. There are magazines for every taste, some entirely flippant, others with useful and reliable information. The same goes for books – millions of them! They range from the most erudite and deeply researched volumes, such as specialist encyclopaedia and academic tomes, to ranting polemics and commercial pap.

It is therefore always important to make an assessment of the quality of the information or opinions provided. You actually do this all the time without even noticing it. We have all learned not to be so gullible as to believe everything that we read. A more conscious approach entails reviewing the evidence that has been presented in the arguments. When no evidence is provided, on what authority does the writer base his/her statements? It is best to find out who are the leading exponents of the subject you are studying.

Television broadcasts, films, radio programmes, recordings of all sorts provide information in an audio-visual non-written form. The assertion that the camera cannot lie is now totally discredited, so the same precautions need to be taken in assessing the quality of the data presented. There is a tendency, especially in programmes aimed at a wide public, to oversimplify issues.

Common pitfall: The powerful nature of films and television can easily seduce one into a less critical mood. Emotions can be aroused that cloud one's better judgement. Repeated viewings help to counter this.

The Internet and CD-ROMs combine written and audio-visual techniques to impart information.

You cannot always be present at an event, but other people might have experienced it. Their accounts may be the nearest you can get to an event. Getting information from several witnesses will help to pin down the actual facts of the event.

> It is good practice, and is especially necessary with secondary data, to compare the data from different sources. This will help to identify bias, inaccuracies and pure imagination. It will also show up different interpretations that have been made of the event or phenomenon.

Quantitative and qualitative data and levels of measurement

The other main categories applied to data refer not to their source but to their nature. Can the data be reduced to numbers or can they be presented only in words? It is important to make a distinction between these two types of data because it affects the way that they are collected, recorded and analysed. Numbers can provide a very useful way of compressing large amounts of data, but if used inappropriately, lead to spurious results.

Much information about science and society is recorded in the form of numbers (e.g. temperatures, bending forces, population densities, cost indices, etc.). The nature of numbers allows them to be manipulated by the techniques of statistical analysis. This type of data is called **quantitative data**. In contrast, there is a lot of useful information that cannot be reduced to numbers. People's opinions, feelings, ideas and traditions need to be described in words. Words cannot be reduced to averages, maximum and minimum values or percentages. They record not quantities, but qualities. Hence they are called **qualitative data**. Given their distinct characteristics, it is evident that when it comes to analysing these two forms of data, quite different techniques are required.

Quantitative data

Quantitative data have features that can be measured, more or less exactly. Measurement implies some form of magnitude, usually expressed in numbers. As soon as you can deal with numbers, then you can apply mathematical procedures to analyse the data. These might be extremely simple, such as counts or percentages, or more sophisticated, such as statistical tests or mathematical models.

Some forms of quantitative data are obviously based on numbers: population counts, economic data, scientific measurements, to mention just a few. There are, however, other types of data that initially seem remote from quantitative measures but that can be converted to numbers. For example, people's opinions about fox hunting might be difficult to quantify, but if, in a questionnaire, you give a set choice of answers to the questions on this subject, then you can count the various responses and the data can then be treated as quantitative.

Typical examples of quantitative data are census figures (population, income, living density, etc.), economic data (share prices, gross national product, tax regimes, etc.), performance data (e.g. sport statistics, medical measurements, engineering calculations, etc.) and all measurements in scientific endeavour.

Qualitative data

Qualitative data cannot be accurately measured and counted, and are generally expressed in words rather than numbers. The study of human beings and their societies and cultures requires many observations to be made that are to do with identifying, understanding and interpreting ideas, customs, mores, beliefs and other essentially human activities and attributes. These cannot be pinned down and measured in any exact way. These kinds of data are therefore descriptive in character, and rarely go beyond the nominal and ordinal levels of measurement. This does not mean that they are any less valuable than quantitative data; in fact their richness and subtlety lead to great insights into human society.

Words, and the relationships between them, are far less precise than numbers. This makes qualitative research more dependent on careful definition of the meaning of words, the development of concepts and the plotting of interrelationships between variables. Concepts such as poverty, comfort, friendship, etc., while elusive to measure, are nonetheless real and detectable.

Typical examples of qualitative data are literary texts, minutes of meetings, observation notes, interview transcripts, documentary films, historical records, memos and recollections, etc. Some of these are records taken very close to the events or phenomena whereas others may be remote and highly edited interpretations. As with any data, judgements must be made about their reliability. Qualitative data, because they cannot be dispassionately measured in a standard way, are more susceptible to varied interpretations and valuation. In some cases even, it is more interesting to see what has been omitted from a report than what has been included.

You can best check the reliability and completeness of qualitative data about an event by obtaining a variety of sources of data relating to the same event. This is called triangulation.

The distinction between qualitative and quantitative data is one of a continuum between extremes. You do not have to choose to collect only one or the other. In fact, there are many types of data that can be seen from both perspectives. For example, a questionnaire exploring people's political attitudes may provide a rich source of qualitative data about their aspirations and beliefs, but might also provide useful quantitative data about levels of support for different political parties. What is important is that you are aware of the types of data that you are dealing with, either during collection or analysis, and that you use the appropriate levels of measurement.

Measurement of data

There are different ways of measuring data, depending on the nature of the data. These are commonly referred to as **levels of measurement – nominal, ordinal, interval** and **ratio**.

Nominal level

The word 'nominal' is derived from the Latin word *nomen*, meaning 'name'. Nominal measurement is very basic and unrefined. Its simple function is to divide the data into separate categories that can then be compared with each other. By first giving names to or labelling the parts or states of a concept, or by naming discrete units of data, we are then able to measure the concept or data at the simplest level. For example, many theoretical concepts are conceived on a nominal **level of quantification**. 'Status structure', as a theoretical concept, may have only two states: either a group of individuals have one or they do not (such as a collection of people waiting for a bus). Buildings may be classified into many types, for example commercial, industrial, educational, religious, etc. Many **operational definitions** are on a nominal level, for example sex (male or female), marital status (single, married, separated, divorced or widowed). This applies in the same way for some types of data, for example dividing a group of children into boys and girls, or into fair-haired, brown-haired or black-haired children, and so on.

> *In effect, different states of a concept or different categories of data which are quantified at a nominal level can only be labelled, and it is not possible to make statements about the differences between the states or categories, except to say that they are recognized as being different.*

We can represent nominal data by certain graphic and statistical devices. Bar graphs, for example, can be appropriately used to represent the comparative measurement of nominal data. By measuring this type of data, using statistical techniques, it is possible to locate the mode, find a percentage relationship of one sub-group to another or of one sub-group to the total group, and compute the chi-square. We will discuss the mode and chi-square (in Chapter 10); they are mentioned here merely to indicate that nominal data may be processed statistically.

Ordinal level

If a concept is considered to have a number of states, or the data have a number of values that can be rank-ordered, it is assumed that some meaning is conveyed by the relative order of the states. The ordinal level of measurement implies that an entity being measured is quantified in terms of being more than or less than, or of a greater or lesser order than. It is a comparative entity and is often expressed by the symbols < or >.

For anyone studying at school or at university, the most familiar ordinal measures are the grades which are used to rate academic performance. An A always means more than a B, and a B always means more than a C, but the difference between A and B may not always be the same as the difference between B and C in terms of academic achievement. Similarly, we measure level of education grossly on an ordinal scale by saying individuals are unschooled, or have an elementary school, a secondary school, a college or a university education. Likewise, we measure members of the workforce on an ordinal scale by calling them unskilled, semi-skilled or skilled.

> *Most of the theoretical concepts in the social sciences seem to be at an ordinal level of measurement.*

In summary, 'ordinal level of measurement' applies to concepts that vary in such a way that different states of the concept can be rank-ordered with respect to some characteristic. The ordinal scale of measurement expands the range of statistical techniques that can be applied to data. Using the ordinal scale, we can find the mode and the median, determine the percentage or percentile rank, and test by the chi-square. We can also indicate relationships by means of rank correlation.

Interval level

The interval level of measurement has two essential characteristics: it has equal units of measurement and its zero point, if present, is arbitrary. Temperature scales are one of the most familiar types of interval scale. In each of the Fahrenheit and Celsius scales, the gradation between each degree is equal to all the others, and the zero point has been established arbitrarily. The Fahrenheit scale clearly shows how arbitrary is the setting of the zero point. At first, the zero point was taken by Gabriel Fahrenheit to be the coldest temperature observed in Iceland. Later he made the lowest temperature obtainable with a mixture of salt and ice, and took this to be 0 degrees. Among the measurements of the whole range of possible temperatures, taking this point was evidently a purely arbitrary decision. It placed the freezing point of water at 32 degrees, and the boiling point at 212 degrees above zero.

> *Although equal-interval theoretical concepts like temperature abound in the physical sciences, they are harder to find in the social sciences.*

Though abstract concepts are rarely inherently interval-based, operational measures employed to quantify them often use quantification at an interval level. For example, attitudes are frequently measured on a scale like this:

Unfavourable −4 −3 −2 −1 0 +1 +2 +3 +4 Favourable

If it is assumed that the difference between +2 and +4 is the same as the difference between say 0 and −2, then this can be seen as an attempt to apply an interval level of quantification to this measurement procedure. This is quite a big assumption to make! The tendency for some social scientists to assume the affirmative is probably because some of the most useful summary measures and statistical tests require quantification on an interval level (e.g. for determining the mode, mean, standard deviation, t-test, F-test and product moment correlation).

> ***Common pitfall:*** Doubts are frequently raised about the precision of responses to questionnaires. Are the meanings intended by the researcher's questions equivalent to those understood by the respondent? Is the formulaic choice of answers given compatible with what the respondent wishes to reply?

I am sure you remember your reaction to attitude quizzes, where the answer 'it all depends' seems more appropriate to a question than any of the multiple choice answers offered.

Ratio level

The ratio level of measurement has a true zero, that is, the point where the measurement is truly equal to nought – the total absence of the quantity being measured. We are all familiar with concepts in physical science which are both theoretically and operationally conceptualized at a ratio level of measurement. Time, distance, velocity (a combination of time and distance), mass and weight are all concepts that have a zero state in an interval scale, both theoretically and operationally. So, there is no ambiguity in the statements 'twice as far', 'twice as fast' and 'twice as heavy'. Compared with this, other statements which use this level of measurement inappropriately are meaningless (e.g. 'twice as clever', 'twice as prejudiced' or 'twice the prestige'), since there is no way of knowing where zero clever, zero prejudice or zero prestige are.

A characteristic difference between the ratio scale and all other scales is that the ratio scale can express values in terms of multiples of fractional parts, and the ratios are true ratios. A metre rule can do that: a metre is a multiple (by 100) of a centimetre distance, a millimetre is a tenth (a fractional part) of a centimetre. The ratios are 1:100 and 1:10. Of all levels of measurement, the ratio scale is amenable to the greatest range of statistical tests. It can be used for determining the geometric mean, the harmonic mean, the percentage variation and all other statistical determinations.

In summary, one can encapsulate this discussion in the following simple test for various kinds of concept and data measurement:

If you can say that

- one object is different from another, you have a **nominal** scale;
- one object is bigger, better or more of anything than another, you have an **ordinal** scale;
- one object is so many units (degrees, inches) more than another, you have an **interval** scale;
- one object is so many times as big or bright or tall or heavy as another, you have a **ratio** scale.

How data relates to theory

There is a hierarchy of expressions, going from the general to the particular, from abstract to concrete, that makes it possible to investigate research problems couched in theoretical language. The briefest statement of the research problem will be the most general and abstract, while the detailed analysis of components of the research will be particular and concrete.

- **Theory** – the abstract statements that make claims about the world and how it works. Research problems are usually stated at a theoretical level.
- **Concepts** – the building blocks of the theory which are usually abstract and cannot be directly measured.
- **Indicators** – the phenomena which point to the existence of the concepts.
- **Variables** – the components of the indicators which can be measured.
- **Values** – the actual units or methods of measurement of the variables. These are data in their most concrete form.

Note that each theory may have several concepts, each concept several indicators, each indicator several variables, and each variable several values. To clarify these terms, consider this example, which gives only one example of each expression:

Theory – poverty leads to poor health

Concept – poverty

Indicator – poor living conditions

Variable – provision of sanitary facilities

Value – numbers of people per WC

Being aware of levels of expression will help you to break down your investigations into manageable tasks. It will enable you to come to overall conclusions about the abstract concepts in your research problem based on evidence rooted in detailed data at a more concrete level.

Theory

Although the word 'theory' is rather imprecise in its meaning, in research it refers to a statement that expresses what is going on in the situation, phenomenon or whatever is being researched. Theories can range from complex large-scale systems developed in academic research, to informal guesses or hunches about specific situations. In research it is common to refer to existing theories, either to challenge them or to develop them by refining them or applying them to new situations. Novel theories are only developed successfully after much research and testing. A theory is expressed in theoretical statements, for example 'taking examinations leads to stress'.

Research activities can be divided into two categories:

1 Those that verify theory.

2 Those that generate theory.

In both cases it is necessary to break down the theoretical statements in such a way as to make them researchable and testable. As mentioned above, several steps are required to achieve this.

Concepts

A concept is a general expression of a particular phenomenon (e.g. cat, human, anger, speed, alienation, socialism, etc.). Each one of these represents an idea, and the word is a label for this idea.

We use concepts all the time as they are an essential part of understanding the world and communicating with other people. Many common concepts are shared by everyone in a society, although there are variations in meaning between different cultures and languages. For example, the concept 'respect' will mean something different to a streetwise rapper than to a noble lord. There are other concepts that are only understood by certain people, such as experts, professionals and specialists, for example dermatoglyphics, milfoil, parachronism, anticipatory socialization, etc.

> **Common pitfalls:** Sometimes, concepts can be labelled in an exotic fashion, often in order to impress or confuse, for example, a 'domestic feline mammal' instead of a 'cat'. This is called jargon, and should be avoided.

It is important to define concepts in such a way that everyone reading the work has got the same idea of what is meant. This is relatively easy in the natural sciences where precise definition is usually possible (e.g. acceleration, radio waves, elements). In the social sciences this may be much more difficult. Human concepts such as fidelity, dishonesty, enthusiasm, and even more technical concepts such as affluence, vagrancy and dominance, are difficult to pin down accurately, as their meanings are often based on opinions, emotions, values, traditions, etc.

> *It is essential to carefully formulate definitions when using concepts that are not precise in normal usage. You will be able to find definitions of the concepts that you are planning to use in your investigations from your background reading.*

Because definitions for non-scientific and non-technical concepts can vary in different contexts, you may have to decide on which meaning you want to give to those concepts. Rarely, you might even have to devise your own definition for a particular word.

Indicators

Many concepts are rather abstract in nature, and difficult or even impossible to evaluate or measure. Take 'anger' as an example. How will you detect anger in a person? The answer is to look for indicators – those perceivable phenomena that give an indication that the concept is present. What, in this case might these be? Think of the signs that might indicate anger – clenched fists, agitated demeanour, spluttering, shouting, wide-open eyes, stamping, reddened face, increased heart-beat, increased adrenaline production, and many others. Again, you can see what indicators were used in previous studies – this is much easier and more reliable than trying to work them out for yourself. For more technical subjects, indicators are usually well defined and universally accepted, for example changes of state like condensation, freezing, magnetism.

Variables

If you want to gauge the extent or degree of an indicator, you will need to find a measurable component. In the case of anger above, it would be very difficult to measure the redness of a face or the degree of stamping, but you could easily measure a person's heartbeat. You could even ask the subject how angry he/she feels.

In the natural sciences, the identification of variables is usually more simple. Temperature, density, speed and velocity are examples. Some of these may be appropriate to social science, particularly in quantitative studies, for example number of people in crowds, frequency and type of activities, etc.

Values

The values used are the units of measurement. In the case of heartbeat, it would be beats per minute, and the level of anger felt could be declared on a scale 1–10. Obviously the precision that is possible will be different depending on the nature of the variable and the type of values that can be used. Certain scientific experiments require incredibly accurate measurement, while some social phenomena (e.g. opinions) might only be gauged on a three-point scale such as 'agree', 'neutral', 'disagree'.

Questions to ponder

❝ What are the essential differences between primary and secondary data, and how does this relate to where and how you would find them? ❞

Primary data is first-hand data, observed or collected directly from the field. Secondary data is interpreted primary data. You can elaborate on this by giving examples. There is plenty of scope to describe where and how you would find the different types of data, for example by doing experiments, surveys, etc. for primary data, and archive searches, official statistics, etc. for secondary data. Keep making the distinction between the immediacy of primary data and the second-hand nature of secondary data.

❝ Can all data be measured in the same way? If not, describe the different ways. Can both quantitative and qualitative data be measured in all these ways? If not, explain why not and what consequences this has. ❞

This obviously relates to the levels of measurement (nominal, ordinal, etc.) which you can describe and give examples of. The main point to be made is that qualitative data is limited in how it can be measured (i.e. only nominal and ordinal levels of measurement), which limits the types of statistical test that can be carried out on them.

❝ Describe how values relate to theoretical statements. ❞

They are at the opposite ends of the scale of abstraction. Values are the most concrete notions (e.g. metres, seconds, etc.). You will have to explain the sequence of values, indicators, concepts and theoretical statements, and how they relate in **levels of abstraction**. Give examples to make your points clear (e.g. using the example of the theory given above, 'taking exams leads to stress', one concept is 'stress') An indicator of stress might be 'raised heartbeat', for which a value could be 'beats per minute'. You can then point out the relationship between the values and the theory.

Taking it *FURTHER*

More about theory

Theory underlies all of our understanding of the world. Animals cannot theorize, which sets them apart from humans. From an early age we use observations of the world around us to make sense of what we experience and to predict what will happen and what the results of our actions might be. Scientific research is all about theories and their ability to explain phenomena and reveal the 'truth'.
   Consider the following list of criteria for judging the quality of theory:

1. A theoretical system must permit deductions that can be tested empirically; that is, it must provide the means for its confirmation or rejection. One can test the validity of a theory only through the validity of the propositions (hypotheses) that can be derived from it. If repeated attempts to disconfirm its various hypotheses fail, then greater confidence can be placed in its validity. This can go on indefinitely, until possibly some hypothesis proves untenable. This would constitute indirect evidence of the inadequacy of the theory and could lead to its rejection (or, more commonly, to its replacement by a more adequate theory that can incorporate the exception).
2. Theory must be compatible with both the observation and previously validated theories. It must be grounded in empirical data that have been verified and must rest on sound postulates and hypotheses. The better the theory, the more adequately it can explain the phenomenon under consideration, and the more fact it can incorporate into a meaningful structure of ever-greater generalizibility.
3. Theories must be stated in simple terms; that is, theory is best that explains the most in the simplest way. This is the law of parsimony. A theory must explain the data adequately and yet must not be so comprehensive as to be unwieldy. On the other hand, it must not overlook the variables simply because they are difficult to explain. (Mouly, quoted in Cohen and Manion, 1994, pp. 15–16)

This sounds all very well for the natural sciences, but some of these conditions cannot be achieved in the social sciences. In point 2, it may be impossible to ground the theory on empirical data that have been verified in the sense of measurement and repeated observations. Following this, it may be difficult therefore to test objectively the validity of its various hypotheses as demanded in point 1.

What is important to stress, though, is the relationship between developing theory and previously validated theory, as mentioned in point 2. The theoretical background to one's inquiries will determine how one looks at the world. As Quine (1969) argued, our experience of the world of facts does not impose any single theory on us. Theories are underdetermined by facts, and our factual knowledge of the external world is capable of supporting many different interpretations of it. The answer to the question 'what exists?' can only receive the answer 'what exists is what theory posits'. Since there are different theories, these will posit different things. There will always be more than one logically equivalent theory consistent with the evidence we have. This is not because the evidence may be insufficient, but because the same facts can be accommodated in different ways by alterations in the configuration of the theory (Hughes and Sharrock, 1997, pp. 88–91).

One philosopher of science expressed it this way: 'it is generally agreed … that the idea of a descriptive vocabulary which is applicable to observations, but which is entirely innocent of theoretical influences, is unrealizable' (Harré, 1972, p. 25). Therefore, one can argue that phenomena cannot be understood, and research cannot be carried out, without a theoretical underpinning:

> Models, concepts and theories are self-confirming in the sense that they instruct us to look at phenomena in particular ways. This means that they can never be disproved but only found to be more or less useful. (Silverman, 1998, p. 103).

It follows, then, that all theories must, by their very nature, be provisional. However sophisticated and elegant a theory is, it cannot be all-encompassing or final. The fact that it is a theory, an abstraction from real life, means that it must always be subject to possible change or development and, in extreme cases, even replacement.

References to more information

What counts as data, and what to do with it, is a big subject in research and gets dealt with exhaustively in most books about academic writing, which can be overwhelming at this stage of your studies.

Below are some useful other ways of looking at this aspect, without getting too deeply into technicalities. If you have other books about research to hand, check the index to see what they have to say about data.

Seale, C. (ed.) (2004) *Researching Society and Culture* (2nd edn). London: Sage. A well-explained section on theories, models and hypotheses appears in Chapter 5.

Preece, Roy (1994) *Starting Research: An Introduction to Academic Research and Dissertation Writing*. London: Pinter.
The first part of Chapter 4 extends some of the issues discussed above.

Leedy, Paul D. (1989 and later editions) *Practical Research: Planning and Design*. London: Collies Macmillan.
Chapter 5/II provides a rather nice philosophical approach to the nature of data.

Blaxter, L., Hughes, C. and Tight, M. (1996) *How to Research*. Buckingham: Open University Press.
The first part of Chapter 10 provides another angle on data and its forms.

6	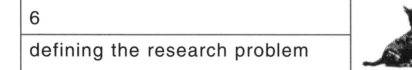
defining the research problem	

In all research projects, on whatever subject, there is a need to define and delineate the **research problem** clearly. The research problem is a general statement of an issue meriting research. Its nature will suggest appropriate forms for its investigation. Here are several forms in which the research problem can be expressed to indicate the method of investigation.

The research problem in some social science research projects using the **hypothetico-deductive method** is expressed in terms of the testing of a particular **hypothesis**. It is therefore important to know what makes good hypotheses and how they can be formulated. However, it is not appropriate to use the hypothetico-deductive method, or even scientific method, in every research study. Much research into society, design, history, philosophy and many other subjects cannot provide the full criteria for the formulation of hypotheses and their testing, and it is inappropriate to try to fit such research into this method. What are the alternative ways of stating the research problem in a researchable form?

Hypotheses and their formulation

Hypotheses are nothing unusual; we make them all the time. They are hunches or reasonable guesses made in the form of statements about a cause or situation, referred to as **causal statements**. If something happens in our everyday life, we tend to suggest a reason for its occurrence by making rational guesses. When a particular hypothesis is found to be supported, we have a good chance of taking the right action to remedy the situation. Many of the greatest discoveries in science were based on hypotheses: Newton's theory of gravity, Einstein's general theory of relativity and a host of others.

You will encounter hypotheses in your background reading, sometimes overt and clearly stated, and at other times, in less scholarly documents, hidden in the text or only hinted at. If you use one in your own research study, a hypothesis should arise naturally from the research problem, and should appear to the reader to be reasonable and sound.

There are two grounds on which a hypothesis may be justified: logical and empirical. Logical justification is developed from arguments based on concepts and theories and premises relating directly to the research problem; empirical justification is based on reference to other research found in the literature.

There are important qualities of hypotheses which distinguish them from other forms of statement. According to Kerlinger (1970), hypotheses are:

- assertions (not suggestions)
- limited in scope
- statements about the relationships between certain variables
- clear in their implications for testing the relationships
- compatible with current knowledge
- expressed as economically as possible using correct terminology

A good hypothesis is a very useful aid to organizing the research effort. It specifically limits the inquiry to the interaction of certain variables; it suggests the methods appropriate for collecting, analysing and interpreting the data; and the resultant confirmation or rejection of the hypothesis through empirical or experimental testing gives a clear indication of the extent of knowledge gained.

While a hypothesis, as described above, is tested in order to provide evidence to support, or to reject, the existence of the stated relationships between the variables, another type of hypothesis, called a **null hypothesis**, starts with an assumption that the relationships do not exist, and maintains that the assumptions are correct if they are not refuted by the results of the tests. Note that null hypotheses always take the form of statistical predictions.

It is often appropriate to balance an alternative hypothesis against a null hypothesis. If the null hypothesis is rejected, then the logical alternative is the alternative hypothesis. The alternative hypothesis is not specific and is not directly tested. An example will illustrate this:

Null hypothesis: People with more than the national average annual personal income do not have more than the national average annual personal spending.

Alternative hypothesis: People with more than the national average annual personal income have more than the national average personal spending.

Formulating hypotheses

Hypotheses can be very varied in nature, ranging from concrete to abstract and from narrow to wide in scope, range and inclusiveness. In order to formulate a useful researchable hypothesis, one needs to have a thorough knowledge of the background to the subject and the nature of the problem or issue which is being addressed. The hypothesis is developed from the result of a successive division and delineation of the problem, and provides a focus around which the research will be carried out.

Researchers work on two levels of reality, the operational level and the conceptual level. On the operational level, they work with events in observable terms, involving the reality necessary to carry out the research. On a conceptual level, events are defined in terms of underlying communality with other events on a more abstract level. Researchers move from single specific instances to general ones and thereby gain an understanding of how phenomena operate and variables interrelate, and vice versa to test whether the conceptual generalizations can be supported in fact.

The formulation of the hypothesis is usually made on a conceptual level, in order to enable the results of the research to be generalized beyond the specific conditions of the particular study. This widens the applicability of the research.

Operationalizing hypotheses

It is one of the fundamental criteria of a hypothesis that it is testable. However, a hypothesis formulated on a conceptual level cannot be directly tested; it is too abstract. It is therefore necessary to convert it to an operational level. This is called **operationalization**. It consists of reversing the conceptionalization process described above.

Often, the first step is to break down the main hypothesis into two or more sub-hypotheses. These represent components or aspects of the main hypothesis and together should add up to its totality. Each sub-hypothesis will intimate a different method of testing and therefore implies different research methods that might be appropriate.

The operationalization of the sub-hypotheses follows four steps in the progression from the most abstract to the most concrete expressions by defining concepts, indicators, variables and values, as described in Chapter 5.

> *Although the term 'hypothesis' is used with many different meanings in everyday and even academic situations, it is advisable to use it in your research only in its strictest scientific sense. This will avoid you being criticized of sloppy, imprecise use of terminology.*

Alternatives to hypotheses

Question or questions

The method of investigating the problem may be expressed through asking a question or a series of questions, the answers to which require scrutiny of the problem from one or more directions. Here is an example:

Four broad, interrelated research questions are raised about the representation of contemporary art in the media and the agenda for public debate which this implies. These questions are:

• What are the characteristics of the overall representation of contemporary art issues in the media?

• What agenda for contemporary art does this imply, and how does this relate to broad values of contemporary art and media?

- How does this representation differ in coverage presented in different types of media (e.g. television)?

- What role is played by specialist journalists, and specifically art correspondents, in shaping this representation?

Obviously, the question or questions should be derived directly from the research problem, and give a clear indication of the subject to be investigated and imply the methods which will be used. Often the form of the questions can be similar to that of hypotheses: a main question is divided into sub-questions which explore aspects of the main question.

Propositions

Focusing a research study on a **proposition** (a theoretical statement that indicates the clear direction and scope of a research project), rather than on a hypothesis, allows the study to concentrate on particular relationships between events, without having to comply with the rigorous characteristics required of hypotheses. Consider this example:

The main research problem was formulated in the form of three interrelated propositions:

- Specifically designed public sector housing provided for young single people to rent has been, and continues to be, designed according to the recommendations and standards in the design guidance for young persons' housing.

- The relevant design guidance is not based on accurate perceptions of the characteristics of young single people.

- From these two propositions the third one should follow: there is a mismatch between the specifically designed public sector housing provided for single young people and their accommodation requirements.

Statement of intent to investigate and evaluate critically

Not all research needs to answer a question or to test a hypothesis. Especially at masters degree level or in smaller studies, a more exploratory approach may be used. The subject and scope of the exploration can be expressed in a statement of intent. Again, this must be derived from the research problem, imply a method of approach and indicate the outcome. An example of this form of research definition is:

This study examines the problems in career development of women lawyers in the British legal establishment. It focuses on the identification of specific barriers (established conventions, prejudices, procedures, career paths) and explores the effectiveness of specific initiatives that have been aimed at breaking down these barriers.

Definition of research objectives

When a research problem has been identified, in order to indicate what measures will be taken to investigate the problem or provide means of overcoming it, it is necessary to formulate a definition of the research objectives. This should be accompanied by some indication of how the research objectives will be achieved.

The following example indicates how it is proposed to provide an adequate assessment of the relationship between the design of security systems in public buildings and the resulting restrictions to the accessibility of these buildings to the general public. The research problem previously highlighted a lack of such methods of assessment.

To overcome this problem it is necessary to:

- Propose a method of measurement by which the extent of incorporation of security systems can be assessed. This will enable an objective comparison to be made between alternative design proposals in terms of the extent of incorporation of security features. There is a need to identify and categorize the main security systems advocated in past studies of publicly accessible buildings in order to establish the general applicability of the methods of measurement proposed.

- Propose a method of measurement by which the extent of public accessibility to buildings can be assessed. This will enable an objective comparison to be made between different buildings in terms of the extent of their accessibility in use. In order to arrive at a method of measurement, a more comprehensive interpretation of accessibility needs to be developed so that the measures proposed will not be confined to any one particular type of public building.

- Assess the extent of accessibility achieved after the incorporation of security systems, by a study of public buildings in use. To achieve this, a number of publicly accessible buildings need to be examined.

Taking it *FURTHER*

The objectives of research

How you define the research problem is a crucial part of the design of a research project. A good way to help you to decide what the nature of the problem will be and therefore what the nature of the research will be, is to decide on the objectives of the research. When reading about research already completed, look to see where the objectives of the research are explained, as these will give you a strong indication of the nature of the research efforts.

Reynolds (1977, pp. 4–11) listed five things which he believed most people expected scientific knowledge to provide. These, together with one that I have added myself, can conveniently be used as the basis for a list of the possible objectives of research:

- Categorization
- Explanation
- Prediction
- Creating understanding
- Providing potential for control
- Evaluation

Categorization involves forming a typology of objects, events or concepts. This can be useful in explaining what 'things' belong together and how. One of the main problems is to decide which is, or are, the most useful methods of categorization, depending on the reasons for attempting the categorization in the first place. Following from this is the problem of determining what criteria to use to judge the usefulness of the categorization. Two obvious criteria are mentioned by Reynolds (1977): that of exhaustiveness, by which all items should be able to be placed into a category, without any being left out; and that of mutual exclusiveness, by which each item should, without question, be appropriately placed into only one category. Finally, it should be noted that the typologies must be consistent with the concepts used in the theoretical background to the study.

There are many events and issues which we do not fully, or even partly, understand. The objective of providing an explanation of particular phenomena has been a common one in many forms of research. An **explanation** is an attempt to describe how and why things work.

On the basis of an explanation of a phenomenon it is often possible to make a **prediction** of future events related to it. In the natural sciences these predictions are often made in the form of abstract statements, for example, given C1, C2, ,..., Cn: if X, then Y. More readily understood are predictions made in text form. For example, if a person disagrees with a friend about his attitude towards an object, then a state of psychological tension is produced.

While explanation and prediction can reveal the inner workings of phenomena – what happens and when – they do not always provide a **sense of understanding** of phenomena – how or why they happen. A complete explanation of a phenomenon will require a wider study of the processes which surround the phenomenon and influence it or cause it to happen.

A good level of understanding of a phenomenon might lead to the possibility of finding a way to **control** it. Obviously, not all phenomena lend themselves to this.: For example, it is difficult to imagine how the disciplines of astronomy or geology could include an element of control. However, all of technology is dependent on the ability to control the behaviour, movement or stability of things. Even in society there are many attempts, often based on scientific principles, to control events such as crime, poverty, the economy, etc., though the record of success is more limited than in the natural sciences, and perhaps there are cases of attempting the impossible. The problem is that such attempts cannot be truly scientific as the variables cannot all be controlled, nor can one be certain that all relevant variables have been considered. The crucial issue in control is to understand how certain variables affect one another, and then be able to change the variables in such a way as to produce predictable results.

Evaluation is making judgements about the quality of objects or events. Quality can be measured either in an absolute sense or on a comparative basis. To be useful, the methods of evaluation must be relevant to the context and intentions of the research. For example, level of income is a relevant variable in the evaluation of wealth, while degree of marital fidelity is not. Evaluation goes beyond measurement, as it implies allotting values to objects or events. It is the context of the research which will help to establish the types of value that should be used.

> *Research can have several legitimate objectives, either singly or in combination. The main, overriding objective must be that of gaining useful or interesting knowledge.*

Questions to ponder

❝ What are hypotheses and why and how are they used in research? ❞

Describe how they are specific statements that are open to testing. You can list the necessary qualities of a good hypothesis. They are obviously used as a focus for research efforts and to test theory – you can expand on this by giving examples. How they are used is a good lead-in to explaining scientific method – there is plenty to write about that.

❝ When is the use of a hypothesis to formulate the research not appropriate? ❞

As you will have explained in the previous answer, scientific method comes with a list of assumptions about the nature of facts and theory. Much research in social science does not conform to the strictures of natural science, being more qualitative in nature and dedicated to gaining an understanding of events, often from a specific viewpoint. You can give several examples where the alternatives to hypotheses would be more appropriate (e.g. when examining the mores of a pop idol's fan club).

❝ Discuss the relative merits of the alternatives to the use of a hypothesis. ❞

Developing from the points made in the previous answer, you should go through the range of alternative choices outlined in this chapter, and by using simple examples, explain how research can be carried out in different ways in response to its formulation. For example, a research question with its sub-questions can focus the research to a narrowly defined topic and clearly identifies the aims (i.e. finding answers to the questions).

Further reading

Hypotheses and alternative ways of setting out the research problem form the foundation of research projects. The clarity with which they are formulated greatly influence the quality of the research.

Seale, C. (ed.) (2004) *Researching Society and Culture*. (2nd edn). London: Sage.
Chapter 6 is devoted to what is a social problem.

Look also at the following for more debate about the workings of hypotheses:
Chalmers, A. (1982) *What is This Thing Called Science*. (2nd edn). Milton Keynes: Open University Press.

Preece, Roy (1994) *Starting Research: An Introduction to Academic Research and Dissertation Writing*. London: Pinter.
See pp. 60–70.

For some really sophisticated reading about hypotheses and the logic behind testing them, see:
Trusted, J. (1979) *The Logic of Scientific Inference*. London: Methuen.

7	
sampling	

A census is a survey of all of the cases in a population. An example of this is a National Census, where everyone in the nation is asked to return a questionnaire. A census is a very costly and time-consuming project.

If you want to get information about a large group of people or organizations, it is normally impossible to get all of them to answer your questions – it would take much too long and be far too expensive. The solution is to just ask some of them and hope that the answers they give are representative (or typical) of the ones the rest would give. If their answers really are the same as the others would give, then you need not bother to ask the rest; rather, you can draw conclusions from those answers which you can then relate to the whole group. This process of selecting just a small group of people from a large group is called sampling. There are several things you must consider in selecting a **sample**, so before discussing the different methods of data collection, let us first deal with the issue of sampling.

A representative sample?

When conducting any kind of survey to collect information, or when choosing some particular cases to study in detail, the question inevitably arises: how representative is the information collected of the whole population? In other words, how similar are the characteristics of the small group of cases that are chosen to those of all the cases in the whole type group.

To be able to make accurate judgements about a population from a sample, the sample should be as representative as possible.

When we talk about population in research, it does not necessarily mean a number of people. **Population** is a collective term used to describe the total quantity of things (or cases) of the type which is the subject of your study. So a population can consist of objects, people or even events (e.g. schools, miners, revolutions). A complete list of cases in a population is called a **sampling frame**. This list may be more or less accurate. A sample is a number of cases selected from the sampling frame that you want to subject to closer study.

> *Common pitfall:* It is not always possible to obtain a representative sample.

You might not know what the characteristics of the population are, or you might not be able to reach sectors of it. Non-representative samples cannot be used to make accurate generalizations about the population.

For example, if you wish to survey the opinions of the members of a small club, there might be no difficulty in getting information from each member, so the results of the survey will represent those of the whole club membership. However, if you wish to assess the opinions of the members of a large trade union, apart from organizing a national ballot, you will have to devise some way of selecting a sample of the members whom you can question, and who are a fair representation of all the members of the union. Sampling must be done whenever you can gather information from only a fraction of the population of a group that you want to study. Ideally, you should try to select a sample which is free from bias. You will see that the type of sample you select will greatly affect the reliability of your subsequent generalizations.

There are basically two types of sampling procedure:

1 **Probability sampling** – based on random selection.

2 **Non-probability sampling** – based on non-random selection.

Probability sampling techniques give the most reliable representation of the whole population, while non-probability techniques, relying on the judgement of the researcher or by accident, cannot be used to make generalizations about the whole population.

Probability sampling

This is based on using random methods to select the sample. Populations are not always quite as uniform or one-dimensional as, say, a particular type of component in a production run, so simple random selection methods are not always appropriate. The selection procedure should aim to guarantee that each element (person, group, **class**, type, etc.) has an equal chance of being selected and that every possible combination of the elements also has an equal chance of being selected.

The first question asked should be about the nature of the population: is it homogeneous or are there distinctly different types of case within it, if there are different types within the population, how are they distributed (e.g. are they grouped in different locations, found at different levels in a hierarchy or are all mixed up together)? Different sampling techniques are appropriate for each.

The next question to ask is: which process of randomization will be used? The following gives a guide to which technique is suited to the different population characteristics.

Simple random sampling is used when the population is uniform or has common characteristics in all cases (e.g. medical students, international airports, dairy cows). A simple form of random selection would be to pick names from a hat or, for samples from larger populations, assigning a number to each case on the sampling frame and using random numbers generated by computer or from random number tables to make the selection.

Systematic sampling is an alternative to random sampling and can be used when the population is very large and of no known characteristics (e.g. the population of a town) or when the population is known to be very uniform (e.g. cars of a particular model being produced in a factory). The method of systematic selection involves the selection of units in a series (e.g. on a list or from a production line) according to a predetermined system. There are many possible systems. Perhaps the simplest is to choose every *nth* case on a list, for example, every tenth person in a telephone directory or list of ratepayers, or every hundredth model off the production line. In using this system, it is important to pick the first case randomly (i.e. the first case on the list is not necessarily chosen). The type of list is also significant: not everyone in the town owns a telephone or is a ratepayer.

Simple stratified sampling should be used when cases in the population fall into distinctly different categories or strata (e.g. a business whose workforce is divided into the three categories of production, research and management). With the presence of distinctly different strata in a population, in order to achieve simple randomized sampling, an equally sized randomized sample is obtained from each stratum separately to ensure that each is equally represented. The samples are then combined to form the complete sample from the whole population.

Proportional stratified sampling is used when the cases in a population fall into distinctly different categories (strata) of a known proportion of that population (e.g. a university in which the proportions of the students studying arts and sciences is 61 per cent and 39 per cent, respectively). When the proportions of the different strata in a population are known, then each stratum must be represented in the same proportions within the overall sample. In order to achieve proportional randomized sampling, a randomized sample is obtained from each stratum separately, sized according to the known proportion of each stratum in the whole population, and then combined as previously to form the complete sample from the population.

Cluster sampling is used in cases when the population forms clusters by sharing one or some characteristics but are otherwise as heterogeneous as possible, for example travellers using main railway stations. They are all train travellers, with each cluster experiencing a distinct station, but individuals vary as to age, sex, nationality, wealth, social status, etc. Also known as **area sampling**, cluster sampling is used when the population is large and spread over a large area. Rather than enumerating the whole population, it is divided into segments, and then several segments are chosen at random. Samples are subsequently obtained from each of these segments using one of the above sampling methods.

Multi-stage cluster sampling is an extension of cluster sampling, where clusters of successively smaller size are selected from within each other. For example, you might take a random sample from all UK universities, then a random sample from subjects within those universities, then a random sample of modules taught in those subjects, then a random sample of the students doing those modules.

Non-probability sampling

Non-probability sampling is based on selection by non-random means. This can be useful for certain studies, but it provides only a weak basis for generalization.

Accidental sampling (or convenience sampling) involves using what is immediately available (e.g. studying the building you happen to be in, examining the work practices in your firm, etc.). There are no ways of checking to see if this kind of sample is in any way representative of others of its kind, so the results of the study can be applied only to that sample.

Quota sampling is used regularly by reporters interviewing on the streets. It is an attempt to balance the sample interviewed by selecting responses from equal numbers of different respondents (e.g. equal numbers from different political parties). This is an unregulated form of sampling as there is no knowledge of whether the respondents are typical of their parties. For example, Labour respondents might just have come from an extreme left-wing rally.

Theoretical sampling is a useful method of getting information from a sample of the population that you think knows most about a subject. A study on homelessness could concentrate on questioning people living on the street. This approach is common in qualitative research where statistical inference is not required.

Purposive sampling is where the researcher selects what he/she thinks is a 'typical' sample based on specialist knowledge or selection criteria.

Systematic matching sampling is used when two groups of very different size are compared by selecting a number from the larger group to match the number and characteristics of the smaller one.

Snowball sampling is where the researcher contacts a small number of members of the target population and gets them to introduce him/her to others (e.g. of an exclusive club or an underground organization).

Sample size

Having selected a suitable sampling method, the remaining problem is to determine the sample size. The first impression is that the bigger the sample size, the more possibility there is of representing all the different characteristics of the population. It is generally accepted that conclusions reached from the study of a large sample are more convincing than those from a small one.

The preference for a large sample must be balanced against the practicalities of the research resources, that is, cost, time and effort.

If the population is very homogeneous, and the study is not very detailed, then a small sample will give a fairly representative view of the whole. The greater the accuracy required in the true representation of the population, then the larger the sample must be. The amount of variability within the population (technically known as the **standard deviation**) is also significant. Obviously, in order that every sector of a diverse population is adequately represented, a larger sample will be required than if the population were more homogeneous.

Common pitfall: If statistical tests are to be used to analyse the data, there are usually minimum sample sizes specified from which any significant results can be obtained. The size of the sample should also be in direct relationship to the number of variables to be studied.

A simple method of clarifying the likely size of sample required in a study is to set up a table which cross-references the variability in the population with the number of variables you wish to study. Figure 7.1 shows a table for a study of the effect of the number of drinks on driving performance around a course delineated by bollards. Dixon (1987) suggests that for a very simple survey, at least five cases are required in each cell (i.e. $12 \times 5 = 60$). Obviously, if the variables are split into smaller units of measurement (i.e. the number of drinks is increased), then the overall size of the sample must be increased. Dixon also suggests that at least 30 cases are required for even the most elementary kinds of analysis.

Sampling error

No sample will be exactly representative of a population. If different samples, using identical methods, are taken from the same population, there are bound to be differences in the mean (average) values of each sample owing to the chance selection of different individuals. The measured difference between the mean value of a sample and that of the population is called the **sampling error**, which will lead to bias in the results. **Bias** is the unwanted distortion of the results of a survey due to parts of the population being more strongly represented than others.

Variable A (Values) Number of drinks	Variation in population (standard deviation) Number of bollards collided with		
	1	2	3
1	At least five cases in each of these cells		
2			
3			
4			

Figure 7.1   Variables and Variability – drinking and driving
Adapted from Dixon, 1987, p. 152.

Factors that can lead to sampling error include:

- the use of non-probability sampling
- an inadequate sampling frame
- non-response by sectors of the sample

Taking it *FURTHER*

Multiple case study selection
When you wish to study several case studies you are faced with the problem of how to choose them. The most common reason for selecting more than one case study is so that several cases can be compared. You will need to know what the characteristics are of the population of possible case studies and devise a sampling frame. Depending on your research objectives you may wish to compare extreme examples e.g. successful and unsuccessful businesses, or wish to compare similar samples e.g. best retirement homes. The selection of case studies will then be based on this decision, using either probability sampling methods or non-probability methods.

Questions to ponder

" Why do researchers use sampling procedures? What factors must you examine when deciding on an appropriate sampling method? "

Usually in order to select a representative sample from a population, but sometimes just to select a manageable number of cases, even if they are not representative. The sorts of factor meant here are the characteristics of the population and practical matters such as location, distribution and number of cases.

" What are the two basic types of sampling procedure, and what are the differences between them? When is it appropriate to use them? "

This obviously refers to probability and non-probability sampling methods. The main difference is the random and non-random element. You can elaborate on this by explaining the consequences this has. Use your imagination to devise examples of where the different procedures can be appropriately used, for example snowball sampling techniques when you cannot approach the cases yourself because they belong to a private network.

" What are the critical issues which determine the appropriate sample size? "

Just read what it says in the chapter above! Mention variability within the population, the number of variables studied, and practical issues among other things.

References to more information

Sampling is a big subject in social research, and all research methods textbooks will have a section on it. Here are two books that are entirely devoted to the subject:

Scheaffer, R. (1996) *Elementary Survey Sampling* (5th edn). Belmont, CA: Duxbury.

Fink, A. (1995) *How to Sample in Surveys*. Volume 6 of *The Survey Kit*. London: Sage.

8	
data collection methods	

Data (the plural form of datum) are the raw materials of research. You need to mine your subject in order to dig out the ore in the form of data, which you can then interpret and refine into the gold of conclusions. So, how can you, as a prospector for data, find the relevant sources in your subject?

Although we are surrounded by data, in fact, bombarded with them every day from the television, posters, radio, newspapers, magazines and books, it is not so straightforward to collect the correct data for our purposes. It needs a plan of action that identifies and uses the most effective and appropriate methods of data collection.

> *Whatever your branch of social science, collecting secondary data will be a must. You will inevitably need to ascertain what is the background to your research question/problem, and also get an idea of the current theories and ideas. No type of project is done in a vacuum, not even a pure work of art.*

Collecting primary information is much more subject-specific. Consider whether you need to get information from people, in single or large numbers, or whether you will need to observe and/or measure things or phenomena. You may need to do several of these. For example, in healthcare you may be examining both the people and their treatments, or in education you may be looking at both the education system or perhaps the building, and the effects on the pupils.

> ***Common pitfall:*** You are probably wasting your time if you amass data that you are unable to analyse, either because you have too much, or because you have insufficient or inappropriate analytical skills or methods to make the analysis.

I say 'probably' because research is not a linear process, so it is not easy to predict exactly how much data will be 'enough'. What will help you to judge the type of and amount of data required is to decide on the methods that you will use to analyse it. In turn, the decision on the appropriateness of analytical methods must be made in relation to the nature of the research problem and the specific aims of the research project. It should be evident in your overall argument what links the research question/problem with the necessary data to be collected and the type of analysis that needs to be carried out in order to reach valid conclusions.

Collecting secondary data

All research studies require **secondary data** for the background to the study. Others rely greatly on them for the whole project, for example when doing a historical study (i.e. of any past events, ideas or objects, even the very recent past) or a nationwide study that uses official statistics.

> *Wherever there exists a body of recorded information, there are subjects for study. An advantage of using this kind of data is that it has not been produced for the specific purposes of social research, and can therefore be the basis of a form of unobtrusive inquiry.*

Many of the prevailing theoretical debates (e.g. postmodernism, post-structuralism) are concerned with the subjects of language and cultural interpretation, with the result that these issues have frequently become central to sociological studies. The need has therefore arisen for methodologies that allow analysis of cultural texts to be compared, replicated, disproved and generalized. From the late 1950s, language has been analysed from several basic viewpoints: the structural properties of language (notably Chomsky, Sacks, Schegloff), language as an action in its contextual environment (notably Wittgenstein, Austin and Searle) and sociolinguistics and the 'ethnography of speaking' (Hymes, Bernstein, Labov and many others).

However, the meaning of the term 'cultural texts' has been broadened from that of purely literary works to that of the many manifestations of cultural exchange, be they formal, such as opera, television news programmes, cocktail parties, etc., or informal, such as how people dress or converse. The main criterion for cultural texts is that one should be able to 'read' some meanings into the phenomena. Texts can therefore include tactile, visual and aural aspects, even smells and tastes. They can be current or historical and may be descriptive or statistical in nature. Any of them can be quantitative or qualitative in nature.

Here are some examples of documentary data that come from a wide range of sources:

- Personal documents
- Oral histories
- Commentaries
- Diaries
- Letters
- Autobiographies
- Official published documents
- State documents and records
- Official statistics
- Commercial or organizational documents
- Mass media outputs
- Newspapers and journals
- Maps
- Drawings, comics and photographs
- Fiction
- Non-fiction
- Academic output
- Journal articles and conference papers
- Lecture notes
- Critiques
- Research reports
- Textbooks
- Artistic output
- Theatrical productions – plays, opera, musicals
- Artistic critiques
- Programmes, playbills, notes and other ephemera
- Virtual outputs
- Web pages
- Databases

Several problems face the researcher seeking historical and recorded data. The main problems are:

- locating and accessing them
- authenticating the sources
- assessing credibility
- gauging how representative they are
- selecting methods of interpreting them

Locating historical data can be an enormous topic. Activities can involve anything from unearthing city ruins in the desert to rummaging through dusty archives in an obscure library or downloading the latest government statistical data from the Internet. Even current data may be difficult to get hold of. For instance, much current economic data are restricted and expensive to buy. It is impossible to give a full description of sources, as the detailed nature of the subject of research determines the appropriate source, and, of course, the possible range of subjects is enormous. However, here are some of the principle sources.

Libraries and archives: these are generally equipped with sophisticated catalogue systems which facilitate the tracking down of particular pieces of data or enable a trawl to be made to identify anything which may be relevant. International computer networks can make remote searching possible. See your own library specialists for the latest techniques. Apart from these modernized libraries and archives, much valuable historical material is contained in more obscure and less organized collections, in remote areas and old houses and institutions. The attributes of a detective are often required to track down relevant material, and that of a diplomat to gain access to private or restricted collections.

Museums, galleries and collections: these often have efficient cataloguing systems that will help your search. However, problems may be encountered with searching and access in less organized and restricted or private collections. Larger museums often have their own research departments that can be of help.

Government departments and commercial/professional bodies: these often hold much statistical information, both current and historic.

The Internet: rapidly expanding source of information of all types.

The field: not all historical artefacts are contained in museums. Ancient cities, buildings, archaeological digs, etc. are available for study *in situ*. Here, various types of observation will be required to record the required data.

Authentication of historical data can be a complex process, and is usually carried out by experts. A wide range of techniques are used, for example textual analysis, carbon dating, paper analysis, locational checks, cross-referencing, and many others. Authentication of modern or current material requires a thorough check of sources.

> *Common pitfall:* '[Documents] should never be taken at face value. In other words, they must be regarded as information that is context specific and as data which must be contextualized with other forms of research. They should, therefore, only be used with caution.' (Forster, 1994, p. 149)

Credibility of data refers to its freedom from error or bias. Many documents are written in order to put across a particular message and can be selective of the truth. Much important contextual data can be missing from such documents as reports of spoken events, where the pauses, hesitations and gestures are not recorded.

> *The degree of representativeness of the documents should be assessed. This will enable judgements of the generalizability of any conclusions drawn from them to be made.*

The wealth of purely statistical data contained in the archives, especially those of more recent date, provides a powerful resource for research into many issues. You will often find, however, that the data recorded is not exactly in the form that you require. For example, when making international comparisons on housing provision, the data might be compiled in different ways in the different countries under consideration. In order to extract the exact data you require, you will have to extrapolate from the existing data.

Collecting primary data

This entails going out and collecting information by observing, recording and measuring the activities and ideas of real people, or perhaps watching animals, or inspecting objects and experiencing events. This process of collecting **primary data** is often called survey research.

You should only be interested in collecting data that is required in order to investigate your research problem. Even so, the amount of relevant information you could collect is likely to be enormous, so you must find a way to limit the amount of data you collect to achieve your aims. The main technique for reducing the scope of your data collection is to study a sample, that is a small section of the subjects of your study, or to select one or several case studies. Most of the data collection methods described below are suitable for qualitative research, the collecting of data is then often combined with ongoing analysis. Some of the methods also lend themselves to quantitative research. The nature of the questions and form of answers sought are the central issue here.

Self-completion questionnaires

Asking questions is an obvious method of collecting both quantitative and qualitative information from people. Using a questionnaire enables you to organize the questions and receive replies without actually having to talk to every respondent. As a method of data collection, the questionnaire is a very flexible tool, but you must use it carefully in order to fulfil the requirements of your research. While there are whole books on the art of questioning and questionnaires, it is possible to isolate a number of important factors to consider before deciding to use a questionnaire.

Before examining its form and content, let's briefly consider why you might choose this form of data collection, and the ways in which you could deliver the questionnaire.

The advantages of self-completion questionnaires:

- They are cheap to administer.
- They are quick to administer.
- They are an easy way to question a large number of cases covering large geographical areas.
- The personal influence of the researcher is eliminated.
- Embarrassing questions can be asked with a fair chance of getting a truthful reply.
- Variability between different researchers or assistants is eliminated.
- They are convenient for respondents.
- Respondents have time to check facts and think about their answers, which tends to lead to more accurate information.
- They have a structured format.
- They can be designed to assist in the analysis stage.
- They are particularly suitable for quantitative data but can also be used for qualitative data.

The disadvantages of self-completion questionnaires:

- They require a lot of time and skill to design and develop.
- They limit the range and scope of questioning – questions need to be simple to follow and understand so complex question structures are not possible.
- Yet more forms to fill in! They can be unpopular, so they need to be as short as possible.
- Prompting and probing are impossible, and this limits the scope of answers and the possibility of getting additional data.
- It is not possible to ascertain if the right person has responded.
- Not everyone is able to complete questionnaires.
- Response rates can be low.

There are two basic methods of delivering questionnaires, personally and by post. The advantages of personal delivery are that you can help respondents to overcome difficulties with the questions, and that you can use personal persuasion and reminders to ensure a high response rate. You can also find out the reasons why some people refuse to answer the questionnaire, and you can check on responses if they seem odd or incomplete. Obviously, there are problems both in time and geographical location that limit the scope and extent to which you can use this method of delivery.

> *Personal involvement in delivery and collection of questionnaires enables you to devise more complicated questionnaires.*

The rate of response for postal questionnaires is difficult to predict or control, particularly if there is no system of follow-up. The pattern of non-response can have a serious effect on the validity of your sample by introducing bias into the data collected. Mangione (1995, pp. 60–1) rates responses like this:

Over 85% – excellent
70–85% – very good
60–70% – acceptable
50–60% – barely acceptable
Below 50% – not acceptable

Here are some simple rules for devising a questionnaire. It is not always easy to carry them out perfectly:

- Establish exactly which variables you wish to gather data about, and how these variables can be assessed. This will enable you to list the questions you need to ask (and those that you don't) and to formulate the questions precisely in order to get the required responses.
- Clear instructions are required to guide the respondent on how to complete the questionnaire.
- The language must be unmistakably clear and unambiguous and make no inappropriate assumptions. This requires some clear analytical effort.
- In order to get a good response rate, keep questions simple and the questionnaire as short as possible.
- Clear and professional presentation is another essential factor in encouraging a good response. Vertical format is best, and answers should be kept close to questions.
- Consider how you will process the information from the completed forms. This may influence the layout of the questionnaire, for example by including spaces for codes and scoring.

It is a good idea to pre-test the questionnaire on a small number of people before you use it in earnest. This is called a **pilot study**.

> If you can, test a pilot study on people of a similar type to those in the intended sample to anticipate any problems of comprehension or other sources of confusion.

It is good practice when sending out or issuing the questionnaire to courteously invite the recipients to complete it, and encourage them by explaining the purpose of the survey, how the results could be of benefit to them, and how little time it will take to complete. Include simple instructions on how to fill in the questionnaire. Some form of thanks and appreciation of their efforts should be included at the end. If you need to be sure of a response from a particular person, send a preliminary letter, with a reply-paid response card, to ask if he/she is willing to complete the questionnaire before you send it.

There are basically two types of question:

1 **Closed-format questions** Where the respondents must choose from a choice of given answers.

2 **Open-format questions** Where the respondents are free to answer in their own words and style.

The advantages of closed-format questions are:

- They are quick to answer.
- They are easy to code.
- They require no special writing skills from respondent.

The disadvantages are:

- There is a limited range of possible answers.
- It is not possible to qualify answers.

Types of question can be listed as:

- Single answer (e.g. nationality) – yes/no.
- Multiple answer (e.g. select from a list).
- Rank order (e.g. number items on a list by preference).

- Numerical (e.g. number of miles, age, etc.).
- Lickert style (e.g. rate the extent to which you agree with a statement: strongly agree, agree, undecided, disagree, strongly disagree).
- Semantic differential (e.g. choose from a range of qualities: very good, good, mediocre, poor, very poor).

A **coding frame** is usefully devised and incorporated into the questionnaire design to make coding and data handling simpler and consistent later on during analysis. Responses are assigned a code, usually in the form of a number, which is used for keying the responses into a computer format.

The advantages of open-format questions are:

- They permit freedom of expression.
- Bias is eliminated because respondents are free to answer in their own way.
- Respondent's can qualify their responses.

The disadvantages are:

- They are more demanding and time-consuming for respondents.
- They are difficult to code.
- Respondents' answers are open to the researcher's interpretation.

Coding categories will need to be devised according to the types of response gained. The results of a pilot survey will help to predict these.

Interviews (structured, semi-structured and unstructured)

While questionnaire surveys are relatively easy to organize and prevent the personality of the interviewer affecting the results, they do have certain limitations. They are not suitable for questions that require probing to obtain adequate information, as they should only contain simple, one-stage questions (i.e. questions whose answers do not lead on to further specific questions). It is often difficult to get responses from the complete sample; questionnaires tend to be returned by the more literate sections of the population.

The use of interviews to question samples of people is a very flexible tool with a wide range of applications. Three types of interview are often mentioned:

1 **Structured interview** – standardized questions read out by the interviewer according to an interview schedule. Answers may be closed-format.

2 **Unstructured interview** – a flexible format, usually based on a question guide but where the format remains the choice of the interviewer, who can allow the interview to 'ramble' in order to get insights into the attitudes of the interviewee. No closed-format questions are used.

3 **Semi-structured interview** – one that contains structured and unstructured sections with standardized and open-format questions.

> *Because of their flexibility, interviews are a useful method of obtaining information and opinions from experts during the early stages of your research project.*

Although suitable for quantitative data collection, interviews are particularly useful when qualitative data is required. There are two main methods of conducting interviews: face-to-face and by telephone.

Face-to-face interviews can be carried out in a variety of situations: in the home, at work, outdoors, on the move (e.g. while travelling). They can be used to question members of the general public, experts or leaders, or specific segments of society, such as elderly or disabled people, ethnic minorities, both singly and in groups. Interviews can be used for a variety of subjects, both general or specific, and even, with the correct preparation, for very sensitive topics. They can be one-off interviews or repeated several times over a period to track developments. As the interviewer, you are in a good position to judge the quality of the responses, to notice if a question has not been properly understood and to encourage the respondent to be full in his/her answers. Using visual signs, such as nods, smiles, etc. helps to get good responses.

Telephone interviews avoid the necessity of travelling to the respondents and all the problems associated with contacting people personally. Telephone surveys can be carried out more quickly than face-to-face interviews, especially if the questionnaire is short (20–30 minutes at the most). However, you cannot use visual aids to explain questions and there are no visual clues such as eye contact, smiling, puzzled looks between you and the interviewee. Voice quality is an important factor in successful telephone interviews. You should speak steadily and clearly, using standard pronunciation and sounding competent and confident.

For interviewing very busy people, you can pre-arrange a suitable time to ring. Modern communications technology is making it more and more difficult to talk with an actual person on the phone!

> *The most important point when you set up an interview is to know exactly what you want to achieve by it, how you are going to record the information, and what you intend to do with it.*

Although there is a great difference in technique for conducting interviews 'cold' with the general public and interviewing officials or experts by appointment, in both cases the personality and bearing of the interviewer is of great importance. You should be well prepared in the groundwork (i.e. writing letters to make appointments, explaining the purpose of the interview), in presenting the interview (with confidence, friendliness, good appearance, etc.) and in the method of recording the responses (tape recording, writing notes, completing forms, etc.).

There are several types of question that can be used to gain information on facts, behaviour, beliefs and attitudes. Kvale (1996) lists nine types:

- Introducing
- Follow-up
- Probing
- Specifying
- Direct

- Indirect
- Structuring
- Silence
- Interpreting

Interviews can be audio-recorded in many instances in order to retain a full, un-interpreted record of what was said. However, in order to analyse the data, the recording will have to be transcribed.

> **Common pitfall:** Transcription is a lengthy process. Bryman (2004, p. 331) reckons that five or six hours are required for every hour of speech. It therefore results in a huge amount of paperwork that needs to be analysed.

The main advantage of recording and transcribing interviews is that it makes it easier to check exactly what was said – memories cannot be relied upon! And repeated checking is possible. The raw data is also available for checks against researcher bias and for secondary or different analysis by others. Short-cuts to full transcription are either to transcribe only the particularly useful sections of the interviews in full, or to record in note form what was said, similar to notes taken during an interview, perhaps already employing a pre-determined coding system.

Standardized tests

A wide range of **standardized tests** have been devised by social scientists and psychologists to measure people's abilities, attitudes, aptitudes, opinions, etc. A well-known example of one of these is the IQ or intelligence test. The objective of the tests is usually to measure the abilities of the subjects according to a standardized scale, so that easy comparisons can be made. One of the main problems is to select or devise a suitable scale for measuring the often rather abstract concepts under investigation, such as attitude (e.g. to school meals, military service, capital punishment, etc.).

> It is safer to use tried-and-tested standard scales, of which there are several, each taking different approaches according to the results aimed at.

One of the most common standardized tests is the **Lickert scale**, using a summated rating approach. There is also, among others, the Thurlstone scale, which aims to produce an equal interval scale, and the Guttman scale, which is a unidimensional scale where items have a cumulative property.

Here is an example of a Lickert scale so that you get the idea of what it is like:

Strongly agree   1   2   3   4   5   Strongly disagree

The 'questions' are expressed as statements (e.g. the 'Labour Party still represents the workers') and the respondent is asked to ring one of the numbers in the scale 1–5. Another way of expressing the same thing is just to use words:

Strongly agree/tend to agree/neither agree nor disagree/tend to disagree/ strongly disagree

at the head of five columns situated to the right of the list of statements, and ask the respondent to tick the column that most reflects his/her opinion. You can use any dichotomous combination you like, such as like/dislike, want/not want, probable/improbable. You just have to be careful that there are gradations of the opinion or feelings, unlike accept/ reject, which is either one or the other. As an alternative to five, you can have three or seven stages. (It is best to keep to odd numbers so that you get a middle value.)

You can see that a score is automatically given by the response, so you can easily count the number of different scores to analyse the results.

> *A useful precaution to prevent oversimplification of responses is to ask many questions about the same topic, all from different angles.*

This form of triangulation helps to build up a more complete picture of complex issues. You can then also weight the results from the different questions – that is, give more importance to those that are particularly crucial by multiplying them by a chosen factor.

Detached and participant observation

This is a method of recording conditions, events and activities through looking rather than asking. As an activity, as opposed to a method, observation is of course required in many research situations, for example, observing the results of experiments, the behaviour of models and even observing the reactions of people to questions in an interview. Observation can also be used for recording the nature or condition of objects or events visually, for example through photography, film or sketching. This is sometimes referred to as **visual ethnography.** The visual materials may be a source of data for analysis, or can be used as a prompt for interviewee reaction.

Observation can be used to record both quantitative and qualitative data. There is a range of levels of involvement in the observed phenomena. Gold (1958) classifies these as follows:

- **Complete observer** – the observer takes a detached stance by not getting involved in the events, and uses unobtrusive observation techniques and remains 'invisible' either in fact or in effect (i.e. by being ignored).
- **Observer-as-participant** – the researcher is mainly an interviewer doing some degree of observation but very little participation.

- **Participant-as-observer** – the researcher engages fully in the life and activities of the observed, who are aware of his/her observing role.
- **Complete participant** – the researcher takes a full part in the social events but is not recognized as an observer by the observed. The complete participant is a covert observer.

> *Observation can record whether people act differently from what they say or intend.*

People can sometimes demonstrate their understanding of a process better by their actions than by verbally explaining their knowledge. For example, a machine operator will probably demonstrate more clearly his/her understanding of the techniques of operating the machine by working with it than by verbal explanation.

Observation is not limited to the visual sense. Any sense (e.g. smell, touch, hearing) can be involved, and these need not be restricted to the range perceptible to the human senses. A microscope or telescope can be used to extend the capacity of the eye, just as a moisture meter can be used to increase sensitivity to the feeling of dampness. You can probably think of instruments that have been developed in every discipline to extend the observational limits of the human senses.

On the one hand, observations of objects can be a quick and efficient method of gaining preliminary knowledge or making a preliminary assessment of its state or condition. For example, after an earthquake, a quick visual assessment of the amount and type of damage to buildings can be made before a detailed survey is undertaken. On the other hand, observation can be very time-consuming and difficult when the activity observed is not constant (i.e. much time can be wasted waiting for things to happen, or so much happens at once that it is impossible to observe it all and record it). Instrumentation can sometimes be devised to overcome the problem of infrequent or spasmodic activity (e.g. automatic cameras and other sensors).

Here are a few basic hints on how to carry out observations:

- Make sure you know what you are looking for. Events and objects are usually complicated and much might seem to be relevant to your study. Identify the variables that you need to study and concentrate on these.
- Getting access is more difficult in closed, as opposed to open, settings. You will need to use friends and other contacts to gain access to organizations, and will invariably have to get clearance for the research from senior management.

- Make sure you can explain clearly what your aims and methods are and how much of a person's time you will be taking up. You may need to negotiate and offer some return (e.g. a short report) for permission to be granted. Be honest.
- Devise a simple and efficient method of recording the information accurately. Rely as much as possible on ticking boxes or circling numbers, particularly if you need to record fast-moving events. Obviously, when observing static objects, you can leave yourself more time to notate or draw the data required. Record the observations as they happen. Memories of detailed observations fade quickly.
- Use instrumentation when appropriate or necessary. Instruments that make an automatic record of their measurements are to be preferred in many situations.
- If possible, process the information as the observations progress. This can help to identify critical matters that need to be studied in greater detail, and others that prove to be unnecessary.
- If you are doing covert observations, use a 'front' to explain your presence, and plan in advance what to do if your presence is discovered, to avoid potentially embarrassing or even dangerous situations! Beware of transgressing the law.
- In overt observation, try to allay worries that you might be a snooping official or inspector by stressing your role as a researcher, your high level of competence, and your ability to retain confidentiality.
- Make sure you observe ethical standards and obtain the necessary clearances with the relevant authorities (see Chapter 12).

Personal accounts and diaries

This is a method of qualitative data collection. Personal accounts and diaries provide information on people's actions and feelings by asking them to give their own interpretation, or account, of what they experience. Accounts can consist of a variety of data sources: people's spoken explanations, behaviour (such as gestures), personal records of experiences and conversations, letters and diaries. As long as the accounts are authentic, there is no reason why they cannot be used to explain people's actions.

Since the information must come directly from the respondents, you must take care to avoid leading questions, excessive guidance and other factors which may cause distortion. You can check the authenticity of the accounts by cross-checking with other people involved in the events, examining the physical records of the events (e.g. papers, documents, etc.) and checking with the respondents during the account-gathering process. You will need to transform the collected accounts into working documents that can be coded and analysed.

Taking it **FURTHER**

Focus groups

Focus groups are a type of group interview, which concentrates in-depth on a particular theme or topic with an element of interaction. The group is often made up of people who have particular experience or knowledge about the subject of the research, or those who have a particular interest in it (e.g. consumers or customers). It can be quite difficult to organize focus groups due to the difficulty of getting a group of people together for a discussion session.

The interviewer's job is a delicate balancing act. He/she should be seen more as a moderator of the resulting discussion than as a dominant questioner, one who prompts the discussion without unduly influencing its direction. Reticent speakers might need encouragement in order to limit dominant speakers. The moderator should also provide a suitable introduction and conclusion to the session, offering information about the research, the topics, what will happen with the data collected and express thanks to the members of the group.

According to Bryman (2004, pp. 247–8), there are several reasons for holding focus groups:

- To develop an understanding about why people think the way they do.
- Members of the group can bring forward ideas and opinions not foreseen by the interviewer.
- Interviewees can be challenged, often by other members of the group, about their replies.
- The interactions found in group dynamics are closer to the real-life process of sense-making and acquiring understanding.

The common size of group is around six to ten people. Selection of members of the group will depend on whether you attempt to get a cross-section of people, a proportional membership (e.g. a proportionate number of representatives reflecting the size of each section of the population), or a convenient natural grouping (e.g. just those who show an interest in the subject).

Common pitfall: Although a lot of information is produced in a short time by a focus group, noting down what is said can be difficult due to the number of people involved and the heat of the discussion.

It is important to know not only what was said, but who said it and how. It is therefore best to tape-record the interview and transcribe it later, which can be a lengthy task. Analysis of the data is not easy due to the dual aspects of what people say and how they say it in interaction with the others.

Questions to ponder

" When and why might you want to collect secondary data? Give some examples of research topics to illustrate your points. "

Two main responses come to mind. First, you need to collect secondary data when you prepare the background for a research project in order to build a basis for the work and, second, when primary data is not available, particularly in the case of historical studies. You can easily devise some examples of topics to illustrate these, and probably think of a few more reasons for collecting secondary data (because they are there! e.g. government statistics).

" Devise four really bad questions for a questionnaire and explain what is wrong with them and why. How can they be improved? "

There are usually examples of ambiguous or puzzling questions in textbooks about questionnaires. A simple example is 'Do you smoke more than 10 cigarettes in a ... day, week, month, year? – Underline one period'. I can see what the questioner is getting at – the frequency of smoking – but anyone smoking more than 10 a day could underline any of the periods! What about non-smokers? A better version could be: Approximately how many cigarettes do you smoke in a year... 0, 20, 100, 500, more than 1,000?

" Can anyone really do observation in a detached fashion? What can be done to avoid getting involved in the situation being observed? "

This brings up the debate about **positivism, relativism** and **realism** (see Chapter 2). You can take a stance with particular reference to social science research, and give examples where it might be easier to be a detached observer and not. Obviously, if you need to participate in order to be accepted in the situation studied, it will be more difficult to remain detached. Give examples of how to avoid getting involved. One way is to be a covert observer, where involvement is impossible (though you might still get caught up in the emotions of the actions).

References to more information

There are hundreds of books about data collection methods. Your own textbooks will give you plenty of information about these – after all, that is what they are about! You should also consult your **library catalogue** for books that deal specifically with how to do research in your own subject branch of social studies (e.g. management, healthcare, education, etc).

I do not include general textbooks on social science research methods here, only more specific books about different methods. You should consult your recommended textbooks by looking up the relevant section.

Fowler, F.J. (2001) *Survey Research Methods* (3rd edn). London: Sage.
This book goes into great detail into all aspects of the subject of doing surveys. Good on sampling, response rates, methods of data collection – particularly questionnaires and interviews. Use it selectively to find out more about the particular methods you want to use. This book will also be useful later for analysis, and has section on ethics too.

Aldridge, A. (2001) *Surveying the Social World: Principles and Practice in Survey Research*. Buckingham: Open University Press.
Another comprehensive book – find what you need by using the contents list and index.

Fink, A. (1995) *The Survey Kit*. London: Sage.
Nine volumes covering all aspects of survey research! This must be the ultimate.

Here are some books specifically on questionnaires, in order of usefulness:

Peterson, R.A. (2000) *Constructing Effective Questionnaires*. London: Sage.

Gillham, W.E. and William, E.C. (2000) *Developing a Questionnaire*. London: Continuum.

Dillman, D.A. (2000) *Mail and Internet Surveys*: *The Tailored Design Method* (2nd edn). Chichester: Wiley.

Frazer, L. (2000) *Questionnaire Design and Administration*: *A Practical Guide*. Chichester: Wiley.

And a few on interviewing, again in order of usefulness at your stage of work:

Keats, D.M. (2000) *Interviewing: A Practical Guide for Students and Professionals*. Buckingham: Open University Press.

Jaber, F. (ed.) (2002) *Handbook of Interview Research: Context and Method*. London: Sage.

Wengraf, T. (2001) *Qualitative Research Interviewing: Biographic, Narrative and Semi-structured*. London: Sage.

And a couple on case studies, the simplest first:

Nisbet, J.D. and Watt, J. (1982) *Case Study*. Rediguide No. 26. Oxford: TRC Rediguides.

Yin, R.K. (2003) *Case Study Research: Design and Methods* (3rd edn). Thousand Oaks, CA: Sage.

9	
experimental design	

The world around us is so complicated that it is often difficult to observe a particular phenomenon without being disturbed by all the other events happening around us. Wouldn't it be useful to be able to extract that part of the world from its surroundings and study it in isolation. You can often do this by setting up an experiment in which only the important factors (variables) that you want to consider are selected for study. Experiments are used in many subject areas, but particularly those that are based on things or the interaction between things and people (things include systems or techniques as well as objects or substances).

Generally, experiments are used to examine causality (causes and effects). It manipulates one or more independent variable (that which supplies causes) and measures the effects of this manipulation on dependent variables (those which register effects), while at the same time controlling all other variables. This is used to find explanations of 'what happens if, why, when and how'. It is difficult to control all the other variables, some of which might be unknown, that might have an effect on the outcomes of the experiment.

In order to combat this problem, random sampling methods are used to select the experimental units (the things that are being experimented on, such as materials, components, persons, groups, etc.). This process, called **random assignment**, neutralizes the particular effects of individual variables and allows the results of the experiment to be generalized.

The design of the experiments depends on the type of data required, the level of reliability of the data required, and practical matters associated with the problem under investigation. There are many locations where experiments can be carried out, but the laboratory situation is the one that provides the greatest possibilities for control. With this approach, the collection and analysis of data are inextricably linked. The preliminary data on which the experiments are based are used to create new data, which, in its turn, can be used for further analysis.

> ***Common pitfall:*** There is plenty of scope for setting up experiments that so simplify, and even falsify, the phenomenon extracted from the real world that completely wrong conclusions can be reached.

Checks should be carried out on experiments to test whether the assumptions made are valid. A control group can be used to provide a 'baseline' against which the effects of the experimental treatment may be evaluated. The control group is one that is identical (as near as possible) to the experimental group, but does not receive experimental treatment. For example, in a medical experiment, the control group will be given placebo pills instead of the medicated pills. As you can see in this example, experiments are not only a matter of bubbling bottles in a laboratory. They can involve people as well as things – only it is more difficult to control the people!

Laboratory and field experiments

What are the significant differences between doing experiments in the contrived setting of a laboratory and those done in a real-life setting? Social science is concerned with what is happening in the real world, so isn't the laboratory the wrong place to do social experiments?

Laboratory experiments have the advantage of providing a good degree of control over the environment, and of studying the effects on the subjects involved. With the aid of some deception, the subjects might not even be aware of what effects they are being tested for. Despite the artificiality of the setting, this can provide reliable data that can be generalized in the real world. However, according to arguments by leading academics (see Robson, 2002, pp. 111–23), the disadvantages of laboratory experiments are that they may:

- lack experimental realism – the conditions may appear to be artificial and not involve the subjects in the same way as in a realistic setting
- lack mundane realism – real-life settings are always much more complicated and ambiguous than those created in a laboratory
- lead to bias through demand characteristics – the expectation of the subjects that certain things are demanded of them and their reaction to the knowledge that they are being observed
- lead to bias through experimenter expectancy – the often unwitting reactive effects of the experimenters that lead to a biased view of the findings to support the tested hypothesis

It is not always easy to distinguish between laboratory and field experiments.

Realistic simulations of rooms in a laboratory or the use of normal settings as laboratories for the purposes of experiments make it difficult to know where to draw the line. There may also be a sense of artificiality in a natural setting when people are organized for the purposes of the experiment, or people are just aware that they are subjects of investigation.

In field experiments, planned interventions and innovations are the most useful strategies for natural experiments as they provide possibilities to apply relatively reliable experimental designs, involving control groups and getting information prior to the interventions. External validity (generalizability to the real world) is obviously more easily achieved when the experiments are carried out in normal life settings. Subjects are also more likely to react and behave normally rather than being affected by artificial conditions. In most cases, it is also easy to obtain subjects to take part in the research as they need not make any special effort to attend at a particular time and place. However, the move out of the confined and controllable setting of the laboratory raises some problems:

- faulty randomization
- lack of validity
- ethical issues
- lack of control
- types of experiment

It is important to explain the different kinds of experiment that can be set up, and the strength of the conclusions that can be drawn from the observations. Campbell and Stanley (1963, pp. 171–246) divided experiments into four general types:

1 Pre-experimental designs.

2 True experimental designs.

3 Quasi-experimental designs.

4 Correlational and ex post facto designs.

To explain how they work, here is a brief summary of these different designs, and each is illustrated with an example of studying the same simple phenomenon (the effect of a revision course on a group's exam results).

Pre-experimental designs

One-shot case study (after only): This is the most primitive type of design where observations are carried out only after the experiment, lacking any control or check.

Example: A group does the revision course and the exam results are reviewed. Do good results mean that the course was effective?

One-group pre-test – post-test (before–after): Here the subject (group) is examined before the experiment takes place.

Example: The group does the exam before taking the revision course and the results are reviewed. The group does the course and a further exam is taken. These exam results are compared with the previous ones. Better results in the second exam may lead to the conclusion that the course was effective.

Static group comparison (before–after): Similar to the previous design except that a control group is introduced.

Example: Two groups are selected at random. The experimental group does the revision course, the control group does not. Both groups take the exam and the results are compared. If the control group does less well, we might conclude that the course enhances exam success.

Common pitfall: The trouble with pre-experimental designs is the lack of control of the variables, which can seriously affect the outcomes. For example, what happens if some of the groups are already well prepared for the exam or are not interested in learning?

True experimental designs

Pre-test – post-test control group (before–after): This is the commonest true experimental design.

Example: Two groups are selected in the same random procedure and both do the exam (pre-test). One group does the revision course, the other does not. The groups are examined again and the exam results are compared. Best results are gained if both samples achieve identical results in the pre-test exam.

Solomon four-group (before–after): This is a refinement of the previous design, using four samples, which additionally tests the effects of the pre-test.

Example: Four groups are selected in the same random procedure. Two do a pre-test exam; one of these then does the revision course. Of the other two, one does the course and all four then do the exam. The results are compared. It will be detectable if the pre-test exam affected their subsequent performance by comparing them with those that did not do the pre-test exam.

Post-test only – control group design (after only): This is used when a pre-test is not possible, for example in a one-off situation like an earthquake, or during a continuous development, or if the pre-test would destroy the material. In this case, let us assume that only one set of exam questions is allowed.

Example: Two groups are selected in the same random procedure. One does the revision course, the other does not. Both do the exam and the results are compared. The validity of this test critically depends on the randomness of the sample.

Quasi-experimental designs

Non-randomized control group, pre-test – post-test: When random selection cannot be achieved, the control group and the experimental group should be matched as nearly as possible.

Example: Two classes from the same year group do a pre-test exam. One class does the revision course, the other does not. Both do the exam and the results are compared.

Time-series experiment: Identical experiments are repeated. Then one variable is changed to produce a new outcome, and the new experiment is repeated, to check if the variable consistently creates the changed outcome.

Example: A group not taking the course is repeatedly examined. The same group does the revision course and is again repeatedly examined. The danger with this design is that, over time, other unknown factors might affect the results (e.g. with all the practice, the pupils may just get better at doing exams).

Control group, time-series: The same process as above, but with a parallel control group, which does not undergo the variable change.

Example: As above but with a parallel group that does not do the revision course and is used to compare outcomes.

Correlational and ex post facto designs

Correlational is a design that is prone to misuse. After a correlation between two factors is statistically proved, a claim is made that one factor has caused the other. Life is rarely so simple! There may be many other factors that have not been recognized in the research, one or some of which could be the cause or could have contributed to the cause.

Ex post facto is not really an experimental approach in that the investigation begins after the event has occurred so no control over the event is possible. The search for the cause of the event (e.g. a plane crash or the outbreak of an unknown disease) relies on the search for, and analysis of, relevant data. The most likely cause has to be discovered from among all possible causes, so there are many opportunities to search in the wrong area!

Ex post facto *is a common form of scientific investigation, and needs the skills of a detective in addition to those of a scientist.*

Taking it **FURTHER**

Internal and external validity

In order for the experiments to be of any use, it must be possible to generalize the results beyond the confines of the experiment itself. For instance, in the revision course example, that introducing the course in all schools will improve exam results everywhere. For this to be the case, the experiment should really reflect the situation in the real world, that is, it should possess both **internal validity** (the extent to which causal statements are supported by the study) and **external validity** (the extent to which findings can be generalized to populations or to other settings).

Cohen and Manion (1994, pp. 170–2) have listed the factors that cause a threat to internal and external validity, and which are worth summarizing briefly here.

First, those affecting internal validity:

- **History** – unnoticed interfering events between pre-test and post-test observations may affect the results.
- **Maturation** – when studied over time, the subjects of the experiment may change in ways not included in the experimental variables (e.g. samples deteriorate with age).
- **Statistical regression** – the tendency for extreme results in the tests to get closer to the mean In repeat tests.
- **Testing** – pre-tests can inadvertently alter the original properties of the subject of experiment.
- **Instrumentation** – faulty or inappropriate measuring instruments and short-comings in the performance of human observers lead to inaccurate data.
- **Selection** – bias may occur in the samples due to faulty or inadequate sampling methods.
- **Experimental mortality** – drop-out of experimental subjects (not necessarily through death!) during the course of a long-running experiment tends to result in bias in what remains of the sample.

And second, those affecting external validity:

- **Vague identification of independent variables** – subsequent researchers will find it impossible to replicate the experiment.
- **Faulty sampling** – if the sample is only representative of what (or who) is available in the population, rather than of the whole population, the results cannot be generalized to the whole population.
- **Hawthorne effect** – people tend to react differently if they know that they are the subject of an experiment.
- **Inadequate operationalization of dependent variables** – faulty generalization of results beyond the scope of the experiment (e.g. in the above examples illustrating experimental designs, predicting the effects of any revision course while using only one course in the experiment).
- **Sensitization to experimental conditions** – subjects can learn ways of manipulating the results during an experiment.
- **Extraneous factors** – these can cause unnoticed effects on the outcome of the experiment, reducing the generalizability of the results.

The level of sophistication of the design and extent of control determines the internal validity of the experimental design. The extent of the legitimate generalizability of the results gives a rating for the external validity of the design.

Questions to ponder

" What are the relative advantages and disadvantages of laboratory and field experiments? "

The main point here is the control over the variables, which is easier in a laboratory setting. However, when dealing with people, they may behave very differently in an artificial setting so a field experiment might give more reliable results. Anyway, not every phenomenon can be made to happen in a laboratory. Again, it will be useful to illustrate your points with examples. Make as many different advantage/disadvantage comparisons as possible using factors such as the importance of context, complexity, non-repeatability, etc.

" True experiments should conform to certain rules. What are these? "

Refer to the notes given in this chapter. The presence of a control group is significant, as is the control over all variables that affect the phenomenon.

" Why are quasi-experiments still useful, even if they do not produce results that are as reliable as true experiments? Provide examples to illustrate your points. "

Basically, true experiments are not possible in many social settings, while quasi-experiments can produce useful information. You could take each type of quasi-experiment from the list above (pp. 105–6) and provide an imaginary example to point out its usefulness in the context.

References to more information

Apart form consulting your textbooks, here are some books dedicated to experimental methods. Again, check them under your own subject headings.

McKenna, R.J. (1995) *The Undergraduate Researcher's Handbook: Creative Experimentation*. Needham Heights, MA: Allyn & Bacon.

Cohen, L. and Manion, L. (1994) *Research Methods in Education*. London: Routledge.
Chapter 8 gives a comprehensive explanation about experiments. Most books on research methods have a chapter devoted to experiment design. (Chapter numbers may be different in later editions.)

Lewis-Beck, M.S. (ed.) (1993) *Experimental Design and Methods*. London: Sage. An international handbook of quantitative applications in the social sciences.

Dean, A. (1999) *Design and Analysis of Experiments*. New York: Springer.

Montgomery, D.C. (1997) *Design and Analysis of Experiments* (4th edn). New York: Wiley.

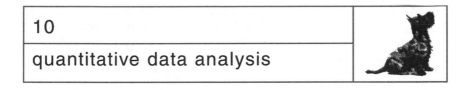

10	
quantitative data analysis	

Managing data

Raw data

The results of your survey, experiments, archival studies, or whatever methods you used to collect data about your chosen subject, are of little use to anyone if they are merely presented as raw data. It should not be the duty of the reader to try to make sense of them, and to relate them to your research questions or problems. It is up to you to use the information that you have collected to make a case for arriving at some conclusions. How exactly you do this depends exactly on what kinds of question you raised at the beginning of the dissertation, and the directions you have taken in order to answer them.

Types of variable

Just a reminder at this point about the levels of measurement related to variables. Investigate each variable to determine whether it belongs to one of the following types:

- **Nominal** or categorical – a name or a category that cannot be rank-ordered. The simplest of these is a dichotomous variable, that is one that can have only two categories (e.g. male, female).
- **Ordinal** – variables that can be put in rank order (e.g. put in order of size, such as s, m, l, xl in clothing sizes, where the difference between sizes cannot be accurately calculated).

- **Interval** – where the measured interval between variables can be accurately gauged (e.g. the finishing times of a race).
- **Ratio** – where the values are measured and relate to a fixed nought value.

> *Sorting the variables according to their levels of measures is important since the possible degree of statistical analysis differs for each.*

The data you have collected might be recorded in different ways that are not easy to read or to summarize. Perhaps they are contained in numerous questionnaire responses, in hand-written laboratory reports, recorded speech, as series of photographs or observations in a diary. It can be difficult for even you, who has done the collecting, to make sense of it all, let alone someone who has not been involved in the project.

The question now is how to grapple with the various forms of data so that you can present it in a clear and concise fashion, and how you can analyse the presented data to support an argument that leads to convincing conclusions. In order to do this you must be clear about what you are trying to achieve.

Creating a data set

In order to manipulate the data, it should be compiled in an easily read form. Organizing your data as part of the collection process has already been mentioned in Chapter 8, but further compilation may be needed before analysis is possible. Robson (2002, pp. 393–98) describes three possible ways to enter data into the computer:

1 **Direct automatic entry** – data is entered on to a database or other computer readable format as it is collected during the research.

2 **Automatic creation of computer file for import into analysis program** – using an optical reading device to read questionnaire responses.

3 **Manual keying-in of data** – using the keyboard to convert the collected data into a suitable format for the analysis program, commonly on to a spreadsheet.

> *The fewer steps required in the creation of data sets, the fewer possibilities there are for errors to creep in. Adding codes to response choices on the questionnaire sheet will simplify the transfer of data.*

The use of rows and columns on a spreadsheet is the most common technique. A row is given to each record or case and a column is given to each variable, allowing each cell to contain the data for the case/variable. In the case of SPSS, the type of variable heading each column will need to be defined on entry, for example integers (whole numbers), real numbers (numbers with decimal points), categories (nominal units, such as gender, of which 'male' and 'female' are the elements). Missing data can either be indicated by a blank cell, or a signal code can be inserted (avoid using 0). You may need to distinguish between genuine missing data and a 'don't know' response.

Accuracy check

It is important to check on the accuracy of the data entry. One way is for two people to do the entry separately and compare the result, although this is a time-consuming method! Alternatively, proofreading, by comparing the entered data with the data set, should uncover mistakes. Use categorical variables wherever possible as the computer program will warn you if you enter an invalid value. Robson (2002, p. 398) also suggests carrying out a frequency analysis on each variable column to highlight 'illegal' or unlikely codes, and box plots for continuous variables to highlight extreme values. Cross-tabulation of the values for two variables will reveal impossible, conflicting or unlikely combinations of values. For large data sets, scattergrans (see pages 116–17) can be used to identify extreme values that could indicate a mistake.

Common pitfall: Don't forget to keep copies of the original checked data set, as these are the raw materials for your analysis. You may want to create altered sets for different analytical purposes, for example with combined variables or simplified values.

Analysis according to types of data

There are several reasons why you may want to analyse data. Some of these are the same as the reasons for doing the study in the first place. You will want to use analytical methods so that you can:

- measure
- make comparisons
- examine relationships
- make forecasts
- test hypotheses

- construct concepts and theories
- explore
- control
- explain

Quantitative analysis of numerical data

Quantitative analysis deals with numbers and uses mathematical operations to investigate the properties of data. The levels of measurement used in the collection of the data (i.e. nominal, ordinal, interval and ratio) are an important factor in choosing the type of analysis that is applicable, as is the number of cases involved. Statistics is the name given to this type of analysis, and is defined in this sense as:

> The science of collecting and analysing numerical data, especially in, or for, large quantities, and usually inferring proportions in a whole from proportions in a representative sample. (*Oxford Encyclopaedic Dictionary*)

Most surveys result in quantitative data (e.g. numbers of people who believed this or that, how many children of what age do which sports, levels of family income, etc.). However, not all quantitative data originates from surveys. For example, **content analysis** is a specific method of examining records of all kinds (e.g. documents or publications, radio and television programmes, films, etc.).

One of the primary purposes of doing research is to describe the data and to discover relationships among events in order to describe, explain, predict and possibly control their occurrence.

Statistical methods are a valuable tool to enable you to present and describe the data and, if necessary, to discover and quantify relationships. And you do not even have to be a mathematician to use these techniques, as user-friendly computer packages (such as Excel and SPSS – Statistical Package for the Social Sciences) will do all the presentation and calculations for you. However, you must be able to understand the relevance and function of the various **displays** and tests in relationship to your own data sets and the kind of analysis required.

The range of statistical tests is enormous, so only the most frequently used tests are discussed here.

Check with your course description and lecture notes to see which tests are relevant to your studies in order to avoid getting bogged down in unnecessary technicalities.

If you intend to carry out some testing as part of a research project, it is always advisable to consult somebody with specialist statistical knowledge in order to check that you will be doing the right thing before you start. Also, attend a course, usually made available to you at your college or university, in the use of SPSS or any other program you intend to use.

An important factor to be taken into account when selecting suitable statistical tests is the number of cases for which you have data. Generally, statistical tests are more reliable the greater the number of cases. Usually, you need 20 cases or more to make any sense of the analysis, although some tests are designed to work with less. On this issue always consult the instructions for the particular tests you want to use. It may affect your choice.

Parametric and non-parametric statistics

The two major classes of statistics are parametric and non-parametric statistics. You need to understand the meaning of a parameter in order to appreciate the difference between these two types. A **parameter** is a constant feature of a population (i.e. the things or people you are surveying) that it shares with other populations. The most common one is the **'bell'** or **Gaussian** curve of normal frequency distribution. This parameter reveals that most populations display a large number of more or less 'average' cases with extreme cases tailing off at each end. For example, most people are of about average height, with those who are extremely tall or small being in a distinct minority. The distribution of people's heights shown on a graph would take the form of the normal or Gaussian curve. Although the shape of this curve varies from case to case (e.g. flatter or steeper, lopsided to the left or right), this feature is so common among populations that statisticians take it as a constant – a basic parameter. Calculations of **parametric statistics** are based on data that conform to a parameter, usually a Gaussian curve.

> *Not all data are parametric, that is, populations sometimes do not behave in the form of a Gaussian curve.*

Data measured by nominal and ordinal methods will not be organized in a curve form. Nominal data tend to be in the dichotomous form of either/or (e.g. this is a cow or a sheep or neither), while ordinal data can be displayed in the form of a set of steps (e.g. the first, second and third positions on the winner's podium). For those cases where this parameter is absent, non-parametric statistics may be applicable.

Non-parametric statistics are tests that have been devised to recognize the particular characteristics of non-curve data, and to take into account these singular characteristics by specialized methods. In general, these types of test are less sensitive and powerful than parametric tests; they need larger samples in order to generate the same level of significance.

Statistical tests (parametric)

There are two classes of parametric statistical tests: **descriptive statistics**, which quantify the characteristics of parametric numerical data, and inferential statistics, which produce predictions through inference based on the data analysed. Distinction is also made between the number of variables considered in relation to each other:

- **Univariate analysis** – analyses the qualities of one variable at a time.
- **Bivariate analysis** – considers the properties of two variables in relation to each other.
- **Multivariate analysis** – looks at the relationships between more than two variables.

Univariate analysis (descriptive)

A range of properties of one variable can be examined using the following measures:

- **Frequency distribution** – usually presented as a table, this simply shows the values for each variable expressed as a number and as a percentage of the total of cases. Alternative ways of presentation are a bar chart, histogram or pie chart, which are easier to read at a glance.
- **Measure of central tendency** – is one number that denotes what is commonly called the 'average' of the values for a variable. There are several measures that can be used:
  - **Arithmetic mean** – this is the arithmetic average calculated by adding all the values and dividing by their number. This can be calculated for ordinal, interval and ratio variables.
  - **Mode** – the value that occurs most frequently. The only measure that can be used with nominal variables, as well as all the others.
  - **Median** – the mid-point in the distribution of values, that is the mathematical middle between the highest and lowest value. It is used for ordinal, interval and ratio variables.

- **Measures of dispersion** (or variability) – all of the above measures are influenced by the nature of dispersion of the values (how values are spread out or bunched up) and the presence of solitary extreme values. To investigate the dispersion, the following measures can be made:
  - **Range** – the distance between the highest and lowest value.
  - **Interquartile range** – the distance between the value that has a quarter of the values less than it (first quartile or 25th percentile) and the value that has three-quarters of the values less than it (third quartile or 75th percentile).
  - **Variance** – the average of the squared deviations for the individual values from the mean.
  - **Standard deviation** – the square root of the variance.
  - **Standard error** – the standard deviation of the mean score.

> *These measures do not mean much on their own unless they are compared with some expected measures or those of other variables.*

Charts and diagrams

SPSS provides a choice of **display** options to illustrate the measures listed above. The most basic is a summary table of descriptive statistics that gives figures for all of the measures. More graphical options, which make comparisons between variables simpler, are:

- **Bar graph** – this shows the distribution of nominal and ordinal variables. The categories of the variables are along the horizontal axis (x axis) and the values are on the vertical axis (y axis). The bars should not touch each other.
- **Histogram** – a bar graph with the bars touching to produce a shape that reflects the distribution of a variable.
- **Frequency polygon** (or frequency curve) – a line that connects the tops of the bars of a histogram to provide a pure shape illustrating distribution.
- **Pie chart** – this shows the values of a variable as a section of the total cases (like slices of a pie). The percentages are also usually given.
- **Standard deviation error bar** – this shows the mean value as a point and a bar above and below that indicates the extent of one standard deviation.
- **Confidence interval error bar** – this shows the mean value as a point and a bar above and below that indicates the range in which we can be (probabilistically) sure that the mean value of the population from which the sample is drawn lies. The level of confidence can be varied, but it is commonly set at 95 per cent.
- **Box and whisker plot** – this gives more detail of the values that lie within the various percentiles (10th, 25th, 50th, 75th and 90th). Individual values that are outside this range can be pinpointed manually if they are judged to be important.

Charts and diagrams are far easier to understand quickly by the non-expert than are results presented as numbers.

Normal and skewed distributions

Normal distribution is when the mean, median and mode are located at the same value. This produces a symmetrical curve. Skewedness occurs when the mean is pushed to one side of the median. When it is to the left, it is known as negatively skewed, and to the right, positively skewed. The curve is lopsided in these cases. If there are two modes to each side of the mean and median points, then it is a bimodal distribution. The curve will have two peaks and a valley inbetween.

Bivariate analysis

Bivariate analysis considers the properties of two variables in relation to each other. The relationship between two variables is of common interest in the social sciences, for example: Does social status influence academic achievement? Are boys more likely to be delinquents than girls? Does age have an effect on community involvement? There are various methods for investigating the relationships between two variables.

An important aspect is the different measurement of these relationships, such as assessing the direction and degree of association, statistically termed **correlation coefficients**. The commonly used coefficients assume that there is a linear relationship between the two variables, either positive or negative. In reality, this is seldom achieved, but degrees of correlation can be computed – how near to a straight line the relationship is.

Scattergrams

Scattergrams are a useful type of diagram that graphically shows the relationship between two variables by plotting variable data from cases on a two-dimensional matrix. If the resulting plotted points appear in a scattered and random arrangement, then no association is indicated. If, however, they fall into a linear arrangement, a relationship can be assumed, either positive or negative. The closer the points are to a perfect line, the stronger the association. A line that is drawn to trace this notional line is called **the line of best fit** or **regression line**. This line can be used to predict one variable value on the basis of the other.

It is quite possible to get forms of relationships between variables that are not represented in a straight line, for example groupings or curved linear arrangements. The strength of the scattergrams is that these are clearly shown, thus needing some discussion and possible explanation. For these relationships, statistical tests that assume linearity should not be used.

Contingency tables

Cross-tabulation (contingency tables) is a simple way to display the relationship between variables that have only a few categories. The cells made by the rows show the relationships between each of the categories of the variables in both number of responses and percentages. In addition, the column and row totals and percentages are shown. These can be conveniently produced by SPSS from the data compiled on a matrix. Patterns of association can be detected if they occur. As an alternative, the display can be automatically presented as a bar chart.

The choice of appropriate statistical methods of bivariate analysis depends on the levels of measurement used in the variables. Here are some of the most commonly used:

- **Pearson's correlation coefficient (r)** should be used for examining relationships between interval/ratio variables. The r value indicates the strength and direction of the correlation (how close the points are to a straight line). +1 indicates a perfect positive association and −1 a perfect negative association. Zero indicates a total lack of association.
- **Spearman's rho (p)** should be used either when both variables are ordinal, or when one is ordinal and the other is interval/ratio.
- **Spearman rank correlation coefficient** and **Kendall's Tau** are both used with ordinal data.
- **Phi (Φ)** should be used when both variables are dichotomous (e.g. yes/no).
- **Cramer's V** is used when both variables are nominal and with positive values.
- **Eta** is employed when one variable is nominal and the other is interval/ratio. It expresses the amount of variation in the interval/ratio variable that is due to the nominal variable.

Check with your lecture notes and course guide to see how many of these statistical tests you need to be familiar with.

Statistical significance

As most analysis is carried out on data from only a sample of the population, the question is raised as to how likely is it that the results indicate the situation for the whole population. Are the results simply occasioned by chance or are they truly representative, that is are they **statistically significant?** The process of testing statistical significance to generalize from a sample to the population as a whole is known as **statistical inference**.

The most common statistical tool for this is known as the **chi-square test.** This measures the degree of association or linkage between two variables by comparing the differences between the **observed values** and **expected values** if no association were present, that is those that would be a result of pure chance. This is commonly referred to as the *p-value* (*p* standing for *probability*). The probability values are sometimes given in reports of quantitative research (e.g. $p = 0.03$ meaning that probability is less than 3 in 100).

A common acceptable maximum *p-value* in social science research is 0.05, but if the researcher wants to be particularly cautious, a maximum of 0.01 is chosen. The value of chi-square is affected by sample size, that is, the bigger the sample, the greater the chance that it will be representative. In addition, for reliable results, the chi-squared calculations require that the minimum expected values of at least 20 per cent of the cells in the contingency table should be greater than 5.

Analysis of variance

The above tests are all designed to look for relationships between variables. Another common requirement is to look for differences between values obtained under two or more different conditions, for example a group before and after a training course, or three groups after different training courses. There are a range of tests that can be applied depending on the number of groups.

For a single group, say the performance of students on a particular course compared with the mean results of all the other courses in the university, you can use:

- **Chi-square** as a test of 'goodness of fit'.
- **One-group t-test**, which compares the means of the results from the sample compared with the population mean.

For two groups, for example comparing the results from the same course at two different universities, you can use:

- **Two-group *t*-test**, which compares the means of two groups. There are two types of test, one for paired scores (i.e. where the same persons provided scores under each condition) or for unpaired scores, where this is not the case.

For three or more groups, for example the performance of three different age groups in a test, it is necessary to identify the dependent and independent variables that will be tested. A simple test using SPSS is:

- **ANOVA** (analysis of variance) – this tests the difference between the means of results gained under different conditions. One-way analysis of variance is applicable when there is one dependent variable (e.g. an exam mark) and one independent variable (e.g. a new study course) and no matter how many groups or tests are involved. For more complex situations, when more than one independent variable is involved and a single variable, then multiple-way or factorial ANOVA should be used.

Multivariate analysis

Multivariate analysis looks at the relationships between more than two variables.

First, let us look at the effect of a third variable in the relationship between two variables. Elaboration analysis method, devised by Paul Lazarfeld and his colleagues (1972), is a set of techniques that involves a set of steps that has been clearly formulates by Marsh (1982, pp. 84–97):

1 Establish a relationship between two variables (e.g. income and level of education).

2 Subdivide the data on the basis of the values of a third variable (e.g. men and women).

3 Review the original two-variable relationship for each of the subgroups (e.g. income and education among men, and income and education among women).

4 Compare the relationship found in each sub-group with the original relationship.

When presented in tabular form, the initial table (step 1) is called the zero order contingency table, for example one which shows a significant positive relationship between two variables. However, this may be a spurious result in that the result is actually influenced more by another variable that has not been taken into account. Therefore, a separate table (conditional table) is set up to test the influence of this variable on the two original ones (step 3 above).

If the two tables show a similar significant relationship between the two original variables, this is called replication – the original relationship remains. If neither table shows a significant relationship (zero-order correlation) between the two variables, the original relationship was either spurious, meaning that the test variable actually caused the association between the original variables, or that the test variable is an intervening variable, one that varies because of the independent variable and in turn effects the dependent variable.

If one of the conditional tables demonstrates the association but the other one does not, then it shows a limitation to the association of the original pair of variables, or provides a specification of the conditions under which association occurs.

> *The elaboration method is a good place to start in multivariate analysis, but its limitation is that it shows what could be happening, but not how and how much the third variable is contributing to the correlation.*

You can continue the process of producing tables for fourth and fifth variables, but this quickly becomes unwieldy. It is also difficult to get enough data in each table to achieve significant results. There are better ways to understand the interactions between large numbers of variables and the relative strength of their influence, for example **regression** techniques such as multiple regression and logistic regression.

Multiple regression

Multiple regression is a technique used to measure the effects of two or more independent variables on a single dependent variable measured on interval or ratio scales, for example the effect on income due to age, education, ethnicity, area of living, and gender. Thanks to computer programs such as SPSS, the complicated mathematical calculations required for this analysis are done automatically. Note that it is assumed that there are interrelationships between the independent variables as well, and this is taken into account in the calculations. The result of multiple regression – the combined correlation of a set of independent variables with the dependent variable – is termed multiple R. The square of this, multiple R2, indicates the amount of variance in the independent variable due to the simultaneous action of two or more independent variables.

Logistic regression

Logistic regression is a development of multiple regression that has the added advantage of holding certain variables constant in order to assess the independent influence of key variables of interest. It is suitable for assessing the influence of independent variables on a dependent variable measured in a nominal scale (for example, whether students' decisions to do a masters degree were determined by a range of considerations such as cost, future job prospects, level of enjoyment of student life, amount of interest in the subject, etc. (see Field, 2000 for details). The statistic resulting is an odds ratio (e.g. a student who was interested in the subject was 2.1 times as likely to do a masters than one that was not, assuming all the other variables were held constant.

Path analysis

The detailed effect of the different interrelationships between independent variables on each other and subsequently on the dependent variable is not investigated in multiple regression analysis. Theories about the types and extent of these interrelationships between independent variables and the effect of these on the dependent variable can be tested with path analysis. It requires the researcher to make guesses about how the system of variables works, and then test if these guesses are correct. The path coefficients for pairs of independent variables can be calculated and mapped to show how much changes in each independent variable influence the others and what effect these have on the dependent variable.

Factor analysis

Factor analysis is an exploratory technique used widely in the social sciences to build reliable, compact scales for measuring social and psychological variables. It is used to package information and for data reduction. Although based on complex mathematical calculations (SPSS will do the calculations for you), the idea behind the technique is simple. This is that if a number of variables correlate with each other, they must have something in common. This common thing is called a factor, a 'super-variable' one that encompasses other variables. This simplifies the explanation of the effects of a set of independent variables on a dependent variable.

Factor analysis starts with a matrix of correlations. Large matrices containing numerous variables are notoriously difficult to interpret. Factor analysis makes this easier by identifying clusters of variables that show a high degree of correlation. These clusters can be reduced to a factor. For example, the level of intelligence may be a factor in the exam results of a wide variety of students studying a range of subjects at different educational establishments over years of results. Factors of this type often represent latent (or unobserved) variables – abstract or theoretical constructs that are not directly observable but must be deduced from several other observable variables. Factor analysis is used to examine the relationship between the latent and observed variables.

Multi-dimensional scaling

Multi-dimensional scaling (MDS) is similar to factor analysis in that it reduces data by seeking out underlying relationships between variables. The difference is that MDS does not require metric data, that is data measured on the interval or ratio scale. Much data about attitudes and cognition are based on ordinal measurement. By using graphical displays to chart the associations between sets of items (people, things, attitudes, etc.) the strength of association can be easily portrayed. The relationships between three variables can be plotted as a triangle – each point representing a variable and the distance between them representing the strength of association. Points closer together have a higher correlation than those further apart. A similar approach can be used for four variables, although the number of interrelationships (six) means that a three-dimensional display will provide a better picture of the correlation strengths.

Obviously, it is impossible to increase the number of dimensions to match that of the variables, so a two-dimensional map based on a matrix is conventionally used to plot a large number of variables. The stress value can be calculated to gauge the amount of distortion required to reduce the display to two dimensions. The pattern of values distributed on the map is then inspected in order to identify any clusters or arrays that reveal patterns of association.

Cluster analysis

Cluster analysis is a descriptive tool that explores relationships between items on a matrix – which items go together in which order. It measures single link and complete link clustering based on data entered on to a dissimilarity matrix. The result of the analysis is a more closely measured grouping than that achieved visually by MDS (see Bernard, 2000, pp. 645–48 for a more detailed explanation). This method does not label the clusters.

Structural equation modelling

Unlike factor analysis, structural equation modelling (SEM) is a confirmatory tool, and has become ever more popular in the social sciences for the analysis of non-experimental data in order to test hypotheses. Its strength is that it provides the opportunity to estimate the extent of error in the model, such as the effects of measurement error. SEM goes a step further than factor analysis by enabling the researcher to test structural (regression) relationships between factors (i.e. between latent variables).

Analysis of variance

Just as ANOVA measured the differences between two variables, the program called **MANOVA** (multiple analysis of variance) enables you to do many types of analysis of variance with several nominal and interval variables together. It is particularly appropriate when the dependent variable is an interval measure and the predicting variables are nominal. It is also able to detect differences on a set of dependent variables instead of just one.

Statistical tests (non-parametric)

Statistical tests built around discovering the means, standard deviations, etc. of the typical characteristics of a Gaussian curve are clearly inappropriate for analysing non-parametric data that does not follow this pattern. Hence, non-parametric data cannot be statistically tested in the ways listed above.

Non-parametric statistical tests are used when:

- the sample size is very small
- few assumptions can be made about the data
- data is rank-ordered or nominal
- samples are taken from several different populations

According to Siegel and Castellan (1988, p. 36), the tests are acknowledged to be much easier to learn and apply, and their interpretation is often more direct than with parametric tests.

Detailed information about which tests to use for particular data sets can be obtained from specialized texts on statistics and your own expert statistical advisor. The levels of measurement of the variables, the number of samples, whether they are related or independent are all factors that determine which tests are appropriate. Here are some tests that you may encounter:

- **Komogarov–Smirnov** is used to test a two-sample case with independent samples, the values of which are ordinal.
- **Kruskal–Wallis test** is a non-parametric equivalent of the analysis of variance on independent samples, with variables measured on the ordinal scale.
- **Friedman test** is the equivalent of the above but with related samples.
- **Cramer coefficient** gives measures of association of variables with nominal categories.
- **Spearman** and **Kendall** provide a range of tests to measure association, such as rank-order correlation coefficient, coefficient of concordance and agreement for variables measured at the ordinal or interval levels.

Common pitfalls: This is perhaps a good place to warn you that computer statistical packages (e.g. SPSS) will not distinguish between different types of parametric and non-parametric data. In order to avoid producing reams of impressive looking, though meaningless, analytical output, it is up to you to ensure that the tests are appropriate for the type of data you have.

Quantitative analysis of text

Content analysis

Content analysis is an examination of what can be counted in the text. It was developed from the mid-1900s chiefly in America, and is a rather positivistic attempt to apply order to the subjective domain of cultural meaning. A quantitative approach is taken by counting the frequency of phenomena within a case in order to gauge its importance in comparison with other cases. As a simple example, in a study of racial equality, one could compare the frequency of the appearance of black people in television advertisements in various European countries.

> *Much importance is given to careful sampling and rigorous categorization and coding in order to achieve a level of objectivity, reliability and generalizability and the development of theories.*

There are five basic stages to this method:

1 Stating the research problem, that is, what is to be counted and why. This will relate to the subject of the study and the relevant contents of the documentary source.

2 Employing sampling methods in order to produce representative findings. This will relate to the choice of publications (e.g. magazine titles), the issues or titles selected and the sections within the issues or titles that are investigated.

3 Retrieving the text fragments. This can be done manually, but computer-based search systems are more commonly used when the text can be digitalized.

4 Quality checks on **interpretation**. This covers issues of:

- the units of analysis (can the selected stories or themes really be divided from the rest of the text?)

- classification (are the units counted really all similar enough to be counted together?)

- combination of data and formation of '100 per cents' (how can the units counted be weighted by length/detail/authoritativeness and how is the totality of the elements to be calculated?)

5 Analysis of the data (what methods will be used?).

Content frames and coding

This is a preliminary analytical method that tabulates the initial results of content analysis in a content frame. A single publication or article is analysed in order to establish codes that can be used as the basis for the units of measurement to be counted. It is essentially a questionnaire that is filled in by the analyst. A separate content frame is devised to investigate each general question, and each column in the frame is headed by a sub-question that is a component of the general one. The answers to these sub-questions provide the codes that suggest appropriate units of measurement.

Tabulation of results

The numerical data that forms the results of a content analysis are most conveniently presented in tabular form. The units of measurement are listed and the number of appearances noted, together with the percentage of the total.

> *Checks should be made on the reliability and validity of the use of the content frame and coding. As the researcher must make many personal judgements about the selection and value of the contents of the publications, other researchers should check these against their own judgements to check on inter-rater reliability.*

What content analysis on its own cannot do is to discover the effects that the publications have on their reader. Other research methods (e.g. questionnaires, interviews, etc.) must be used to gain this type of information. What content analysis can uncover, however, is how the communications are constructed and which styles and conventions of communication are used by authors to produce particular effects. It allows large quantities of data to be analysed in order to make generalizations.

Taking it ***FURTHER***

Discussion of results

Both spreadsheet and statistical programs will produce very attractive results in the form of charts, graphs and tables that you can integrate into your project report or dissertation to back up your argument. The important issue is that you have carried out the appropriate analysis related to what you want to demonstrate or test. Explain what data you have collected, perhaps supplying a sample to show its form (e.g. a returned questionnaire), the reasons for doing the particular tests for each section of the investigation, and then present the results of the tests.

Common pitfall: Graphs, tables and other forms of presentation always need to be explained. Do not assume that the reader knows how to read them and that they are self-explanatory in relation to your argument.

Spell out in words the main features of the results and explain how these relate to the parts of the sub-problems or sub-questions that you are addressing. Now draw conclusions. What implications do the results have? Are they conclusive or is there room for doubt? Mention the limitations that might affect the strength of the result, for example a limited number of responses, possible bias or time constraints. Each conclusion will only form a small part of the overall argument, so you need to fit everything together like constructing a jigsaw puzzle. The full picture should clearly emerge at the end. It is best to devote one section or chapter to each of the sub-problems or sub-questions. Leave it to the final chapter to draw all the threads together in order to answer the main issue of the dissertation.

Tip: Computer programs provide you with enormous choice when it comes to presenting graphs and charts. It is best to experiment to see which kind of presentation is the clearest.

Consider whether you will be printing in monochrome or colour, as different coloured graph lines will lose their distinctiveness when reduced to shades of grey. It is also a good idea to set up a style that you maintain throughout the dissertation.

Questions to ponder

❝ Univariate analysis essentially describes the properties of one variable. What sorts of description are used? ❞

This is a pretty straightforward question. Refer to the list of descriptive statistics relevant to the properties of one variable, such as frequency distribution, arithmetic mean, etc. You can also mention the ways that these can be displayed, apart from simple numerical statements. You can also expand the answer by suggesting how the descriptions are used to gain understanding of the data.

❝ What does statistical significance mean, and what importance does this have on the usefulness of the results obtained from bivariate analysis? ❞

It is a measure of how much the sample selected is likely to be representative of the population from which it has been drawn. This is obviously important when one wants to make generalizations from the sample to the population. You will need to explain what bivariate analysis is, and mention the chi-square test and explain about probability values. Your textbook will provide you with more information.

❝ Why is multivariate analysis inherently rather complicated? How can these complications be tackled? ❞

Pretty obvious really! Because the interaction of more than two variables is bound to be more complicated than just two. There is also the question of which of the variables are independent and dependent and which are intervening. The second half of the question can be answered by explaining the different statistical tests, such as multiple and logistic regression, path analysis, etc.

References to more information

For a more detailed, though straightforward, introduction to statistics, see:

Preece, R. (1994) *Starting Research: An Introduction to Academic Research and Dissertation Writing.* London: Pinter, Chapter 7.

Diamond, I. and Jeffries, J. (2000) *Beginning Statistics: An Introduction for Social Scientists.* London: Sage.
This book emphasizes description, examples, graphs and displays rather than statistical formula. A good guide to understanding the basic ideas of statistics.

For a comprehensive review of the subject, see below. I have listed the simplest text first. The list could go on for pages with ever increasing abstruseness. You can also browse through what is available on your library shelves to see if there are some simple guides there.

Wright, D.B. (2002) *First Steps in Statistics.* London: Sage.

Kerr, A., Hall, H. and Kozub, S. (2002) *Doing Statistics with SPSS.* London: Sage.

Byrne, D. (2002) *Interpreting Quantitative Data.* London: Sage.

Bryman, Alan (2001) *Quantitative Data Analysis with SPSS Release 10 for Windows: A Guide for Social Scientists.* London: Routledge.

Siegel, S. and Castellan, N.J. (1988) *Nonparametric Statistics for the Behavioral Sciences.* New York: McGraw-Hill.

And for a good guide of how to interpret official statistics, look at Chapter 26 on data archives in:
Seale, C. (ed.) (2004) *Researching Society and Culture* (2nd edn). London: Sage.

11	
qualitative data analysis	

Doing research is not always a tidy process where every step is completed before moving on to the next step. In fact, especially if you are doing it for the first time, you often need to go back and reconsider previous decisions or adjust and elaborate on work as you gain more knowledge and acquire more skills. But there are also types of research in which there is an essentially reciprocal process of data collection and data analysis.

Qualitative research is the main one of these. Qualitative research does not involve counting and dealing with numbers but is based more on information expressed in words – descriptions, accounts, opinions, feelings, etc. This approach is common whenever people are the focus of the study, particularly small groups or individuals, but can also concentrate on more general beliefs or customs. Frequently, it is not possible to determine precisely what data should be collected as the situation or process is not sufficiently understood. Periodic analysis of collected data provides direction to further data collection. Adjustments to what is examined further, what questions are asked and what actions are carried out is based on what has already been seen, answered and done. This emphasis on reiteration and interpretation is the hallmark of qualitative research.

> *The essential difference between quantitative analysis and qualitative analysis is that with the former, you need to have completed your data collection before you can start analysis, while with the latter, analysis is often carried out concurrently with data collection.*

With qualitative studies, there is usually a constant interplay between collection and analysis that produces a gradual growth of understanding. You collect information, you review it, collect more data based on what you have discovered, then analyse again what you have found. This is quite a demanding and difficult process, and is prone to uncertainties and doubts.

Bromley (1986, p. 26) provides a list of ten steps in the process of qualitative research, summarized as follows:

1 Clearly state the research issues or questions.

2 Collect background information to help understand the relevant context, concepts and theories.

3 Suggest several interpretations or answers to the research problems or questions based on this information.

4 Use these to direct your search for evidence that might support or contradict these. Change the interpretations or answers if necessary.

5 Continue looking for relevant evidence. Eliminate interpretations or answers that are contradictory, leaving, hopefully, one or more that are supported by the evidence.

6 'Cross-examine' the quality and sources of the evidence to ensure accuracy and consistency.

7 Carefully check the logic and validity of the arguments leading to your conclusions.

8 Select the strongest case in the event of more than one possible conclusion.

9 If appropriate, suggest a plan of action in the light of this.

10 Prepare your report as an account of your research.

The strong links between data collection and theory building are a particular feature of qualitative research. Different stress can be laid on the balance and order of these two activities.

> **Common pitfall:** According to grounded theory, the theoretical ideas should develop purely out of the data collected, the theory being developed and refined as data collection proceeds. This is an ideal that is difficult to achieve because without some theoretical standpoint, it is hard to know where to start and what data to collect!

At the other extreme some qualitative researchers (e.g. Silverman, 1993) argue that qualitative theory can first be devised and then tested through data collected by field research, in which case the feedback loops for theory refinement are not present in the process. However, theory testing often calls for a refinement of the theory due to the results of the analysis of the data collected. There is room for research to be pitched at different points between these extremes in the spectrum.

According to Robson (2002, p. 459), 'the central requirement in qualitative analysis is clear thinking on the part of the analyst', where the analyst is put to the test as much as the data! Although it has been the aim of many researchers to make qualitative analysis as systematic and as 'scientific' as possible, there is still an element of 'art' in dealing with qualitative data. However, in order to convince others of your conclusions, there must be a good argument to support them. A good argument requires high-quality evidence and sound logic. In fact, you will be acting rather like a lawyer presenting a case, using a quasi-judicial approach such as used in an inquiry into a disaster or scandal.

Qualitative research is practised in many disciplines, so a range of methods has been devised to cater for the varied requirements of the different subjects. Bryman (2004, pp. 267–8) identifies the main approaches:

- **Ethnography and participant observation** – the immersion of the researcher into the social setting for an extended period in order to observe, question, listen and experience the situation in order to gain an understanding of processes and meanings.
- **Qualitative interviewing** – asking questions and prompting conversation in order to gain information and understanding of social phenomena and attitudes.
- **Focus groups** – asking questions and prompting discussion within a group to elicit qualitative data
- **Discourse and conversation analysis** – a language-based approach to examine how versions of reality are created.
- **Analysis of texts and documents** – a collection and interpretation of written sources.

Steps in analysing the data

Qualitative data, represented in words, pictures and even sounds, cannot be analysed by mathematical means such as statistics. So how is it possible to organize all this data and be able to come to some conclusions about what they reveal? Unlike the well-established statistical methods of analysing quantitative data, qualitative data analysis is still in its early stages. The certainties of mathematical formulae and determinable levels of probability are not applicable to the 'soft' nature of qualitative data, which is inextricably bound up with human feelings, attitudes and judgements. Also, unlike the large amounts of data that are often collected for quantitative analysis, which can be readily managed with the available standard statistical procedures conveniently incorporated in computer packages, there are no such standard procedures for codifying and analysing qualitative data.

However, there are some essential activities that are necessary in all qualitative data analysis. Miles and Huberman (1994, pp. 10–12) suggest that there are three concurrent flows of action:

- data reduction
- data display
- conclusion drawing/verification

The activity of data display is important. The awkward mass of information that you will normally collect to provide the basis for analysis cannot be easily understood when presented as extended text, even when coded, clustered, summarized, etc. Information in text is dispersed, sequential rather than concurrent, bulky and difficult to structure. Our minds are not good at processing large amounts of information, preferring to simplify complex information into patterns and easily understood configurations.

> *If you use suitable methods to display the data in the form of matrices, graphs, charts and networks, you not only reduce and order the data, but can also analyse it.*

Preliminary analysis during data collection

When you conduct field research it is important that you keep a critical attitude to the type and amount of data being collected, and the assumptions and thoughts that brought you to this stage. It is always easier to structure the information while the details are fresh in the mind, to identify gaps and to allow new ideas and hypotheses to develop to challenge your assumptions and biases.

> **Common pitfall:** Raw field notes, often scribbled and full of abbreviations, and tapes of interviews or events need to be processed in order to make them useful. Much information will be lost if this task is left too long.

The process of data reduction and analysis should be a sequential and continuous procedure, simple in the early stages of the data collection, and becoming more complex as the project progresses. To begin with, one-page summaries can be made of the results of contacts (e.g. phone conversations or visits). A standardized set of headings will prompt the ordering of the information – contact details, main issues, summary of information acquired, interesting issues raised, new questions resulting from these. Similar one-page forms can be used to summarize the contents of documents.

Typologies and taxonomies

As the data accumulates, a valuable step is to organize the shapeless mass of data by building typologies and taxonomies. These are technical words for the nominal level of measurement, that is ordering by type or properties, thereby forming sub-groups within the general category.

> *Even the simplest classification can help to organize seemingly shapeless information and to identify differences In, say, behaviour or types of people.*

For example, children's behaviour in the playground could be divided into 'joiners' and 'loners', or people in the shopping centre as 'serious shoppers', 'window-shoppers', 'passers through', 'loiterers', etc. This can help you to organize amorphous material and to identify patterns in the data. Then, noting the differences in terms of behaviour patterns between these categories can help you to generate the kinds of analysis that will form the basis for the development of explanations and conclusions.

This exercise in classification is the start of the development of a coding system, which is an important aspect of forming typologies. Codes are labels or tags used to allocate units of meaning to the collected data. **Coding** helps you to organize your piles of data (in the form of notes, observations, transcripts, documents, etc.) and provides a first step in conceptualization. It also helps to prevent 'data overload' resulting from mountains of unprocessed data in the form of ambiguous words.

Codes can be used to label different aspects of the subjects of study. Loftland, for example, devised six classes on which to plan a coding scheme for 'social phenomena' (Lofland, 1971, pp. 14–15). These are:

- acts
- activities
- meanings

- participation
- relationships
- settings

The process of coding is analytical, and requires you to review, select, interpret and summarize the information without distorting it.

> Normally, you should compile a set of codes before doing the fieldwork. These codes should be based on your background study. You can then refine them during the data collection.

There are two essentially different types of coding: one that you can use for the retrieval of text sequences, the other devised for theory generation. The former refers to the process of cutting out and pasting sections of text from transcripts or notes under various headings. The latter is a more open coding system which is used as an index for your interpretative ideas, – that is reflective notes or **memos**, rather than merely bits of text.

Several computer programes used for analysing qualitative data (such as Ethnograph and NUDIST) also have facilities for filing and retrieving coded information. They allow codes to be attached to the numbered lines of notes or transcripts of interviews, and for the source of the information/opinion to be noted. This enables a rapid retrieval of selected information from the mass of material collected. However, it does take quite some time to master the techniques involved, so take advice before contemplating the use of these programs.

Pattern coding, memoing and interim summary

The next stage of analysis requires you to begin to look for patterns and themes, and explanations of why and how these occur. This requires a method of pulling together the coded information into more compact and meaningful groupings. Pattern coding can do this by reducing the data into smaller analytical units, such as themes, causes or explanations, relationships among people and emerging concepts, to allow you to develop a more integrated understanding of the situation studied and to test the initial explanations or answers to the research issues or questions. This will generally help to focus later fieldwork and lay the foundations for cross-case analysis in multi-case studies by identifying common themes and processes.

Miles and Huberman (1994, pp. 70–1) describe three successive ways that pattern codes may be used:

1 The newly developed codes are provisionally added to the existing list of codes and checked out in the next set of field notes to see whether they fit.

2 The most promising codes are written up in a memo (described below) to clarify and explain the concept so that it can be related to other data and cases.

3 The new pattern codes are tested out in the next round of data collection.

Actually, you will find that generating pattern codes is surprisingly easy, as it is the way by which we habitually process information. However, it is important not to cling uncritically on to your early pattern codes, but to test and develop, and if necessary reject, them as your understanding of the data progresses, and as new waves of data are produced. Compiling **memos** is a good way to explore links between data and to record and develop intuitions and ideas. You can do this at any time, but it is best done when the idea is fresh!

Remember that memos are written for yourself. The length and style is not important, but it is necessary to label them so that they can be easily sorted and retrieved.

You should continue the activity of memoing throughout the research project. You will find that the ideas become more stable with time until 'saturation' point, that is the point where you are satisfied with your understanding and explanation of the data, is achieved.

It is a very good idea, at probably about one-third of the way through the data collection, to take stock and seek to reassure yourself and your supervisors by checking:

- the quantity and quality of what you have found out so far
- your confidence in the reliability of the data
- the presence and nature of any gaps or puzzles that have been revealed
- what still needs to be collected in relation to your time available

This exercise should result in the production of an **interim summary**, a provisional report a few pages long. This report will be the first time that everything you know about a case will be summarized, and presents the first opportunity to make cross-case analyses in multi-case studies and to review emergent explanatory variables.

Remember, however, that the nature of the summary is provisional and, although perhaps sketchy and incomplete, should be seen as a useful tool for you to reflect on the work done, for discussion with your colleagues and supervisors, and for indicating any changes that might be needed in the coding and in the subsequent data collection work. In order to check on the amount of data collected about each research question, you will find it useful to compile a data accounting sheet. This is a table that sets out the research questions and the amount of data collected from the different informants, settings, situations, etc. With this you will easily be able to identify any shortcomings.

Main analysis during and after data collection

Traditional text-based reports tend to be lengthy and cumbersome when presenting, analysing, interpreting and communicating the findings of a qualitative research project. Not only do they have to present the evidence and arguments sequentially, they also tend to be bulky and difficult to grasp quickly because information is dispersed over many pages. This presents a problem for you, the writer, as well as for the final reader, who rarely has time to browse backwards and forwards through masses of text to gain full information. This is where graphical methods of data display and analysis can largely overcome these problems and are useful for exploring and describing as well as explaining and predicting phenomena. They can be used equally effectively for one case and for cross-case analysis.

Graphical **displays** fall into two categories:

1 Matrices.

2 Networks.

Matrices (or tables)

Matrices are two-dimensional arrangements of rows and columns that summarize a substantial amount of information. You can easily produce these informally, in a freehand fashion, to explore aspects of the data, and to any size. You can also use computer programs in the form of databases and spreadsheets to help in their production.

> You can use matrices to record variables such as time, levels of measurement, roles, clusters, outcomes and effects. If you want to get really sophisticated, the latest developments allow you to formulate three-dimensional matrices.

Networks

Networks are maps and charts used to display data. They are made up of blocks (nodes) connected by links. You can produce these maps and charts in a wide variety of formats, each with the capability of displaying different types of data:

- Flow charts are useful for studying processes or procedures. They are not only helpful in explaining concepts, but their development is a good device for creating understanding.
- Organization charts display relationships between variables and their nature, for example formal and informal hierarchies.
- Causal networks are used to examine and display the causal relationships between important independent and dependent variables, causes and effects.

These methods of displaying and analysing qualitative data are particularly useful when you compare the results of several case studies because they permit a certain standardization of presentation, allowing comparisons to be made more easily across the cases.

> You can display the information on networks in the form of text, codes, abbreviated notes, symbols, quotations or any other form that helps to communicate compactly.

The detail and sophistication of the display can vary depending on its function and on the amount of information available. Displays are useful at any stage in the research process.

The different types of display can be described by the way that information is ordered in them:

Time-ordered displays record a sequence of events in relation to their chronology. A simple example of this is a project programme giving names, times and locations for different kinds of task. The scale and precision of timing can be suited to the subject. Events can be of various types, for example tasks, critical events, experiences, stages in a programme, activities, decisions, etc.

Some examples of types of time ordered-displays are:

- **Events lists or matrices** – showing a sequence of events, perhaps highlighting the critical ones, and perhaps including times and dates.
- **Activity records** – showing the sequential steps required to accomplish a task.
- **Decision models** – commonly used to analyse a course of action employing a matrix with yes/no routes from each decision taken.

Conceptually ordered displays concentrate on variables in the form of abstract concepts related to a theory and the relationships between these. Examples of such variables are motives, attitudes, expertise, barriers, coping strategies, etc. They can be shown as matrices or networks to illustrate taxonomies, content analysis, cognitive structures, relationships of cause and effect or influence. Some examples of conceptually ordered displays are:

- **Conceptually or thematically clustered matrix** – these help to summarize the mass of data about numerous research questions by combining groups of questions that are connected, either from a theoretical point of view or as a result of groupings that can be detected in the data.
- **Taxonomy tree diagram** – these can be used to break down concepts into their constituent parts or elements.
- **Cognitive map** – this is a descriptive diagrammatic plotting of a person's way of thinking about an issue. It can be used to understand somebody's way of thinking or to compare that of several people.
- **Effects matrix** – this plots the observed effects of an action or intervention. It is a necessary precursor to explaining or predicting effects.
- **Decision tree modelling** – this helps to make clear a sequence of decisions by setting up a network of sequential yes/no response routes.
- **Causal models** – these are used in theory building to provide a testable set of propositions about a complete network of variables with causal and other relationships between them, based on a multi-case situation. A preliminary stage in the development of a causal model is to develop causal chains, linear cause-and-effect lines.

Role-ordered displays show people's roles and their relationships in formal and informal organizations or groups. A role defines a person's standing and position by assessing his/her behaviour and expectations within the group or organization. These may be conventionally recognized positions (e.g. judge, mother, machine operator) or more abstract and situation-dependent (e.g. motivator, objector). People in different roles tend to see situations from different perspectives – a strike in a factory will be viewed very differently by the management and the workforce. A role-ordered matrix will help to systematically display these differences or can be used to investigate whether people in the same roles are unified in their views.

Partially ordered displays are useful in analysing 'messy' situations without trying to impose too much internal order on them. For example, a context chart can be designed to show, in the form of a network, the influences and pressures that bear on an individual from surrounding organizations and persons when making a decision to act. This helps us to understand why a particular action was taken.

Case-ordered displays show the data of cases arranged in some kind of order according to an important variable in the study. This allows you to compare cases and note their different features according to where they appear in the order.

> If you are comparing several case studies, you can combine the above displays to make 'meta'-displays that amalgamate and contrast the data from each case.

For example, a case-ordered meta-matrix does this by simply arranging case matrices next to each other in the chosen order to enable you simply to compare the data across the meta-matrix. The meta-matrix can initially be quite large if there are a number of cases. A function of the analysis is to summarize the data in a smaller matrix, giving a summary of the significant issues discovered. Following this a contrast table can also be devised to display and compare how one or two variables perform in cases as ordered in the meta-matrix.

Qualitative analysis of texts and documents

Documentary sources form a large resource of data about society, both historically and of the present. The analysis of the subtleties of text is not a simplistic matter and, as usual in research, there is a wide range of analytical methods that can be applied to documentary sources. Both quantitative and qualitative options are available. Here is a brief summary of the main methods and their characteristics.

Check your course guide and lecture notes to see which are featured as you may not need to know about all of them. If you are going to do some research as part of your assessment, perhaps some of these methods might be applicable to your own project.

Interrogative insertion

By devising and inserting implied questions into a text for which the text provides the answers, the analyst can uncover the logic (or lack of it) of the discourse and the direction and emphasis of the argument as made by the author. This helps to uncover the recipient design of the text – how the text is written to appeal to a particular audience and how it tries to communicate a particular message.

Problem–solution discourse

Problem–solution discourse (PSD) develops interrogative insertion by investigating more closely the implications of statements. Most statements can be read to have one of two implications. The first is the assertion of a fact or a report of a situation, the second is a call for action or a command. This is very commonly found in advertising (e.g. 'Feeling tired? Eat a Mars Bar'). The same, but in a more extended form, is found in reports, instruction manuals, even this SAGE COURSE COMPANION. A full problem–solution discourse will tabulate the results of the analysis of a text under the following categories:

- the situation
- the problem
- the response
- the result and evaluation

The absence of any of the categories in the report will lead to a sense of incompleteness and lack of logical argument. A negative result and evaluation will result in a feeling of incompleteness and may lead either to an apportionment of blame or to a further round of PSD as a response to the new problem posed by the unsatisfactory outcome. Another way of presenting the analysis of PSD is to devise a network in the form of a decision tree that traces the problems and the possible solutions with their implications (very often grouped in threes, and assessed according to desirability, suitability, etc.).

> *Each person involved in the same situation will perceive the problems and solutions differently according to their standpoint and values. Their judgements and attitudes will be revealed by this type of analysis.*

Membership categorization

Membership category analysis (MCA) is a technique that analyses the way people, both writers and readers, perceive commonly held views on social organization, how people are expected to behave, how they relate to each other and what they do in different social situations. Examples of these are the expected relationships between parents and their children, the behaviour of members of different classes of society, or the roles of different people in formal situations. Most of these assumptions are not made explicit in the text. By highlighting what is regarded as normal, assumptions and pre-judgements may be revealed and an understanding of typical characterization can be gained.

The category is the label for the unit being considered. Every person can be categorized in many different ways, but the label chosen brings with it certain expectations (e.g. a factory worker, an executive, a parent). Category modifiers provide some additional meaning to the category (e.g. hard-working parent, militant trade unionist). A membership category device (MCD) is the label given to a particular grouping of categories into a unit, for example parents and children are grouped to make the MDC 'family', bride-to-be and her friends celebrating before the wedding form a 'hen party'.

Standardized relational pairs are expected to perform in particular ways with each other, such as the employee will behave with deference to the boss, the parents will look after their children. The type of expected behaviour is called a category-bound activity. The reader will tend to group people mentioned into membership categories unless it is indicated otherwise, for example parent and child will be expected to belong to the same family, a bride and groom are a wedding couple.

Rhetorical analysis

As I am writing this book, a national election campaign is in full swing. All the politicians are trying to give the impression that they should be believed, and harness the vocabulary and structure of spoken and written language to bolster this impression – clearly demonstrating the use of rhetoric. Rhetorical analysis uncovers the techniques used in this kind of communication.

Rhetoric is used to aim at a particular audience or readership. It may appeal to, and engender belief in, the target audience, but is likely to repel and undermine the confidence of others. For example, a racist diatribe will encourage certain elements on the far-right but repel others.

Any type of partisan writing will contain clear credibility markers, signals that indicate the 'rightness' of the author and the 'wrongness' of others. Typical markers in this kind of text are:

- correct moral position
- alliance with oppressed groups
- privileged understanding of the situation
- deconstruction of alternatives as unbelievable

Even in apparently non-partisan writing, such as scientific reports, where the author is de-personalized, rhetorical techniques are used to persuade the reader about the 'rightness' of the conclusions. Markers to look for are:

- objectivity
- methodical practice
- logicality
- circumspection

> It is impossible to avoid the use of rhetoric in writing. This form of analysis will reveal the effect of the rhetoric used.

If rhetoric is used purposely to target a message or convince an audience, one should be become even more aware of the techniques used in order to uncover the hidden arguments and suggestive language employed.

Semiotics

Semiotics is the 'science of signs'. This approach is used to examine other media (e.g. architecture and design) as well as written texts. Semiotics attempts to gain a deep understanding of meanings by the interpretation of single elements of text rather than to generalize through a quantitative assessment of components. The approach is derived from the linguistic studies of Saussure, in which he saw meanings being derived from their place in a system of signs. Words are only meaningful in their relationship with other words, for example we only know the meaning of 'horse' if we can compare it with different animals with different features.

This approach was further developed by Barthes and others to extend the analysis of linguistic-based signs to more general sign systems in any sets of objects:

> semiotics as a method focuses our attention on to the task of tracing the meanings of things back through the systems and codes through which they have meaning and make meaning. (Slater, 1998, p. 240)

Hence the meanings of a red traffic light can be seen as embedded in the system of traffic laws, colour psychology, codes of conduct and convention, etc. (which could explain why in China a red traffic light means 'go'). A strong distinction is therefore made between denotation (what we perceive) and connotation (what we read into) when analysing a sign. Bryman (2004, p. 393) lists the most important terms that are used in semiotics, summarized as follows:

- **Sign** – a signal denoting something. This consist of a signifier and signified.
- **Signifier** – that which performs as a vehicle for the meaning.
- **Signified** – what the signifier points to.
- **Denotative meaning** – the obvious functional element of the sign.
- **Connotative meaning** – a further meaning associated with a particular social situation.
- **Sign function** – an object that denotes a certain function.
- **Polysemy** – the term that indicates that signs can be interpreted in different ways.
- **Code or sign system** – the generalized meaning instilled in a sign by interested parties.

Discourse analysis

Discourse analysis studies the way that people communicate with each other through language within a social setting. Language is not seen as a neutral medium for transmitting information; it is bedded in our social situation and helps to create and recreate it. Language shapes our perception of the world, our attitudes and identities. While a study of communication can be broken down into four elements (sender, message code, receiver and channel), or alternatively into a set of signs with both syntactical (i.e. orderly or systematic) organization and semantic (i.e. meaningful and significant) relationships, such simplistic analysis does not reflect the power of **discourse**.

It is the triangular relationship between discourse, cognition and society which provides the focus for this form of analysis (van Dijk, 1994, p. 122). Two central themes can be identified: the interpretative context in which the discourse is set, and the rhetorical organization of the discourse. The former concentrates on analysing the social context, for example the power relations between the speakers (perhaps due to age or seniority) or the type of occasion where the discourse takes place (a private meeting or at a party). The latter investigates the style and scheme of the argument in the discourse, for example a sermon will aim to convince the listener in a very different way from a lawyer's presentation in court.

Post-structuralist social theory, and particularly the work of the French theorist Michel Foucault, has been influential in the development of this analytical approach to language. According to Foucault (1972, p. 43), discourses are 'practices that systematically form the objects of which they speak'. He could thus demonstrate how discourse is used to make social regulation and control appear natural.

Taking it *FURTHER*

Hermeneutics

This is not a method for the uninitiated, but it may be useful to know about it, especially if you are reading some research that has been based on this method. Modern hermeneutics is derived from the techniques used to study sacred texts, especially the Bible. It is based on the principles of interpretivism in that it aims to discover the meanings within the text while taking into account the social and historical context in which it was written. Weber's concept of *Verstehen* is closely linked with this approach.

Common pitfall: This form of analysis requires a deep knowledge of the relevant culture and language in order to understand the symbolic references contained in the text.

Phillips and Brown (1993, pp. 1558–67) identify three stages in the process, referred to as 'moments':

- **The social-historical moment** – this stage involves the investigations into the context in which the text is written, produced and read, what it refers to, who it is aimed at and who wrote it and why.
- **The formal moment** – this stage consists of an examination of the structure and formal qualities of the text, using several possible methods such as semiotics or discourse analysis.
- **The interpretation-reinterpretation moment** – in this stage the first two 'moments' are synthesized.

Questions to ponder

" What are the first steps in analysing qualitative data that you can undertake during data collection? Describe some of the techniques involved. "

Apart from making one-page summaries, the process of classification through the generation of typologies and taxonomies forms an important part of analysis that can feed back into subsequent data gathering. After explaining what this involves, you can then go on to discuss the activities of pattern coding and memoing, giving examples of the sorts of code you might use in a particular type of research.

" Explain the difference between matrices and networks. What are the strengths of each? "

These are two major types of display used to present, sort and analyse qualitative data. Matrices are basically tables that can be combined to form meta-matrices. Networks are more like two-dimensional diagrams that form a layout of nodes connected in various ways (influence, cause, association, etc.). You can usefully cite examples when discussing the advantages and disadvantages, for example how a network can clearly show the chain of command in a management structure.

" Describe three different qualitative methods of analysing text. "

This is a pretty straightforward question to answer. You just need to select three of the several methods described in this chapter, for example rhetorical analysis or problem-solving discourse. You will probably need to refer to your textbook to find enough information for a longer answer. Include a discussion of the contexts in which each is suitable for use, and some comparison of their relative merits would provide more evidence of your knowledge and understanding.

References to more information

As you would expect with this big and complex a subject, there are a myriad of books dedicated to explaining all aspects of qualitative data analysis. All the textbooks on social research methods will have sections on qualitative analysis. In the list below, I have tried to explain a bit about the individual book and how it may be of use to you. I have ordered them in what I think is going from simplest to most sophisticated.

Robson, C. (2002) *Real World Research: A Resource for Social Scientists and Practitioner-Researchers* (2nd edn). Oxford: Blackwell.
A brilliant resource book, and should be used as such. Good for getting more detailed information on most aspects of data collection and analysis.

David, M. and Sutton, C. (2004) *Social Research: The Basics*. London: Sage.
See Chapter 16 to start with.

Bryman, A. (2004) *Social Research Methods* (2nd edn). Oxford: Oxford University Press.
Another fantastic book on all aspects of social research. Perhaps it is your set textbook. Part 3 is about qualitative research.

Flick, U. (1998) *An Introduction to Qualitative Research*. London: Sage.
The second half of the book is dedicated to analysing verbal, visual data, with practical advice on documentation, coding, interpretation and analysis. Be selective in picking out what is relevant to you, as a lot of it will not be.

Seale, C. (ed.) (2004) *Researching Society and Culture*. (2nd edn). London: Sage.
This edited book has chapters by various authors, each on one aspect of research. See those on qualitative analysis, choosing whatever is appropriate for your study.

For a really comprehensive, though incredibly dense and rather technical guide to qualitative data analysis, refer to:

Miles, M.B. and Huberman, A.M. (1994) *Qualitative Data Analysis: An Expanded Sourcebook*. London: Sage.
This has a lot of examples of displays that help to explain how they work, but is technically sophisticated so you might find it difficult initially to understand the terminology in the examples.

Your library catalogue will list many more. Try a search using key words, such as data analysis, with management, education (or whatever your particular subject is), to see if there are specific books dedicated to your particular interest. And a few more books if you don't find what you want in the above.

Silverman, D. (1993) *Interpreting Qualitative Data: Methods for Analysing Talk, Text and Interaction*. London: Sage.

Holliday, A. (2001) *Doing and Writing Qualitative Research*. London: Sage.
A general guide to writing qualitative research aimed at students of sociology, applied linguistics, management and education.

Schwandt, T. (1997) *Qualitative Enquiry: A Dictionary of Terms*. Thousand Oaks, CA: Sage.
To help you understand all the technical jargon.

Coffey, A. and Atkinson, P. (1996) *Making Sense of Qualitative Data: Complementary Research Strategies*. London: Sage.

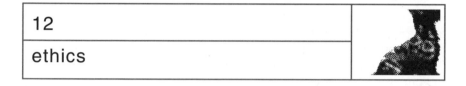

12

ethics

The value of research depends as much on its ethical veracity as on the novelty of its discoveries. How can we believe in the results of a research project if we doubt the honesty of the researchers and the integrity of the research methods used? It is easy to cheat and take short-cuts, but is it worth it? The penalties resulting from discovery are stiff and humiliating. It is also easy to follow the simple guidelines of citation that avoid violations of intellectual property, and which also enhance your status as being well-read and informed about the most important thinkers in your subject.

To treat participants in your research with respect and due consideration is a basic tenet of civilized behaviour. Official concern about the ethical issues in research at any level that involves human subjects is growing. This means that there is a greater need to analyse the methods used in research in detail and to account for the decisions made when seeking official approval. Admittedly, the issues can become quite complicated, with no clear-cut solutions. It is therefore important that you consult with others, especially advisors appointed for that purpose.

Miller and Bell (2002, p. 67) suggest that keeping a constant record of decisions made is a good safeguard against sloppy thinking and inadvertent overlooking of ethical issues.

Using a research diary to document access routes and decisions made throughout the research process is one practical way of developing an ethics checklist. This practice of regular reflection helps ensure that ethical and methodological considerations are continually reassessed.

Ethics are the rules of conduct in research. You must know about ethics if you are required to do some research as part of your assessment. If you have to do an exam, it is likely that you will have a question about research ethics, as this is a really important issue that affects every aspect of research about people.

There are two perspectives from which you can view the ethical issues in research:

1 The values of honesty and frankness and personal integrity.

2 Ethical responsibilities to the subjects of research, such as consent, confidentiality and courtesy.

If you are working with human participants, it is likely that you will have to obtain some kind of ethical approval from your university or organization. It is necessary for you to find out what conditions apply in your situation.

> *While the principles underpinning ethical practice are fairly straightforward and easy to understand, their application can be quite difficult in certain situations. Not all decisions can be clear-cut in the realm of human relations.*

Honesty in your work

First consider those issues which are concerned with research activities generally, and the conduct of researchers in particular. Honesty is essential, not only to enable straightforward, above-board communication, but to engender a level of trust and credibility that promotes debate and the development of knowledge. This applies to all researchers, no matter what the subject. Although honesty must be maintained in all aspects of the research work, it is worth focusing here on several of the most important issues.

Intellectual ownership and plagiarism

Unless otherwise stated, what you write will be regarded as your own work; the ideas will be considered your own unless you say to the contrary. The worst offence against honesty in this respect is called

plagiarism – directly copying someone else's work into your report, thesis etc. and letting it be assumed that it is your own.

> *Using the thoughts, ideas and work of others without acknowledging the source, even if you have paraphrased them into your own words, is unethical. Equally serious is claiming sole authorship of work which is in fact the result of collaboration or amanuensis ('ghosting').*

Citation and acknowledgement

Obviously, in no field of research can you rely entirely on your own ideas, concepts and theories. Therefore standard practices have been developed to permit the originators of the work and ideas to be acknowledged within your own text. This is called **citation**. These methods of reference provide for direct quotations from the work of others and references from a wide variety of sources (such as books, journals, conferences, talks, interviews, television programmes, etc.), and should be meticulously used. You should also acknowledge the assistance of others and any collaboration with others.

Responsibility and accountability of the researcher

You do have responsibilities to fellow researchers, respondents, the public and the academic community. Apart from correct attribution, honesty is essential in the substance of what you write. Accurate descriptions are required of what you have done, how you have done it, the information you obtained, the techniques you used, the analysis you carried out, and the results of experiments – a myriad of details concerning every part of your work.

Data and Interpretations

There is often a temptation to be too selective in the data used and in presenting the results of the analysis carried out. Silently rejecting or ignoring evidence which happens to be contrary to one's beliefs constitutes a breach of integrity. What could be of vital importance in developing a theory could be lost. For example, the hypothetico-deductive method depends on finding faults in theoretical statements in order not only to reject them but to refine them and bring them nearer to the truth.

> *It is difficult, and some maintain that it is impossible, to be free from bias. However, distorting your data or results knowingly is a serious lapse of honesty.*

Scientific objectivity should be maintained (or attained as closely as is practical). If you can see any reason for a possibility of bias in any aspect of the research, it should be acknowledged and explained. If the study involves personal judgements and assessments, the basis for these should be given. The sources of financial support for the research activities should be mentioned, and pressure and sponsorship from sources which might influence the impartiality of the research outcomes should be avoided.

> *It is good practice to admit to limitations of competence and resources. Promising more than you can deliver can be seen as not only foolhardy but also dishonest.*

Where do you stand? – epistemology

There are often lively debates about how research should be carried out, and the value and validity of the results derived from different approaches. The theoretical perspective, or **epistemology**, of the researcher should be made clear at the outset of the research so that the 'ground rules' or assumptions that underpin the research can be understood by the readers and, in some instances, the subjects of the research.

> *Although others might disagree with your epistemology, you should at least make it clear to all as to what it is.*

In many subjects it will initially be a challenging task to become aware of, and understand, all the current and past theoretical underpinnings to relevant research. One of the principal functions of doing background research is to explore just this aspect, and to come to decisions on theory that will form the basis of your research approach. You will have the opportunity to make this clear in your research proposal.

> *Data analysis is an ethical issue and data analysis methods are not ethically neutral. They are founded on both ontological and epistemological assumptions.*

Situations that raise ethical issues

Now let us consider ethics in terms of the personal relationships often involved in research projects. Social research, and other forms of research which study people and their relationships to each other and to the world, needs to be particularly sensitive about issues of ethical behaviour. As this kind of research often impinges on the sensibilities and rights of other people, researchers must be aware of necessary ethical standards which should be observed to avoid any harm which might be caused by carrying out or publishing the results of the research project.

Research aims

The aims of the research can be analysed from an ethical viewpoint. Is the research aimed merely at gaining greater knowledge and understanding of a phenomenon? If so, this kind of quest, seen in isolation, has little or no ethical consequences – the expansion of scientific knowledge is generally regarded as a good thing. The aims of applied research are more easily subjected to ethical investigation. A series of questions can be posed to tease out the ethical issues:

- Are the aims clearly stated?
- Are the aims likely to be achieved by the outcomes of the research?
- Will the results of the research benefit society, or at least not harm it?
- Will there be losers as well as those who gain from the research?
- Are the aims of your research in accordance with the ethical standards proscribed by your university or organization?

> *Aims that are too ambitions and that cannot be achieved by the planned research can be seen as a form of deception, or at least, self-delusion. It is necessary to be realistic.*

Means and ends

How the aims, however laudable, are achieved should also be examined from an ethical viewpoint. 'No gain without pain' is a popular expression, but can this approach be justified in a research project? There are many famous controversies that surround this issue, for example the experiments on animals for developing and testing medicines, or the growing of test areas of GM crops on open farmland.

> There might be several ways that the research aims can be achieved. You should look at the alternatives to see if there are any ethical implications in the choice.

Ethics in relation to other people

Quite obviously, research ethics are principally concerned with the effects of research on people, and, importantly, on those people who get involved in the research process in one way or another. It is the researcher who plans the project who has the responsibility to predict what the effect will be on those people that he/she will approach and involve in the research, as subject, participant, respondent, interviewee, etc.

Use of language

Before going into details about the process of the research, it is worth discussing briefly the important influences of terminology used during the research. Let us look at the use of language first. According to an Open University guide to language and image (1993), there are five aspects to be aware of when writing:

- Age – avoid being patronizing or disparaging.
- Cultural diversity – avoid bias, stereotyping, omission, discrimination.
- Disability – avoid marginalizing, patronizing.
- Gender – avoid male centricity, gender stereotyping.
- Sexual orientation – avoid prejudice, intolerance, discrimination.

The aim is to be as neutral as possible in the use of terminology involving people – who and what they are, and what they do.

> **Common pitfall:** There are many words and phrases in common usage that make unwarranted assumptions and assertions about people, or are at least imprecise and possibly insulting. Acceptable terminology changes with time, so you should be aware that what is used in some older literature is not suitable for use now. It requires you to be constantly aware of the real meaning of terms, and their use within the particular context.

Presentation

How will you present yourself in the role of the researcher? As a student-researcher, you can present yourself as just that, giving the correct impression that you are doing the research as an academic exercise that may reveal useful information or understanding, but do not have the institutional or political backing to cause immediate action. If you are a practitioner embarking on research (e.g. a teacher-researcher, nurse-researcher or social-worker-researcher), then you have a professional status that lends you more authority and possibly power to instigate change. This may influence the attitude and expectations of the people you involve in your project.

Common pitfall: Be aware – how one behaves with people during the research sends out strong signals and might raise unforeseen expectations.

Stopping people in the street and asking them a set of standardized questions is unlikely to elicit much engagement by the subjects. However, if you spend a lot of time with a, perhaps lonely, old person delving into her personal history, the more intimate situation might give rise to a more personal relationship that could go beyond the simple research context. How 'friendly' should you become? Even more expectations can be raised if you are working in a context of deprivation or inequality – will the subjects begin to expect you to do something to improve their situation?

Participants

Participants, **subjects**, respondents, or whatever term you wish to use for the people you will approach for information to help your research, need to be treated with due ethical consideration, both on their own part and on the part of the information they provide. There are a series of issues that need to be considered when you use human participants. Here are some comments on a range of these to take into consideration.

Choosing participants

In some cases, participants themselves choose whether to take part in a survey. If you simply drop off a questionnaire at their house, they are quite free to fill it in or not, assuming that there is nothing in the questionnaire that threatens or otherwise affects a free choice. There are situations, however, where pressure, inadvertent or not, might be exerted on participants.

> *Common pitfall:* Enlisting friends or relatives, people who feel they have an obligation to help you despite reservations they may have, could result in a restriction of their freedom to refuse. Leaving too little time for due consideration might also result in participants regretting their decision to take part.

Freedom from coercion. Reward or not?

Obviously, dishonest means of persuasion, for example posing as an official, making unrealistic and untrue promises, allowing the belief that you have come to help, being unduly persistent, and targeting people in vulnerable situations, must be avoided. Although it is easy to detect crass instances of these, you can sometimes find yourself employing them almost inadvertently if you are not alert to people's situations and reactions.

The question of whether, what and how much to reward the participants is one that is not often posed in research student projects, as the financial means are rarely sufficient to cover such incentives beyond perhaps the inclusion of reply-paid envelopes. However, in funded research this can be a real issue. Some commensurate recompense for time and inconvenience can usually be justified.

Gaining consent

An important aspect about participants' decisions to take part or not is the quality of the information they receive about the research, enabling them to make a fair assessment of the project so that they can give **informed consent**. The form that this information takes depends on the type of respondent, the nature of the research process and the context.

There may be several layers of consent required. When working within an organization, the managers or other people with overall responsibilities may need to be consulted before the individual participants.

> *Common pitfall:* Research can sometimes result in a conflict of interest, say between management and employees or unions. It must be made clear and be agreed at all levels how the investigation will be conducted, how confidentiality will be maintained, and what issues are to be discussed.

This is a particularly sensitive matter in cases where criticism may be made of persons, organizations or systems of work or conditions. There must be some obvious form of protection for those making criticisms and those at the receiving end.

> *Clarity, brevity and frankness are key attributes in providing information on which consent is based.*

Verbal explanations may suffice in informal situations, although a written resumé on a flyer could be useful. Questionnaires should always provide the necessary written information as an introduction. Gaining consent from vulnerable people (this includes children, some old people, the illiterate, foreign language speakers, those who are ill, and even the deceased) requires particular consideration, depending on the circumstances.

> *Notwithstanding any agreement to take part in a research project, participants must have the right to terminate their participation at any time.*

Carrying out the research

Potential harm and gain

Ethical research is aimed at causing no harm and, if possible, producing some gain, not only in the wider field, but for the participants in the project. A prediction must be made by the researcher about the potential of the chosen research methods and their outcomes for causing harm or gain.

> *The implications of involving people in your research are not always obvious, so if there are issues about which you are uncertain, you should consult with experts in the field who have had more experience.*

What sorts of precaution should be taken? Find out how you can avoid risk to participants by recognizing what the risks might be, and choosing methods that minimize these risks.

Other types of harm to avoid are those that may result from the outcomes of the investigation. For example, can the results of the research be harmful in any way to the reputation, dignity or privacy of the subjects? Can it in any way alter the status quo to the disadvantage of the participants, for example by unjustifiably raising their expectations or by souring their relationships with other people?

> *Common pitfall:* Particular care must be taken when the researcher is working in an unfamiliar social situation, for example in an institution or among people of a different cultural or ethnic background. Being aware of the problems is half way to solving them!

Interviews and questionnaires

When recording data, particularly from interviews and open questions, there is a danger of simplifying transcripts, and in the process losing some of the meaning. By cleaning up, organizing, ignoring vocal inflections, repetitions and asides, etc. you start to impose your own view or **interpretation**. This is difficult to avoid as the grammar and punctuation of written text impose their own rules which are different from those of verbal forms. Losing subtleties of humour can misrepresent emotional tone and meaning. Alldred and Gillies (2002, pp. 159–161) point out that speech is a 'messy' form of communication, and by writing it down we tend to make an account 'readable' and interpret 'what was meant'.

> *Common pitfall:* It is easy to impose one's own particular assumptions (e.g. in interviews), especially when questioning people of different backgrounds, culture or social status. Is the content of your interview based, perhaps, on white, western assumptions, or other assumptions inherent in your own cultural milieu?

Participant involvement – experiments, observations, groups

If your research entails close communication between you, the researcher, and the participants, the issues of 'getting involved' and the question of rapport are raised. How will those involved understand your actions and are these in balance with your judgement about your own practice? Your intentions for your research might be to gain as much revealing information as possible, and by 'doing rapport' or faking friendship you might encourage the interviewee to open up. The intimacy between researcher and respondent can resemble friendship. This raises the question: is it taken so far as to deceive in order 'to encourage or persuade interviewees to explore and disclose experiences and emotions which – on reflection – they may have preferred to keep to themselves or even "not-to-know"' (Duncombe and Jessop, 2002, p. 120)?

Sensitive material

Research into human situations, whether it is in the workplace, in social settings, in care institutions or in education, can throw up information that is of a sensitive nature. This means that if the information is revealed, it could do damage to the participants or to other people. Revelations about the treatment of individuals due to the actions of others or due to the workings of an organization may call for action on the part of the researcher that is outside the remit of the project.

Every case must be judged individually, and careful thought must be given to the implications of divulging information to any third party. It may be possible to give advice to the participant about who to contact for help, such as a school tutor, trade union or ombudsman.

It is not advisable to get personally involved as this can lead to unforeseen and unfortunate consequences that can not only cause harm to the participant and other people, but can also endanger your integrity and that of the research project. Take advice from your supervisor or ethics officer if the decisions are difficult.

Honesty, deception and covert methods

An ethically sound approach to research is based on the principle of honesty. This precludes any type of deception and use of covert methods. However, it may be argued that some kinds of information, which can be of benefit to society, can only be gained by these methods, because of obstruction by people or organizations that are not willing to risk being subjected to scrutiny. Injustices might be brought to light that are otherwise obscured by lack of information, such as discrimination, unfair working practices or the neglect of duties.

If the argument is based on the principle of doing good without doing harm, it must be recognized that the prediction of the outcomes of the research are speculative. How can one be sure of the benign consequences of the actions?

> ***Common pitfall:*** The risks involved are such as to make the use of deception and covert methods extremely questionable, and even in some cases dangerous.

Storing and transmitting data

The data that you have collected will be, in many cases, sensitive, that is, it contains confidential details about people and/or organizations. It is therefore important to devise a storage system that is safe and only accessible to you. Paper-based and audio data should be locked away, and computer databases should be protected by a password. If it is necessary to transmit data, make sure that the method of transmission is secure. Emails and file transfers can be open to unauthorized access, so precautions should be taken to use the securest transmission method available.

The Data Protection Act 1998 covers virtually all collections of personal data in whatever form and at whatever scale in the UK. It spells out the rights of the subjects and the responsibilities of the compilers and holders of the data. You can search for a copy of this on the UK government website (www.open.gov.uk) and equivalent regulations on sites in other countries (e.g. www.open.gov.au for Australia, www.usgovsearch. northernlight.com for the USA – a pay-site).

Checking data and drafts

It is normal practice to produce drafts of your work in order for you and others to check it for spelling and grammatical errors and for structure and content. It is appropriate to pass the drafts on to colleagues or supervisors for comment, with the proviso that the content is kept confidential, as in this stage it is not ready for publication and dissemination. It is generally not appropriate, however, to allow sponsors to make comments on a draft because of the danger that they may demand changes to be made to conclusions that are contrary to their interests. This could undermine the intellectual independence of the findings of the report.

> ***Common pitfall:*** It is not practical to let respondents read and edit large amounts of primary data due to the delays it would cause and as they are unlikely to have the necessary skills to judge its validity and accuracy.

Dissemination

You may wish to disseminate your work by publishing the results in the form of conference or journal papers, a website or other types of publication. As this process inevitably involves reducing the length of the material, and perhaps changing the style of the writing for inclusion into professional journals or newspapers, you must be careful that the publication remains true to the original. Oversimplification, bias towards particular results or even sensationalization may result from targeting a particular readership.

> *In most cases, the intellectual ownership of sponsored research remains with the researchers.*

Disposing of records

When the data has been analysed and is no longer needed, a suitable time and method for disposal should be decided. Ideally, the matter will have been agreed with the participants as a part of their informed consent, so the decision will have been made much earlier.

One basic policy is to ensure that all the data is anonymous and non-attributable. This can be done by removing all labels and titles that can lead to identification.

> *When destroying data, make sure that it is disposed of in such a way as to be completely indecipherable. This might entail shredding documents, formatting discs and erasing tapes.*

Taking it **FURTHER**

Ethics policies, permissions and ethics committees

Organizations
All organizations that are involved in research concerning human participants will have set up a code of practice for their researchers. To see typical examples of these types of guidelines, you can refer to the web page produced by the British Educational Research Association (www.bera.ac.uk/guidelines.htms) or the British Sociological Association statement of ethical practice (www.britsoc.co.uk/index). Your university will certainly have set up its own code of practice.

Ethics committees

The role of ethics committees is to oversee the research carried out in their organizations in relation to ethical issues. It is they who formulate the research ethics code of conduct and monitor its application in the research carried out by members of their organizations. Your university or other institution will probably have a system which makes it possible for its research committee to do its job. This, inevitably, involves filling in forms.

Beyond the moral obligations of research, there are forms of behaviour and etiquette desirable in the civilized pursuit of knowledge which should be observed when communicating with people. A considerate and courteous attitude to people will also help to improve their readiness to assist you and provide you with the information you require.

Tip: Remember that you are relying on their cooperation and generosity to make your research possible, and this should be acknowledged in your attitude and behaviour.

You should devise a systematic method of making requests for information, interviews, visits, etc., together with one for confirmation of appointments, letters of thanks, and some follow-up and feedback where appropriate.

Questions to ponder

❝Summarize the major areas in which ethics plays an important role in social research.❞

You could easily write a lot in response to this. Two areas can be highlighted: honesty and integrity in the writing and presentation of the research, and the due consideration for the people involved in the research project. You can then detail the various and numerous aspects within these areas, as is outlined quite briefly in this chapter.

❝What is the difference between being an observer and a participant in a research project? What different ethical issues are associated with these roles?❞

Observing without being involved in the process under examination implies a certain detachment from the events. The issue of whether you are seen to be observing by the subjects is also relevant. Invasion of privacy and lack of consent are two possible major ethical issues here. Taking part in the process raises the concern about how to avoid unduly influencing the proceedings, or being carried away by them. Intimate and sensitive material might be revealed. Numerous other ethical issues are likely to be involved, many of which will be shared by other methods of data collection and handling.

"What precautions must you take to avoid being accused of plagiarism? "

Unlike journalists, it is incumbent on researchers to reveal their sources. It is accepted that all investigation work is at least partly based on previous work, and you must acknowledge the authors of the material you use. As long as you acknowledge your sources, you cannot be accused of plagiarism, although you may be accused of unoriginality! You can run through the different ways in which you can legitimately use other people's writing and thinking, and the accepted forms of citation, reference and acknowledgement.

References to more information

Although ethical behaviour should underlay all academic work, it is in the social sciences (as well as medicine, etc.) that the really difficult issues arise. Researching people and society raises many ethical questions that are discussed in the books below. The first set of books are aimed generally at student and professional researchers, the second set are examples of more specialized books, although the issues remain much the same for whoever is doing research involving human participants.

Oliver, P. (2003) *The Student's Guide to Research Ethics*. Maidenhead: Open
   University Press.
This is an excellent review of the subject, going into detail on all aspects of ethics in research, and providing useful examples of situations where ethical questions are raised. It demonstrates that there are not always simple answers to these questions, but suggests precautions that can be taken to avoid transgressions.

Laine, M. de (2000) *Fieldwork, Participation and Practice: Ethics and Dilemmas
   in Qualitative Research*. London: Sage.
The main purposes of this book are to promote an understanding of the harmful possibilities of fieldwork and to provide ways of dealing with ethical problems and dilemmas. Examples of actual fieldwork are provided that address ethical problems and dilemmas, and show ways of dealing with them.

Mauthner, M. (ed.) (2002) *Ethics in Qualitative Research*. London: Sage.
This book explores ethical issues in research from a range of angles, including: access and informed consent, negotiating participation, rapport, the intentions of feminist research, epistemology and data analysis, and the tensions between being a professional researcher and a 'caring' professional. The book includes practical guidelines to aid ethical decision-making rooted in feminist ethics of care.

Geraldi, O. (ed.) (2000) *Danger in the Field: Ethics and Risk in Social Research*.
   London: Routledge.

Read this if you are going into situations that might be ethically hazardous.

Townend, D. (2000) 'Can the law prescribe an ethical framework for social science research?' in D. Burton (ed.), *Research Training for Social Scientists*. London: Sage.

There are also books about ethics that specialize in certain fields. Here are some examples. You can also search out some in your subject.

Bryson, B. (1987) *The Penguin Dictionary of Troublesome Words* (2nd edn). Harmondsworth: Penguin.

Graue, M.E. (1998) *Studying Children in Context: Theories, Methods and Ethics*. London: Sage.

Royal College of Nursing (1993) *Ethics Related to Research in Nursing*. London: Royal College of Nursing, Research Advisory Group.

Burgess, R.G. (ed.) (1989) *The Ethics of Educational Research*. London: Falmer Press.

Rosnow, R.L. (1997) *People Studying People: Artefacts and Ethics in Behavioral Research*. New York: W.H. Freeman.

part three

study, writing and revision skills*

This section will help you to profit from your lectures and seminars, construct your essays efficiently, develop effective revision strategies and respond comprehensively to the pressures of exam situations. It also provides a guide to writing literature reviews, research proposals and longer research reports or dissertations.

If you are reading this at the beginning of your course, you will find helpful advice on how to consolidate your knowledge of the subject as you are doing your course – it is much easier to revise when you are familiar with the subject! If you have bought this book at a late stage in order to help you cram for the exam or prepare for doing a research project, then some of this advice is too late. However, this is probably not the last course you will be doing in your life, so it will help you in your subsequent studies.

The guidance given here for the longer written assignments will give you a framework on which to base your writing. If the written work is based on research that you have carried out, for example in a dissertation, then you will need to consult the material in the rest of this book for assistance during the research project. I recommend some specialist books at the end for really useful advice on how to set up and organize a whole research project and write a dissertation.

Finally the overall aim of the section is to point you to the keys for academic and personal development. The twin emphases of academic development and personal qualities are stressed throughout. By giving attention to these factors you will give yourself the toolkit you will need to excel in your studies.

---

*Written in collaboration with David McIlroy

13
how to get the most out of your lectures

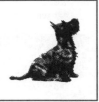

Best quality learning is facilitated when it is set within an overall learning context. Your tutors will provide the context in which you can learn, but it is your responsibility to realize this.

Find your way around your study programme and locate the position of each lecture within this overall framework.

Use of lecture notes

If you can, do some preliminary reading before you enter a lecture. Sometimes, lecture notes are provided in advance (e.g. electronically). If so, print these out and read them. Otherwise use the notes if they are provided at the beginning of the lecture. Supplement these with your own notes as you listen. This will make it easier to learn material the second time round.

Don't overdo it! You are more likely to maintain preliminary reading for a lecture if you set modest targets.

Mastering technical terms

Most subjects require technical terms and the use of them is unavoidable. However, when you have heard a term a number of times it will not seem as daunting as it initially was. Below are some hints to help in mastering the terms you hear in lectures.

- Read lecture notes before the lectures.
- List any unfamiliar terms.
- Read over the listed terms until you are familiar with their sound.
- Try to work out meanings of terms from their context.

- Write out a sentence that includes the new word (do this for each word).
- Meet with other students and test each other with the technical terms.
- Jot down new words you hear in lectures and check out the meaning soon afterwards.

> *Your confidence will greatly increase when you begin to follow the flow of arguments that contain technical terms, and more especially when you can freely use the terms yourself in speaking and writing.*

Developing independent study

The issues raised in lectures are pointers to provide direction and structure for your extended personal study. Your aim should invariably be to build on what you are given, and you should never think of merely returning the bare bones of the lecture material in a coursework essay or exam.

> *It is always very refreshing to a marker to be given work from a student that contains recent studies that the examiner has not previously encountered.*

Note-taking strategy

Note taking in lectures is an art that you will only perfect with practice and by trial and error. The problem will always be to try to find a balance between concentrating on what you hear and making sufficient notes that will enable you to comprehend later what you have heard. Don't become frustrated that you will not understand or remember everything you have heard.

> *By being present at a lecture, and by making some attempt to attend to what you hear, you will already have a substantial advantage over those students who do not attend.*

Guidelines for note taking in lectures

Develop the note-taking strategy that works best for you. Find a balance between listening and writing. Make some use of optimal shorthand (e.g. a few key words may summarize a story).

- Too much writing may impair the flow of the lecture.
- Too much writing may impair the quality of your notes.
- Some limited notes are better than none.
- Good note taking may facilitate deeper processing of information.
- It is essential to 'tidy up' notes as soon as possible after a lecture.
- Reading over notes soon after lectures will consolidate your learning.

Developing the lecture

Lectures are often criticized for being just 'passive learning'. Some lecturers work to devise ways of making a lecture more interactive. For example, they make use of interactive handouts or pose questions during the lecture and form small discussion groups during the session. You can ensure that you are not merely a passive recipient of information by taking steps to develop the lecture yourself.

Here is a list of suggestions to help you take the initiative in developing the lecture content:

- Try to interact with the lecture material by asking questions.
- Highlight points that you would like to develop in personal study.
- Trace connections between the lecture and other parts of your study programme.
- Bring together notes from the lecture and other sources.
- Restructure the lecture outline into your own preferred format.
- Think of ways in which aspects of the lecture material can be applied.
- Design ways in which aspects of the lecture material can be illustrated.
- If the lecturer invites questions, make a note of all the questions asked.
- Follow up on issues of interest that have arisen out of the lecture.

You can contribute to this active involvement in a lecture by engaging with the material before, during and after it is delivered.

14	
how to make the most of seminars	

Seminars are often optional in a degree programme and sometimes poorly attended because they are underestimated.

Not to be underestimated

Lectures do play an important role in an academic programme, but seminars have a unique contribution to learning that will complement lectures. For example, they can:

- identify problems that you had not thought of
- clear up confusing issues
- allow you to ask questions and make comments
- help you develop friendships and teamwork
- enable you to refresh and consolidate your knowledge
- help you sharpen motivation and redirect study efforts
- be an asset to complement other learning activities

Although private study is essential for personal learning and development, you will diminish your learning experience if you neglect seminars. If seminars were to be removed from academic programmes, then something really important would be lost. But, as with most things, a bit of effort will make a lot of difference to the benefits gained. Here is how you can benefit from seminars:

- Do some preparatory reading.
- Familiarize yourself with the main ideas to be addressed.
- Make notes during the seminar.
- Make some verbal contribution, even a question.
- Remind yourself of the skills you can develop.
- Trace learning links from the seminar to other subjects/topics on your programme.
- Make brief bullet points on what you should follow up on.
- Read over your notes as soon as possible after the seminar.
- Continue discussion with fellow students after the seminar has ended.

In seminars you will hear a variety of contributions, and different perspectives and emphases. You will have the chance to interrupt and the experience of being interrupted! You will also learn that you can get things wrong and still survive! It is often the case that when one student admits that he/she does not know some important piece of information, other students quickly follow on to the same admission in the wake of this. If you can, learn to ask questions and not feel stupid. Do speak yourself, even if it is just to repeat something that you agree with. You can also learn to disagree in an agreeable way.

If you are required to give a presentation, here are a few useful hints to make it less stressful and more successful:

- Have a practice run with friends.
- If using visuals, do not obstruct them.
- Check out beforehand that all equipment works.
- Space out points clearly on visuals (large and legible).
- Time talk by visuals (e.g. 5 slides by 15 minute talk = 3 minutes per slide).
- Make sure your talk synchronizes with the slide on view at any given point.
- Project your voice so that all in the room can hear.
- Inflect your voice and do not stand motionless.
- Spread eye contact around audience.
- Avoid twin extremes of fixed gaze at individuals and never looking at anyone.
- It is better to fall a little short of time allocation than run over it.
- Be selective in what you choose to present.
- Map out where you are going and summarize the main points at the end.

Links in learning and transferable skills

When you progress from shallow to deep learning you develop the capacity to make connecting links between themes or topics and across subjects. This also applies to the various learning activities such as lectures, seminars, fieldwork, computer searches and private study. Ask yourself 'what skills can I develop, or improve on, from seminars that I can use across my study programme?' A couple of examples of key skills are the ability to communicate and the capacity to work within a team. These are skills that you will be able to use at various points in your course (transferable), but you are not likely to develop them within the formal setting of a lecture.

A key question that you should bring to every seminar is 'How does this seminar connect with my other learning activities and my assessments?'

15	
revision hints and tips	

Because the subject of social science research methods is a practical one, students on most courses are assessed by having to do a small research project or dissertation rather than doing an exam. Even if you do not have to do an exam, it is not a bad idea to follow the advice below to really be in command of the subject. You will also have developed a very useful personal record of the course in the form of notes that will be really helpful in organizing your writing. If you do need to do an exam, then revision is a must.

Start at the beginning

Strategy for revision should be on your mind from your first lecture at the beginning of your academic semester. You should be like the squirrel that stores up nuts for the winter. Do not waste any lecture, tutorial, seminar, group discussion, etc. by letting the material evaporate into thin air. Get into the habit of making a few guidelines for revision after each learning activity. Keep a folder, or file, or little notebook that is reserved for revision and write out the major points that you have learned. By establishing this regular practice you will find that what you have learned becomes consolidated in your mind, and you will also be in a better position to 'import' and 'export' your material both within and across subjects.

If you do this regularly, and do not make the task too tedious, you will be amazed at how much useful summary material you have accumulated when revision time comes.

Keep organized records

Keep a folder for each subject and divide this topic by topic. You can keep your topics in the same order in which they are presented in your course lectures. Bind them together in a ring binder or folder and use subject dividers to keep them apart. Notes may come from lectures, seminars, tutorials, Internet searches, personal notes, etc. It is also essential that when you remove these for consultation that you return them to their 'home' immediately after use.

> *Academic success has as much to do with good organization and planning as it has to do with ability. The value of the quality material you have accumulated on your academic programme may be diminished if you have not organized it into an easily retrievable form.*

Use past papers

It is essential that you become familiar with previous exam papers so that you will have some idea of how the questions are likely to be framed. Therefore, build up a good range of past exam papers (especially recent ones) and add these to your folder.

> *If you think over previous exam questions, this will help you not only recall what you have deposited in your memory, but also to develop your understanding of the issues. The questions from past exam papers, and further questions that you have developed yourself, will allow you to 'chew the cud'.*

Alternate between methods

It is not sufficient to present outline points in response to an exam question (although it is better to do this rather than nothing if you have run out of time in your exam). Your aim should be to put 'meat on the bones' by adding substance, evidence and arguments to your basic points. You should work at finding the balance between the two methods – outline revision cards might be best reserved for short bus journeys, whereas extended reading might be better employed for longer revision slots at home or in the library. Your ultimate goal should be to bring together an effective, working approach that will enable you to face your exam questions comprehensively and confidently.

> *In revision it is useful to alternate between scanning over your outline points and reading through your notes, articles, chapters, etc. in an in-depth manner. Also, the use of different times of the day and places of study will provide you with the variety that might prevent monotony and facilitate freshness.*

Revising with others

If you can find a few other students to revise with, this will provide another fresh approach to the last stages of your learning. This collective approach will allow you to assess your strengths and weaknesses (showing you where you are going off-track) and to benefit from the resources and insights of others. Before you meet up you can each design some questions for the whole group to address. The group could also go through past exam papers and discuss the points that might provide an effective response to each question. It should not be the aim of the group to provide standard and identical answers for each group member to mimic. Group work is currently deemed to be advantageous by educationalists, and teamwork is held to be a desirable quality by employers.

> *Each individual should aim to use his/her own style and content while drawing on and benefiting from the group's resources.*

Checklist: Good study habits for revision time

✓ Set a date for the 'official' beginning of revision and prepare for 'revision mode'.

✓ Do not force cramming by leaving revision too late.

✓ Take breaks from revision to avoid saturation.

✓ Indulge in relaxing activities to give your mind a break from pressure.

✓ Minimize or eliminate use of alcohol during the revision season.

✓ Get into a good rhythm of sleep to allow renewal of your mind.

✓ Avoid excessive caffeine, especially at night, so that sleep is not disrupted.

✓ Try to adhere to regular eating patterns.

✓ Try to have a brisk walk in fresh air every day (e.g. in the park).

✓ Avoid excessive dependence on junk food and snacks.

16	
exam tips	

Exam nerves are not unusual and it has been concluded that test anxiety arises because of the perception that your performance is being evaluated, that the consequences are likely to be serious and that you are working under the pressure of a time restriction. If you focus on the task at hand rather than on feeding a downward negative spiral in your thinking patterns, this will help you keep your nerves under control. In the run-up to your exams you can practise some simple relaxation techniques that will help you bring stress under control.

> *It is a very good thing if you can interpret your nervous reactions positively, but the symptoms are more likely to be problematic if you interpret them negatively, pay too much attention to them or allow them to interfere with your exam preparation or performance.*

Here are some practices that may help reduce or buffer the effects of exam stress:

- Listening to music.
- Going for a brisk walk.
- Simple breathing exercises.
- Some muscle relaxation.
- Watching a movie.
- Enjoying some laughter.
- Doing some exercise.
- Relaxing in a bath (with music if preferred).

The best choice is going to be the one (or combination) that works best for you – perhaps to be discovered by trial and error. The idea behind all this is, first, stress levels must come down, and second, relaxing thoughts will serve to displace stressful reactions. It has been said that stress is the body's call to take action, but anxiety is a maladaptive response to that call.

It is important that you are convinced that you can control your stress levels. Do not give anxiety a vacuum to work in.

Time management

One of the issues you will need to be clear about before the exam is the length of time you should allocate to each question. Sometimes this can be quite simple, for example if two questions are to be answered in a two-hour paper, you should allow one hour for each question. If it is a two-hour paper with one essay question and five shorter questions, you could allow one hour for the essay and 12 minutes each for the shorter questions. However, you always need to check the weighting of the marks on each question, and you will also need to deduct whatever time it takes you to read over the paper and to choose your questions. More importantly, give yourself some practice on the papers you are likely to face.

Remember to check if the structure of your exam paper is the same as in previous years, and do not forget that excessive time on your 'strongest' question may not compensate for very poor answers to other questions. Also ensure that you read the instructions carefully in the exam.

Task management

Once you have decided on the questions you wish to address, you then need to plan your answers. Some students prefer to plan all outlines and draft work at the beginning, while others prefer to plan and address one answer at a time before proceeding to address the next question. Decide on your strategy before you enter the exam room and stick to your plan. When you have done your draft outline as rough work, you should allocate an appropriate time for each section. This will prevent you from excessive treatment of some aspects while falling short on other parts. Such careful planning will help you achieve balance, fluency and symmetry.

Be aware of time limitations, this will help you to write succinctly, keep focused on the task and prevent you dressing up your responses with unnecessary padding.

Attend to practical details

This short section is designed to remind you of the practical details that should be attended to in preparation for an exam. There are always students who turn up late, or to the wrong venue or for the wrong exam, or do not turn up at all! Check and re-check that you have all the details of each exam correctly noted, and that you take everything that you need with you. What you want to avoid is to arrive late and then have to tame your panic reactions. The exam season is the time when you should aim to be at your best.

> *Turn up to the right venue in good time so that you can quieten your mind and bring your stress under control.*

Art of 'name dropping'

In most topics at university you will be required to cite studies as evidence for your arguments and to link these to the names of researchers, scholars or theorists. It will help if you can use the correct dates or at least the decades, and it is good to demonstrate that you have used contemporary sources, and have done some independent work. A marker will have dozens if not hundreds of scripts to work through and they will know if you are just repeating the same phrases from the same sources as everyone else. There is inevitably a certain amount of this that must go on, but there is room for you to add fresh and original touches that demonstrate independence and imagination.

> *Give the clear impression that you have done more than the bare minimum and that you have enthusiasm for the subject. Also, spread the use of researchers' names across your exam essay rather than compressing them into, for example, the first and last paragraphs.*

| 17 | 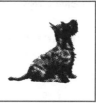 |
| tips on interpreting essay and exam questions | |

Although examiners do not deliberately design questions to trick you or trip you up, they cannot always prevent you from seeing things that were not designed to be there. When one student was asked what the four seasons are, the response given was 'salt, pepper, mustard and vinegar'. This was not quite what the examiner had in mind!

If you write down the question you have chosen to address, and perhaps quietly articulate it with your lips, you are more likely to process fully its true meaning and intent. Think how easy it is to misunderstand a question that has been put to you verbally because you have misinterpreted the tone or emphasis.

> *Be well prepared when you go into the exam room, or address the course work essay, but be flexible enough to structure your learned material around the slant of the question.*

If you are asked to discuss

Students often ask how much of their own opinion they should include in an essay. In a discussion, when you raise one issue, another one can arise out of it. One tutor used to introduce his lectures by saying that he was going to 'unpack' the arguments. When you unpack an object (such as a new desk that has to be assembled), you first remove the overall packaging, such as a large box, and then proceed to remove the covers from all the component parts. After that you attempt to assemble all the parts, according to the given design, so that they hold together in the intended manner. In a discussion your aim should be not just to identify and define all the parts that contribute, but also to show where they fit (or don't fit) into the overall picture.

> *Although the word 'discuss' implies some allowance for your opinion, remember that this should be informed opinion rather than groundless speculation. Also, there must be direction, order, structure and an end project.*

Checklist: Responses to a 'discuss' question

✓ Responses should contain a chain of issues that lead into each other in sequence.

✓ Clear shape and direction are unfolded in the progression of the argument.

✓ Answers should be underpinned by reference to findings and certainties.

✓ Issues where doubt remains should be identified.

✓ The tone of argument may be tentative but should not be vague.

If you are asked to critique

One example that might help clarify what is involved in a critique is the hotly debated topic of the physical punishment of children. It is important, in the interest of balance and fairness, to present all sides and shades of the argument. Therefore, you would look at whether there is available evidence to support each argument, and you might introduce issues that have been coloured by prejudice, tradition, religion and legislation. You would aim to identify emotional arguments, arguments based on intuition and to get down to those arguments that really have solid, evidence-based support. Finally, you would want to flag up where the strongest evidence appears to lie, and you should also identify issues that appear to be inconclusive. It would be expected that you should, if possible, arrive at some certainties.

If you are asked to compare and contrast

When asked to compare and contrast, you should be thinking in terms of similarities and differences. You should ask what the two issues share in common, and what features of each are distinct. Your preferred strategy for tackling this might be to work first through all the similarities and then through all the contrasts (or vice versa). On the other hand, you could discuss the similarities and differences of each point in turn.

> *When you compare and contrast you should aim to paint a true picture of the full 'landscape'.*

If you are asked to evaluate

Some summary questions are presented below to guide you on the best approach to a question that asks you to evaluate a theory or concept in your own academic field of study.

*   Has the theory/concept stood the test of time?
*   Is there a supportive evidence base that would not easily be overturned?
*   Are there questionable elements that have been or should be challenged?
*   Does more recent evidence point to a need for modification?
*   Is the theory/concept robust and likely to be around for the foreseeable future?
*   Could it be strengthened through being merged with other theories/concepts?

It should be noted that the words presented in the above examples might not always be the exact words that will appear on your exam script. For example, you might find 'analyse' or 'outline' or 'investigate', etc. The best advice is to check over your past exam papers and familiarize yourself with the words that are most recurrent.

18	
essay writing	

In essay writing, one of your first aims should be to get your mind active and engaged with your subject. Tennis players like to go out on to the court and hit the ball back and forth just before the competitive match begins. In the same way you can warm up for your essay by tossing the ideas to and fro within your head before you begin to write. This will allow you to think within the framework of your topic, and this will be especially important if you are coming to the subject for the first time. Make a list of the main points that occur to you and put them in a logical order if possible – you can easily change these later. You can also add further points as they occur to you while you write.

Finding major questions

When you are constructing a draft outline for an essay or project, you should ask what is the major question or questions you wish to address. It is useful to make a list of all the issues that spring to mind that you may wish to tackle. Which are the most interesting and address the most important issues? The ability to design a good question is an artform that should be cultivated, and such questions will allow you to impress your assessor with the quality of your thinking.

If you construct your ideas around key questions, this will help you focus your mind and engage effectively with your subject. Your role will be like that of a detective – exploring the evidence and investigating the findings.

Listing and linking the key concepts

All subjects will have central concepts that can sometimes be usefully labelled by a single word. Course textbooks may include a glossary of terms and these provide a direct route to the beginning of efficient mastery of the topic. The central words or terms are the essential raw materials that you will need to build upon. Ensure that you learn the words and their definitions, and that you can go on to link the key words together so that in your learning activities you will add understanding to your basic memory work.

It is useful to list your key words under general headings if that is possible and logical. You may not always see the connections immediately but when you later come back to a problem that seemed intractable, you will often find that your thinking is much clearer.

An adversarial system

In higher education students are required to make the transition from descriptive to critical writing. Think of the critical approach as like a law case that is being conducted in a courtroom, where there is both a prosecution and a defence. Your concern should be for objectivity, transparency and fairness. No matter how passionately you may feel about a given cause, you must not allow information to be filtered out because of your personal prejudice. An essay is not to become a crusade for a cause in which the contrary arguments are not addressed in an even-handed manner. This means that you should show awareness that opposite views are held and you should at least represent these as accurately as possible. The challenge will be to present these in a balanced way and come to some conclusions based on what you have found out.

> *Your role as the writer is like that of the judge in that you must ensure that all the evidence is heard, and that nothing will compromise either party.*

Structuring an outline

It is a basic principle in all walks of life that structure and order facilitate good communication. Therefore, when you have the flow of inspiration in your essay you must get this into a structure that will allow the marker to recognize the true quality of your work. For example, you might plan for:

- an introduction
- three main headings (each of these with several sub-headings)
- a conclusion

In an introduction to an essay you have the opportunity to define the problem or issue that is being addressed and to set it within context. You can also provide a brief guide to the reader on the structure of your essay. Resist the temptation to elaborate on any issue at the introductory stage. The introduction should be written last, as you do not really know what you are introducing before you have actually written it!

Break down the main part of the essay into sections that address the main questions or major issues separately. Use the main points that you drafted out at the beginning. You can then deal with detailed matters under sub-headings. Don't forget to include secondary conclusions for each section.

In the conclusion you should aim to tie your essay together in a clear and coherent manner. It is your last chance to leave an overall impression in your reader's mind. This is your opportunity to identify where the strongest evidence points or where the balance of probability lies. The conclusion to an exam question often has to be written hurriedly under the pressure of time, but with an essay (course work) you have time to reflect on, refine and adjust the content to your satisfaction. Do not underestimate the value of an effective conclusion.

Once you have drafted this outline you can then easily sketch some material under the main headings and sub-headings, after which you will be well prepared for devising the main conclusion and the introduction.

> *A good structure will help you to balance the weight of each of your arguments against each other, and arrange your points in the order that will facilitate the fluent progression of your argument.*

Rest your case: evidence, citations and quotes

It should be your aim to give the clear impression that your arguments are not based entirely on hunches, bias, feelings or intuition. In exams and essay questions it is usually assumed (even if not directly specified) that you will appeal to evidence to support your claims. Therefore, when you write your essay you should ensure that it is liberally sprinkled with citations and evidence. By the time the assessor reaches the end of your work, he or she should be convinced that your conclusions are evidence-based. A fatal flaw to be avoided is to make claims for which you have provided no authoritative source.

> *Give the clear impression that what you have asserted is derived from recognized sources (including up-to-date sources). It also looks impressive if you spread your citations across your essay rather than compressing them into a paragraph or two at the beginning and end.*

It is sensible to vary the expression used so that you are not monotonous and repetitive, and it also aids variety to introduce researchers' names at various places in the sentence (not always at the beginning). It is advisable to choose the expression that is most appropriate. For example, you can make a stronger statement about reviews that have identified recurrent and predominant trends in findings as opposed to one study that appears to run contrary to all the rest. Some examples of how you might introduce your evidence and sources are provided below:

- According to O'Neil (1999) ...
- Wilson (2003) has concluded that ...
- Taylor (2004) found that ...

- It has been claimed by McKibben (2002) that ...
- Appleby (2001) asserted that ...
- A review of the evidence by Lawlor (2004) suggests that ...
- Findings from a meta-analysis presented by Rea (2003) would indicate that ...

> *Credit is given for the use of caution and discretion when this is clearly needed.*

Although it is desirable to present a good range of cited sources, it is not judicious to present these as a 'patchwork quilt' – that is, you just paste together what others have said with little thought for interpretative comment or coherent structure. It is a good general point to aim to avoid very lengthy quotes – short ones can be very effective. Aim at blending the quotations as naturally as possible into the flow of your sentences. Also, it is good to vary your practices – sometimes use short, direct, brief quotes (cite page number as well as author and year), and at times you can summarize the gist of a quote in your own words. In this case you should cite the author's name and year of publication but leave out quotation marks and page number.

> *Use your quotes and evidence in a manner that demonstrates that you have thought the issues through, and have integrated them in a manner that shows you have been focused and selective in the use of your sources.*

In terms of referencing, practice may vary from one discipline to the next, but some general points that will go a long way in contributing to good practice are:

- If a reference is cited in the text, it must be included in the list of references at the end of the essay (and vice versa).
- Names and dates in the text should correspond exactly with the list in the References or **Bibliography**.
- The list of References or Bibliography should be in alphabetical order by the surname (not the initials) of the author or first author.
- Any reference you make in the text should be traceable by the reader (readers should clearly be able to identify and trace the source).

19

writing a literature review

The oft-repeated instruction to 'do a literature review' belies some of the complexities of the task. In order to understand the present 'state of the art' you too need to read what other people have written and make some kind of an assessment of where your research will fit into that body of work.

Swales and Feak (2000, p. 115) explain that literature reviews fall into two basic types: a survey article (an expert's general review of current literature on a particular topic) and a review that forms part of a research paper, proposal, thesis or dissertation. Here, we are obviously concerned with the latter, and in particular with the proposal literature review.

This type of review forms an important introduction to the research project and underpins the argument about why the project is worth doing. It therefore forms a distinctly recognizable section near the beginning of the proposal and leads on to the more specific and practical description of the research activities. Usually, one of the first chapters of a dissertation or thesis consists of a review of the literature relevant to the research subject under consideration. This is a more extended version of what is required for a proposal.

Doing a literature review means not only tracking down all the relevant information, but also taking a critical position on the ideas contained therein.

Critical reading is a skill that needs to be developed.

Assessing the text

Perhaps a better word in this context would be analysis, because the point of the exercise is not just to denigrate or find fault with the style of writing or ideas, but to present a critique, a scrutiny, an analysis, or an examination of them. Providing a description is not enough; your task is to give your own personal and professional appraisal of the content and quality of the text in question. In order to be able to do this, you will have to look at the text from different perspectives to reveal a multi-dimensional view of the work. So, what are these perspectives?

The structure of the argument

You can analyse this by first detecting the conclusion-type words, or so-called conclusion indicators (e.g. therefore, it follows that, etc.), in order to pinpoint the conclusion(s). The main conclusions should normally appear towards the end of the work, though there may be intermediate conclusions scattered throughout. There are then three aspects that need to be examined:

- What evidence is given to support the conclusions?
- Is the evidence credible, that is, does it come from reliable sources?
- Is the logic of the argument sound, that is, what are the steps in the argument that leads from the evidence to the conclusions?

You need to do this kind of analysis coolly, like a judge appraising the argument of a lawyer making a case.

The assumptions upon which the writings and arguments are based

All writing is rooted in theory and based on values, and must be appraised in relation to these. Sometimes these are quite clearly stated at the beginning of the text, sometimes they are obscured or not mentioned. You will need to have some knowledge of the different theoretical positions in your subject in order to be able to detect them and know what they imply. Some common examples of these are: a feminist approach in social science, a Keynesian approach in economics, a Modernist approach in architecture and a Freudian approach in psychology. In each subject there are competing theoretical standpoints with their own values. Only by being aware of these can you make your own considered evaluation of the literature.

The wider context of the work

Intellectual work is carried out in a complex arena where power, politics, fashion, economics, competing orthodoxies and many other factors play influential roles. These can be determining factors in the formulation of views and need to be exposed in order to understand the forces behind them. For example, the forces behind the industrial revolution were formative in the thinking of the day, just as those of the electronic revolution are today.

Comparison with other work

There are no absolute values to which you can appeal in order to make assessments. There are no clear rules about what is right and wrong. Critical reading can, however, be used to make comparisons between texts in order to highlight the different approaches, levels of thoroughness, contradictions, strength of arguments, implications of theoretical stances and accepted values and types of conclusion. This will enable you to group together or divide the various strands in the literature to help you map out the larger picture that forms the background to your project.

Background review for a research project

The review will need to be carried out in four major directions, not just narrowly confined to your specific subject area. Here they are, arranged from the general to the particular, their relative importance depending on the nature of your subject:

- Research theory and philosophy – to establish the intellectual context(s) of research related to your subject.
- History of developments in your subject – to trace the background to present thinking.
- Latest research and developments in your subject – to inform about the current issues being investigated and the latest thinking and practice, to discuss the conflicting arguments, and to detect a gap in knowledge.
- Research methods – to explore practical techniques that have been used, particularly those that might be relevant to your project.

> *Literature reviews do not all follow the same structure, so it is difficult to be prescriptive as to the form it should take. Look at similar reviews to the one you have to do to see the options.*

Research projects usually begin with a review of the background to the research and use this to develop the research problem of the project.

Research proposals should also contain a short review of previous research.

The review should begin with a general outline of the features of the relevant literature.

This gives you a good excuse to introduce literature that supports your introductory statements. Here is a checklist of useful points for you to review the content and form of your literature review, based on a compilation of comments from professors, listed by Swales and Feake (2000, p. 149):

- Make sure that your review is not just a list of previous research papers or other literature, devoid of any assessment of their relative importance and their interconnections. Make an overview of the literature to produce a guide to the rich interplay and major steps in the development of research in your subject.
- Check that the important issues of your research problem are introduced through the analysis of the literature. A simple chronological account of previous research will not give a sufficient thrust to the argument of why your research problem is significant and how it continues the research effort.
- Ensure that the general theoretical background is intimately connected to your examination of the more detailed writings about ideas and specific research that leads up to your own research project. The theory should help the reader understand the attitudes behind the reviewed literature and your own philosophical stance.
- Make links across discipline boundaries when doing an interdisciplinary review, rather than keeping each separate and examined in turn. Many research subjects cannot be hermetically sealed within one discipline, so the connections are there to be exposed. You might even be able to suggest some new links that need to be investigated.
- Ensure that you have included some account of how the previous research was done, so that you have a precedent for your own approach to methodology.

How many references should you have? This depends on the subject and extent of the review. As the literature review part of a research proposal has to be very short and compact due to limitation of space, you are unlikely to be able to cite more than 15–20 authors, 5–10 might even be sufficient in a narrowly defined field. For a literature review chapter of a dissertation or research project, 20–35 references are more likely. The important thing is to select those that are really significant for your work.

> It is a good idea to look at previous proposals or dissertations in your subject area to see what has been successful before.

20	
writing a research proposal	

Before you have to do an undergraduate dissertation or any other research project, you will normally be asked to produce a proposal of what you are planning to research and write about. This will enable your tutor to make sure that the subject is suitable and that the planned project is 'do-able' within the time and resources available.

We have already discussed the literature review that forms a part of the proposal, but what about the rest? Here is a summary of what you need to write.

A proposal is a careful description of what your dissertation or research project will be about and how you intend to carry out the work involved until its completion. It is a really useful document that challenges you to think very carefully about what you are going to do, how you will do it and why. It will be required in order to inform your supervisor of your intentions so that he/she can judge whether:

- the subject and suggested format conforms to the requirements of the course
- it is a feasible project in respect to scope and practicality
- you have identified some questions or issues that are worth investigating
- your suggested methods for information collection and analysis are appropriate
- the expected outcomes relate to the aims of the project

Writing a proposal not only gives you an opportunity to crystallize your thoughts before you embark on the project, but it also allows you to consider how much you will actually be able to achieve within the few weeks/months allowed.

You will not be able to sit down and write your proposal without referring to your background research. A good proposal will indicate how your chosen topic emerges from issues that are being debated within your subject field, and how your work will produce a useful contribution to the debate. At this level of research, you do not have to produce any earth-shattering discoveries, but it is necessary to produce some useful insights through the appropriate application of research theory and methods.

Because the proposal must be quite short (usually not more than one or two sides of paper) a lot of thought needs to be put into its production in order to cover all the matter that needs to be conveyed in an elegantly dense manner. Several redrafts will be needed in order to pare it down to the limited length allowed, so don't panic if you cannot get it all together first time. A really informative proposal will not only impress your supervisor, but will also give you a good guide to the work. It will also help you to focus on the important issues if (and probably, when) you get diverted on to branching paths of investigation later on in the project.

There is a fairly standardized format for writing proposals that, if followed, ensures that you cover all the important aspects that must be included. The following advice will help you to focus on the essential matters and help you to make the hard choices required at this early stage in the project.

The subject title

The subject title summarizes in a few words the entire project. You will probably not be able to formulate this finally until you have completed the proposal, but you will need something to be going on with in order to focus your thinking.

A title should contain the key words of the dissertation subject, that is, the main subjects, concepts or situations. Added to these are normally a few words that delineate the scope of the study. For example:

Temporary housing in the suburbs: the expansion of residential caravan sites in British cities in the 1970s.

Start, therefore, by summing up the core of your chosen subject by its principal concepts. To find these, refer to the background reading you have done. What words are mentioned in the book titles, the chapter headings and the contents lists? These may be quite esoteric, but should represent the very heart of your interest. They should also, when linked together, imply an issue or even a question.

This part of the title will, by its nature, be rather general and even abstract. In order to describe the nature of the project itself, more detail will be required to state its limitations, such as the location, time and extent. Locations can be countries or towns, types of place, or situations. Time might be historical periods, the present, or during specific events.

The previous delineations help to define the extent of the project, but further factors can be added, such as under certain conditions, in particular contexts, etc. A few examples here will give you the general idea:

- in Brazil
- in market towns
- in one-to-one teaching lessons
- in the sixteenth century
- contemporary trends
- during the General Strike
- after motorway accidents
- high-altitude mountaineering

The aims or objectives

The aims or objectives of the project should be summarized in three or four bullet points. This then provides a very succinct summary of the thrust of the research and provides an introduction to the rationale that follows.

> ***Common pitfall:*** If you find it difficult to write your aims, then you have probably not thought sufficiently about what you are actually going to do.

Some useful indicative words you can use are: to explore, to test, to investigate, to explain, to compare, to predict. Ensure that there is an indication of the limits of the project by mentioning place, time, extent, etc. Here is an example:

Social interaction in children's playgrounds in parks.

Aims:

- **to examine the range of social interactions that occur in children's playgrounds in four different parks**

- **to compare the design of the playgrounds and types of park in which they are situated**

- **to explore the possible connections between characteristics of the playgrounds and parks, and types of social interactions**

The background

Anyone reading your proposal for the first time needs to be informed about the context of the project and where it fits in with current thinking. Do not assume that the reader knows anything about the subject, so introduce it in such a way that any intelligent person can understand the main issues surrounding your work. That is the one function of the background section. The other function is to convince your supervisor that you have done the necessary reading into the subject, and that you have reviewed the literature sufficiently. This is why it is necessary to have a good range of references in this section. See Chapter 19 on how to write a literature review.

Defining the research problem

Based on the issues explained and discussed in the background section you should be able to identify the particular part of the subject that you want to investigate.

Common pitfall: Every subject could be studied for a lifetime, so it is important that you isolate just one small facet of the subject that you can manageably deal with in the short amount of time that you are given.

Once you have explained the topic of your study, and argued why it is necessary to do work in this area, it is a good idea briefly to state the research problem in one or two clear sentences. This will be a direct reflection of your title, and will sum up the central question or problem that you will be investigating.

A clear definition of the research problem is an essential ingredient of a proposal; after all, the whole project hinges on this.

The nature of the problem also determines the issues that you will explore, the kind of information that you will collect, and the types of analysis that you will use. The main research problem should grow naturally and inevitably out of your discussion of the background. You can state it clearly as a question, hypothesis, etc. Then explain briefly how it will be broken down into sub-problems, hypotheses, etc. in order to make it practicable to research. There should be a connection between these and the aims or objectives of the project – everything should link up neatly.

The main concepts and variables

Every subject has its own way of looking at things, its own terminology and its own ways of measuring. Consider the differences between analysing the text of a Shakespearean play and the data transmitted back from a space probe. You will certainly be familiar with some of the concepts that are important in your subject – just look at the title you have chosen for examples of these. It will probably be necessary to define the main concepts in order to dispel any doubts as to their exact meaning. There might even be some dispute in the literature about terminology. If so, highlight the nature of the discussion.

A mention of the indicators that are used to make the concepts recognizable will be the first step to breaking down the abstract nature of most concepts. Then a description of the variables that are the measurable components of the indicators can be used to demonstrate how you will actually be able to collect and analyse the relevant data to come to conclusions about the concepts and their nature.

You do not need to write much here, just enough to convince the reader that you are clear as to how you can investigate the abstract concepts with which you might be dealing, for example suitability, success, creativity, quality of life, etc. Even well-known terms might need to be broken down to ensure that the reader understands just how you will study them.

Methods

What exactly will you do in order to collect and analyse the necessary information? This is the practical part of the proposal where you explain what you will do, how you will do it, and why. It is important to demonstrate the way that your research activities relate to the aims or objectives of your project and thus will enable you to come to conclusions relevant to the research problem. Different methods will be required for different parts of the research. At this stage you need not know in detail just how you will implement them, but you should quite easily be able to choose those that seem appropriate for different aspects of your inquiry. Consider the following actions that you might need to take:

- Do a literature search and critical analysis of sources.
- Consult with experts.
- Identify research population(s), situations, possible case studies.
- Select samples – size of sample(s), location of sample(s), number of case studies.
- Collect data (quantitative, qualitative and combination of both) – question-naires, interviews, study of documents, observations, etc.
- Set up experiments or models and run them.
- Analyse data – statistical tests, enumerating and classifying, data displays for data reduction and analysis.
- Evaluate results of analysis – summarizing and coming to conclusions.

It is best to spell out what you intend to do in relation to each sub-problem or question when they require different methods of data collection and analysis. Try to be precise and add reasons for what you are planning to do (i.e. add the phrase 'in order to ...'). This methods section of the proposal can be in the form of a list of actions.

This whole process will need quite a lot of thought and preparation, especially as you will not be familiar with some of the research methods. But time spent now to make informed decisions is well spent. It will make you much more confident that you can plan your project, that you have not overreached yourself, and that you have decided on activities that you will enjoy doing.

Expected outcomes

It is a good idea to spell out to the reader, and to yourself, just what you hope will be achieved by doing all this work. Since the proposal is a type of contract to deliver certain results, it is a mistake to 'promise mountains and deliver molehills'. Although you cannot predict exactly what the outcomes will be (if you could, there would be little point in carrying out the research), you should try to be quite precise as to the nature and scope of the outcomes and as to who might benefit from the information. Obviously you should make sure that the outcomes relate directly to the aims of the research that you described at the beginning of the proposal. The outcomes may be a contribution at a practical and/or theoretical level.

Programme of work

A simple bar chart showing the available time in weeks and the list of tasks you will need to complete, and their sequence and duration, will be a sufficient programme of work. Don't forget to give yourself plenty of time to write up and present your dissertation. You will quickly spot if you have been too ambitious in your intentions if the tasks just will not fit realistically into time allowed. If you see problems ahead, now is the time to adjust your proposal to make it more feasible. Reduce the scope of the investigations by narrowing the problem still further (you can do this by becoming more specific and by reducing the number of sub-problems or questions), being less ambitious with the amount of data to collect, and by simplifying the analytical stages.

21	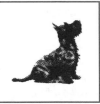
writing up a dissertation or research project	

Your dissertation is probably your first lengthy piece of independent writing. The big question when faced with such a task is how to structure the work so that it forms an integral whole. The structure will provide a guide to the reader, as well as providing a framework for you to fill in as you are writing it. In academic-type writing, the aim is not to tell a story as one might in a novel, but to set up an argument to support a particular view, analysis or conclusion. In fact, argument will pervade all that you write – you will be trying to persuade the reader that what you have done is worthwhile and based on some kind of intellectual process.

Whatever the subject of the inquiry, there has to be a focus, a central issue that is being considered. You should be able to define this quite clearly when you prepare your proposal, by explanation and persuasion.

The body of the dissertation will then revolve around this focal point, perhaps considering it from different perspectives, or examining causes or finding explanations for the situation. At the end you will have to come to some conclusions, and this is where argument is required. You will need to base these conclusions on evidence, and you should produce some reasoned argument about how this evidence leads to your conclusions.

When to start writing up

> *Common pitfal:* To sit down in front of a blank computer monitor with the task of writing a 20,000 word dissertation is a daunting prospect and one to be avoided. It is not difficult to avoid being faced with this situation.

The trick is to gradually amass a collection of notes, observations and data on the issues relevant to your study, which you can then use as a basis for your first draft. This way, you will have started writing your dissertation without even realizing it!

To lessen the anguish of starting writing up late on in the programme, it helps to build up your first draft from an early stage. To be able to do this you will need to prepare a structure for the dissertation as soon as you are clear what you will be doing. You can devise this in outline after you have done some background reading and completed your proposal. The structure will then provide a framework into which you can insert your text. Don't expect either the framework or the text to be the final version. Both will need refining and revising as your work and understanding progresses. Luckily, word processors make revision very quick and easy.

The issue of writing style should be considered at this point. As a dissertation is an academic piece of work, generally a more formal style is adopted. This, at its extreme, avoids the personal pronoun, I, altogether.

> *It is a good idea to raise the issue of style when you discuss your work with your tutor. There may be some indications given in the assignment details – you should read these carefully anyway for instructions on what is expected of you.*

Frame and fill

The framework for your dissertation is most easily created by making a list of possible chapter or section headings. Consult your proposal and plan of work for indications of what these may be. At the very simplest level, the divisions may be like this:

1 Introduction

2 Background

3 The main issues

4 Research methods

5 The research actions and results

6 Conclusions

This assumes that you will use the background reading to clarify the main issues of your research; that you will use one or several research methods to delve more deeply into these issues; that this will produce some data or results that you will present and analyse; and that you will be able to draw some conclusions from this analysis in relation to the main issues explained in point 3. This is a conventional format and can be applied to a study in almost any subject. There are other, unconventional, ways of organizing a dissertation. If you do want to use an unusual structure or even want to develop your own, it is best to discuss this with your supervisor to check that it will be acceptable. The main thing is that you can set up a convincing overall argument that leads from your intentions to your conclusions.

Once you have the main framework, you can elaborate on the contents of each section by inserting sub-headings indicating the aspects that you want to cover in each. Just use your current knowledge and a bit of imagination at first to suggest relevant sub-headings. This will help to establish the thread of your argument. You will be able to reorder, expand or change these as you progress. An example of sub-headings is given below:

Introduction

- The main aims of the dissertation

- A short summary of the context of the study

- The main problems or issues to be investigated

- The overall approach to the project

- A short description of the structure of the dissertation

Background

- Aspects of the subject investigated

- Historical and current context

- Evidence of problems or contentious issues

- Current debate – comparison of different opinions or approaches

- Shortcomings in the level of knowledge

The main issues

- A summary of the main problem or issue and how it can be divided into different aspects or sub-problems

- First aspect/sub-problem described and analysed

- Second aspect/sub-problem described and analysed

- Third aspect/sub-problem described and analysed

Research methods

- General approach to investigation (philosophy?)

- Alternative methods discussed

- Selection and description of methods related to aspects/sub-problems (experiment, survey, modelling, accounts, archival analysis, case study, historical, etc.)

- Selection of samples or case studies (if you are doing a survey or choosing particular examples for detail study), pilot study

- Methods of presentation of results (e.g. charts, graphs, diagrams, spreadsheets, mathematical calculations, commentaries, etc.)

- Analytical methods used (statistical tests – specify which ones, comparisons, coding, systems analysis, **algorithms**, models, diagramming, etc.)

Research actions and results

- Description of actions taken (use a heading for each type of action, for example questionnaires, interviews, observations, textual analysis, etc.), possibly related to the different aspects/sub-problems

- Results of actions (give account of data collected from each of the actions above), again, possibly related to the different aspects/sub-problems

Conclusions

- Conclusions drawn from sets of data in relation to the main issues (this can be separated into sections for each aspect/sub-problem

- Overall conclusions of the dissertation

I have kept the sub-headings as general as possible so that you can apply these or something equivalent in the context of your subject. You will have to use your imagination and judgement to assess if this arrangement actually suits what you want to do. Devise your own sequence if you like, but note the overall pattern of identifying issues from background study, the definition of how you will investigate these, and how you will present the information gained and how this will be analysed to enable you to come to conclusions.

> ***Common pitfall:*** You don't have to start writing your text at the beginning and continue to the end.

Use what notes you have got so far and insert them where they are relevant in order to fill in the framework. If you have the notes already written on computer, then you can simply copy and paste them in a rough order under the appropriate headings and sub-headings. If you have recorded them on paper, now is the time to transfer them into the word processor. You will thus quickly have several pages of (very) rough draft.

However, be warned. Even though it might look pretty impressive, the text will be no more than a series of raw notes, completely unedited, disjointed and incomplete. But it will provide a solid basis for working on to produce a first draft.

Marshalling your notes and drafting your text

You will probably be told what the overall length of your dissertation is required to be. If not, find out by asking your tutor, or consult previous dissertations written in your course. You need to know this in order to determine how long each section should be to get a balanced result. As a guide, 5,000 words are equivalent to about 25 double-space typed pages. Taking the above six-chapter arrangement, a balanced proportion of content might be as follows:

- Introduction – 5%. This serves as a guide to the dissertation for the reader.
- Background – 20%. A review of the literature and information about the context of the study.
- The main issues – 10%. The main points or problems arising from the background that your research will tackle.
- Research methods – 10%. A description of the steps you will take and techniques you will use to investigate the main issues. Reasons for using these methods must also be included.
- The research actions and results – 35%. A record of what you did and what results came out of your investigations. You might split this into two or three sections if you are investigating two or three different issues.
- Conclusions – 15%. An interpretation of the results in the light of the main issues.
- The remaining 5% will be ancillary matter such as the abstract or summary, list of contents, bibliography, etc.

Now you will be ready to start inserting your notes into your structure. How do you get the right notes in the right place? This is where your retrieval techniques will be put to the test. Assuming that your framework gives you enough indication of what you are looking for, search through your notes by keyword or subject. If you do this on the computer, you will be shown a selection of relevant notes, from which you can choose what you think is suitable for that section. You can do this manually with notes on paper. Other useful search parameters may be date or author.

For the introduction, just insert your proposal for now. You will be able to use this, suitably edited, when you have finished the rest of the writing, to explain the nature of the dissertation. You will add more later to explain the structure of the dissertation.

Your proposal will indicate the sorts of area that your background study will need to cover. There are likely to be several aspects of the subject that need looking at, for example historical precedents, conflicting opinions, political/financial/organizational/social aspects, etc.

> At this stage you will need to define the limits of your study clearly – you only have a short time to complete it, so keep it manageable.

Revisions

The nice thing about using a word processor is that you can easily change things after you have written them. This takes off the pressure of getting everything right first time – something that is impossible to do anyway. Once your work is on paper, then you can review it, get a second opinion on it, and discuss it. You cannot do these if it is still all in your head. Hence the importance to get on with writing as soon as possible.

You don't have to finish the dissertation or even a section of it before you revise it. You can use the process to accumulate your written material, adding to the latest version as the information comes in or as you get the writing bug. Regularly reviewing what you have done so far and to what quality will keep you aware of how far you have progressed and what still needs to be done. It also enables you to break down the work into small sections – revising, altering and expanding sections as your understanding develops. The text will thus evolve as a series of small steps that should need no drastic revision at the last moment.

> Regard the making of revisions to be an integral part of the process of doing a dissertation. You will of course have to include some time for this in your time plan.

Revising can be done at different levels. The more general levels are concerned with getting the structure and sequence right. Revision might entail moving around headings and blocks of text. Apart from the content of the text, you may want to try out different page layouts and formatting. At a more detailed level, you might look at the sequence of paragraphs: Does each concentrate on one point? Do they follow each other in the right sequence? At the most detailed level you will be looking at grammar, punctuation, vocabulary and spelling.

I find that it is much easier to review what I have written when it is printed out on paper rather that reading it from the screen – I can get a better overview of the layout, length of sections, and line of the argument. If your eyesight is good, decrease the font size (perhaps 8 point) before printing, both to save paper and to make it easier to have an overall view of the work. You will quickly spot gaps, dislocations in the sequence and imbalances in the length of sections.

It is important to keep track of your revisions – make sure you know what the latest one is! The best way is to save your revision as a new file, clearly labelled with a revision number (e.g. Chapter 3/1, 3/2, etc.) You will thus be able to go back to a previous revision if you change your mind or want to check on some detail. Most word-processing programs also provide a facility for keeping track of revisions.

Coming to conclusions

The whole point of collecting data and analysing it is so that you can come to some conclusions that answer your research questions and achieve the aims of your dissertation project.

> ***Common pitfall:*** The trouble with this part of the dissertation is that it inevitably comes near the end of your project, when you are probably tired from all the work you have already done, when your time is running out, when you have pressures from other commitments such as revision and exams. Let alone all the other things you want to get in before your undergraduate days are over.

To compound it all, the coming to conclusions is a demanding and creative process that requires a lot of clear thinking, perception and meticulous care. All the previous work will be devalued if you do not sufficiently draw out the implications of your analysis and capitalize on the insights that it affords. You cannot rely on the reader to make inferences from your results. It really is up to you to explain vividly how the results of your analysis provide evidence for new insight into your chosen subject and answer the particular research questions that you posed at the beginning of the dissertation.

> *The main point I want to make is that you should allocate some time for this process, and not underestimate its importance.*

Ideally, you will have the research question(s) at the forefront of your mind throughout your time working on your dissertation. However, this is not always possible as you grapple with learning new techniques, methods and the problems of organizing your data collection and analysis. However, you must come back to your research question(s) regularly in order to ensure that you are keeping to the intentions of the project, and will end up with relevant material in order to be able to suggest answers to the questions.

Coming to conclusions is a cumulative process. It is unlikely that the problem you have chosen is simple, with questions raised that can be answered with a simple yes or no. Even if they can, you will be required to describe why it is one or the other and make an argument to support your case. Normally, you will find that the questions have several sub-questions, and even these can be broken down into components requiring separate investigation. Throughout the analysis part of your work you will be able to make conclusions about these fragments of the main issues. The skill is to gather these up at the end in the concluding chapter to fit them together into a 'mosaic' that will present the complete picture of the conclusion to the entire dissertation.

> *Just as you should be able to summarize the main problem that your dissertation addresses in one or two sentences, so you should be able to state the conclusion equally briefly.*

This belies the complexities that lie in between. You can picture your dissertation as having a continuous thread of argument running through it. The beginning and end of the argument is fat and tightly woven but, in between, the separate strands fan out, become twisted and frayed as different aspects are investigated, but manage to web together before reaching the end.

> The secret to success lies in the sound construction of your argument.

References to more information

There are loads of books on advice for students for different aspects of study. I have picked a range of books that will provide more information than was possible in the short summary above. Have a look at them in your library to see what you will find to be most useful before buying.

Let's start with three on studying in general:

King, D. and Evans, K. (2005) *Studying Society: Study Skills in the Social Sciences*. London: Sage.

McIlroy, D. (2003) *Studying at University: How to be a successful student*. London: Sage.

Turner, J. (2002) *How to Study*. London: Sage.

You can quickly get into deep water on the subject of thinking and argument. I would recommend the following to start with:

Brink-Budgen, R. (2000) *Critical Thinking for Students: Learn the Skills of Critical Assessment and Effective Argument* (3rd edn). Oxford: How To Books.

Thouless, R.H. (1974) *Straight and Crooked Thinking* (rev. edn). London: Pan Books. Old, but still entertaining and thought provoking.

Here is one on exams:

McIlroy, D. (2005) *Exam Success*. London: Sage.

These are worth a look for aspects of writing and doing essays and literature reviews:

Taylor, G. (1989) *The Student's Writing Guide for the Arts and Social Sciences*. Cambridge: Cambridge University Press.

Redman, P. (2001) *Good Essay Writing*. London: Sage.

Hart, C. (1998) *Doing a Literature Review*. London: Sage in association with The Open University.

There are books that are solely dedicated to writing academic proposals of all kinds. The principles are the same for all of them, it is the extent and detail that varies. Some will be rather too detailed for your purposes, but you will undoubtedly find something useful. I have put them in order of complexity, with the simplest first. Every book on how to do dissertations will also have a section on writing a proposal.

Jay, R. (2000) *How To Write Proposals and Reports That Get Results*. London: Prentice Hall.

Vithal, R. (1997) *Designing Your First Research Proposal: A Manual for Researchers in Education*. Cape Town: Juta.

Locke, L.F. (1993) *Proposals That Work: A Guide for Planning Dissertations and Grant Proposals* (3rd edn). London: Sage.

Coley, S.M. and Scheinberg, C.A. (1990) *Proposal Writing*. Newbury Park, CA: Sage. Published in cooperation with the University of Michigan.

And if you will be doing a dissertation or research project, try two other books written by me:

Walliman, N. (2004) *Your Undergraduate Dissertation: The Essential Guide for Success*. London: Sage.

Walliman, N. (2005) *Your Research Project: A Step-by-Step Guide for the First-Time Researcher* (2nd edn). London: Sage.

glossary

Accidental sampling Also called convenience sampling. A non-random sampling technique that involves selecting what is immediately available, for example studying the building you happen to be in or examining the work practices of your firm.

Action research Small-scale interventions in the functioning of the real world in order to make a close examination of the effects of such an intervention.

Algorithm A process or set of rules used for calculation or problem solving, especially using a computer. These can be expressed graphically or, more often, as a mathematical formula. An example is a formula that summarizes the interior conditions that lead to the feeling of climatic comfort, with factors such as air temperature, humidity, air movement, amount of clothing, etc.

Area sampling See cluster sampling.

Argument A type of discourse that not only makes assertions but also asserts that some of these assertions are reasons for others. Argument is often based on the rules of logic in order to provide a solid structure.

Authentication Checking on historical data to verify whether it is authentic. Typical techniques used are textual analysis, carbon dating, paper analysis, cross-referencing, etc.

Bell curve See Gaussian curve.

Bias The unwanted distortion of the results of a survey due to parts of the population being more strongly represented than others.

Bibliography A list of key information about publications. These can be compiled on particular subjects or in relation to a particular piece of academic work. There are standard systems for compiling bibliographies (e.g. the Harvard system). Libraries usually compile their own bibliographies to guide students to literature in their particular subject.

Bivariate analysis Considers the properties of two variables in relation to each other.

Case study design   Intensive investigation into one or a few cases in order to generate ad test theory, using both inductive and deductive reasoning.

Categorization   Involves forming a typology of object, events or concepts. This can be useful in explaining what 'things' belong together and how.

Causal statements   These make an assertion that one concept or variable causes another – a 'cause and effect' relationship. This can be deterministic, meaning that under certain conditions an event will inevitably follow, or if the outcome is not so certain, probabilistic, meaning that an event has a certain chance (which may be quantifiable) of following.

Citation   A reference to a source of information or quotation given in a text. This is usually in abbreviated form to enable the full details to be found in the list of references.

Class   A set of persons or things grouped together or graded or differentiated from others. Classes can be formed by collection or division. Classes can be divided into sub-classes to form a hierarchy.

Closed-format questions   Where the respondent must choose from a choice of given answers.

Cluster sampling   Selection of cases in a population that share one or some characteristics but are otherwise as heterogeneous as possible (e.g. travellers using a railway station). Also known as area sampling when random segments are chosen from a large area of population distribution.

Coding   The application of labels or tags to allocate units of meaning to collected data. This is an important aspect of forming typologies and facilitates the organization of copious data in the form of notes, observations, transcripts, documents, etc. It helps to prevent 'data overload' resulting from mountains of unprocessed data in the form of ambiguous words. Coding of qualitative data can form a part in theory building. Codes can also be allocated to responses to fixed-choice questionnaires.

Coding frame   A list of codes that is used to categorize the answers to questionnaire questions in order to facilitate analysis.

Correlation coefficient   The measure of a statistical correlation between two or more variables. There are many types, the 'Pearsonian r' being the most common.

Comparative research   Examines two or more cases to highlight differences and similarities between them, leading to a better understanding of social phenomena and their theoretical basis. Suitable for both qualitative and quantitative methodologies.

Concepts   General expressions of a particular phenomenon, or words that represent an object or an idea. These can be concrete (e.g. dog, cat, house) or abstract, that is, independent of time or place (e.g. anger, marginality, politics). We use concepts to communicate our experience of the world around us.

Consistency   A quality of argument concerned with the compatibility of beliefs, that is a set of beliefs that can be shown to be consistent with each other is said to be consistent.

Constructionism   The belief that social phenomena are in a constant state of change because they are totally reliant on social interactions as they take place. Even the account of researchers is subject to these interactions, therefore social knowledge can only be interdeterminate.

Content analysis   An examination of what can be counted in a text. Developed from the mid-1900s chiefly in America, it is a rather positivistic attempt to apply order to the subjective domain of cultural meaning. A quantitative approach is taken by counting the frequency of phenomena within a case in order to gauge its importance in comparison with other cases.

Control   Having the ability to determine the influences on variables in a phenomenon, for example in an experiment. The crucial issue in control is to understand how certain variables affect one another, and then be able to change the variables in such a way as to produce predictable results. Not all phenomena can be controlled as many are too complex or not sufficiently understood.

Correlation research   Describes the measure of association or the relationships between two phenomena. In order to find meaning in the numerical data, the techniques of statistics are used. What kind of statistical tests are used to analyse the data depends very much on the nature of the data. This form of quantitative research can be broadly classified into relational studies and prediction studies.

Critical realism   A non-empirical (i.e. realist) epistemology that maintains the importance of identifying the structures of social systems, even if they are not amenable to the senses. This will enable the structures to be changed to ameliorate social ills.

Cross-sectional design   Research that often uses survey methods, and surveys are often equated with cross-sectional studies. It entails the collection of quantitative or qualitative data on more than one case, generally using a sampling method to select cases, collected at a single point in time in order to examine patterns of association between variables.

Deduction   The inferring of particular instances from a general law (i.e. the 'theory then research' approach).

Descriptive statistics   A method of quantifying the characteristics of parametric numerical data, for example where the centre is, how broadly data are spread, the point of central tendency, the mode, median and means. These are often explained in relation to a Gaussian (bell) curve.

Discourse   Communication in the form of words as speech or writing or even attitude and gesture.

Discourse analysis   Studies the way people communicate with each other through language in a social setting, where language is not seen as a neutral medium for transmission of information, but is loaded with meanings displaying different versions of reality.

Display   A graphical form of showing data and the interrelationships between variables. Two main forms are matrices and networks.

Ecological validity   The extent to which the findings are applicable to people's everyday, natural social settings.

Empiricism   Knowledge gained by sensory experience (using inductive reasoning).

Epistemology   The theory of knowledge, especially about its validation and the methods used. Often used in connection with one's epistemological standpoint, that is, how one sees and makes sense of the world.

Ethics   The rules of conduct in research. In this book, particularly about conduct with other people and organizations, aimed at causing no harm and providing, if possible, benefits.

Ethnography   An approach used to uncover the shared cultural meanings of the behaviour, actions, events and contexts of a group of people, using an insider's perspective, studied in its natural setting. The focus of the research and detailed research questions emerge and evolve in the course of the involvement. Data collection is usually in phases over an extended time.

Ethnomethodology   The theoretical basis for conversation analysis, which studies how talk and social interaction generate social order.

Evaluation   Making judgements about the quality of objects or events. Quality can be measured either in an absolute sense or on a comparative basis.

Evaluation research   A design that is concerned with the critical assessment of real-life interventions in the social world.

Experience   Actual observation or practical acquaintance with facts or events that results in knowledge and understanding.

Experimental research   A design in which the research strives to isolate and control every relevant condition which determines the events investigated, so as to observe the effects when the conditions are manipulated. Comparisons are made between results from a control group not exposed to the treatment and an experimental group that is.

Explanation   An attempt to describe how and why things work. One of the common objectives of research.

External reality   Acceptance of the reliability of knowledge gained by experience to provide empirical evidence.

External validity   The extent to which findings can be generalized to populations or to other settings.

Falsification   The process by which a hypothesis is rejected as a result of true observational statements which conflict with it.

Fixed designs   A design strategy that calls for a tight pre-specification at the outset and is commonly equated with a quantitative approach. The designs employ experimental and non-experimental methods.

Flexible designs   A design strategy that evolves during data collection and is associated with a qualitative approach, although some quantitative data may be collected. The designs employ, among other things, case study, ethnographic and grounded theory methods.

Focus group   A type of group interview which concentrates in-depth on a particular theme or topic with an element of interaction. The group is often made up of people who have particular experience or knowledge about the subject of the research, or those who have a particular interest in it (e.g. consumers or customers).

Gaussian curve   A graph showing a normal frequency distribution of a population, often known as the 'bell curve'.

Generality   The assumption that there can be valid relationships between the particular cases investigated by the researcher and other similar cases in the world at large.

Generalizability   Refers to the results of the research and how far they are applicable to locations and situations beyond the scope of the study. Especially in qualitative research, there may well be limits to the generalizability of the findings.

Grounded theory   Emphasizes the continuous data collection process interlaced with periodic pauses for analysis. The analysis is used to tease out categories in the data on which the subsequent data collection can be based. This process is called 'coding'. This reciprocal procedure continues until these categories are 'saturated' (i.e. the new data no longer provides new evidence). From these results, concepts and theoretical frameworks can be developed resulting in a gradual emergence and refinement of theory.

Hypothesis   A theoretical statement that has not yet been tested against data collected in a concrete situation, but which it is possible to test by providing clear evidence for support or rejection.

Hypothetico-deductive method   Synonymous with scientific method. Progress in scientific thought by the four-step method of: (1) identification of a problem, (2) formulation of a hypothesis, (3) practical or theoretical testing of the hypothesis, and (4) rejection or adjustment of the hypothesis if it is falsified.

Indicator   A phenomenon which points to the existence of a concept.

Induction   The inference of a general law from particular instances. Our experiences lead us to make conclusions from which we generalize.

Inferential statistics   Statistical analysis that goes beyond describing the characteristics of the data and the examination of correlations of variables in order to produce predictions through inference based on the data analysed. Inferential statistics are also used to test statistically based hypotheses.

Informed consent   Consent given by participants taking part in a research project based on having sufficient information about the purposes and nature of the research and the involvement required.

Interim summary   A short report prepared about one-third of the way through data collection in qualitative research in order to review the quantity and quality of the data, confidence in its reliability, the presence and nature of any gaps or puzzles that have been revealed, and to judge what still needs to be collected in the time available.

Internal reliability   The degree to which the indicators that make up the scale or index are consistent.

Internal validity   The extent to which causal statements are supported by the study. In an experiment it is a measure of the sophistication of the design and extent of control. The values of data gained should genuinely reflect the influences of the controlled variables.

Inter-observer consistency   The degree to which there is consistency in the decisions of several 'observers' in their recording of observations or translation of data into categories.

Interpretation   An integral part of the analysis of data that requires verification and extrapolation in order to make out or bring out the meaning.

Interpretivism   The recognition that subjective meanings play a crucial role in social actions. It aims to reveal interpretations and meanings. This standpoint recognizes the 'embedded' nature of the researcher, and the unique personal theoretical stances upon which each person bases his/her actions. It rejects the assertion that human behaviour can be codified in laws by identifying underlying regularities, and that society can be studied from a detached, objective and impartial viewpoint by the researcher. Attempts to find understanding in research are mediated by our own historical and cultural milieu.

Interrogation   Data gained by asking and probing (e.g. information about people's believe motivations, etc.).

Interval (level of measurement)   The use of equal units of measurement, but without a significant zero value (e.g. the Fahrenheit or Centigrade temperature scales).

Levels of abstraction   The degree of abstraction of a statement based on three levels – theoretical, operational and concrete, the last being the least abstract.

Levels of measurement (or levels of quantification)   The four different types of quantification, especially when applied to operational definitions, namely nominal, ordinal, interval and ratio.

Library catalogue   Bibliographic details of items in a library. The databases are now usually accessed by computer as online public access catalogues (OPACs).

Lickert scale   A format for asking attitude questions using a summated rating approach that indicates the intensity of feeling a subject has about a topic.

Longitudinal design   Consists of repeated cross-sectional surveys to ascertain how time influences the results.

Matrices   Two-dimensional arrangements of rows and columns that summarize substantial amounts of information. They can be used to record variables such as time, levels of measurement, roles, clusters outcomes, effects, etc. Latest developments allow the formulation of three-dimensional matrices.

Measurement   Records of amounts or numbers (e.g. population statistics, instrumental measurements of distance, temperature, mass, etc.).

Measurement validity   The degree to which measures (e.g. questions on a questionnaire) successfully indicate concepts.

Memos   Short analytical descriptions based on the developing ideas of the researcher reacting to the data and development of codes and pattern codes. Compiling memos is a good way to explore links between data and to record and develop intuitions and ideas.

Model   (a) A term used to describe the overall framework that we use to look at reality, based on a philosophical stance (e.g. postmodernism, post-structuralism, positivism, empiricism, etc.).
   (b) A simplified physical or mathematical representation of an object or a system used as a tool for analysis. It may be able to be manipulated in order to obtain data about the effects of the manipulations.

Multi-stage cluster sampling   An extension of cluster sampling, where clusters of successively smaller size are selected from within each other. For example, you might take a random sample from all UK universities, then a random sample from subjects within those universities, then a random sample of modules taught in those subjects, then a random sample of students doing those modules.

Multivariate analysis   Looks at the relationships between more than two variables.

Networks   Maps or charts used to display data, made up of blocks (nodes) connected by links. They can be produced in a wide variety of formats, each with the capability of displaying different types of data (e.g. flow charts, organization charts, causal networks, mind maps, etc.).

Nominal (level of measurement)   The division of data into separate categories by naming or labelling.

Non-parametric statistics   Statistical tests devised to recognize the particular characteristics of data that do not conform to a parameter.

Non-probability sampling   Sampling based on non-random selection. This relies on the judgement of the researcher or by accident and cannot be used to make generalizations about the whole population.

Null hypothesis   A statistically based hypothesis tested by using inferential statistics. A null hypothesis suggests no relationship between two variables.

Objectivism   The belief that social phenomena and their meanings have an existence that is not dependent on social actors. They are facts that have an independent existence.

Observation   Records, usually of events, situations or things, of what you have experienced in your own senses, perhaps with the help of an instrument (e.g. camera, tape recorder, microscope, etc.).

Ontology   A theory of the nature of social entities that is concerned with what there exists to be investigated.

Open-format questions   Questions that the respondents are free to answer in their own words and style.

Operational definition   A set of actions that an observer should perform in order to detect or measure a theoretical concept. Operational definitions should be abstract, that is, independent of time and space.

Operationalization (of a hypothesis)   Breaking down the hypothesis into its components to make it testable, from the most abstract to the most concrete expressions by defining in turn concepts, indicators, variables and values.

Order   The condition in which things are constituted, in an organized fashion, that can be revealed through observation.

Ordinal (level of measurement)   Ordering data by rank without reference to specific measurement (i.e. more or less than, bigger or smaller than).

Parameter   A constant feature of a population that it shares with other populations. The most common one is the 'bell' or 'Gaussian' curve of normal frequency distribution.

Parametric statistics   Statistical calculations based on data that conform to a parameter, usually a Gaussian curve.

Parsimony   The economy of explanation of phenomena, especially in formulating theories.

Participant   Someone who takes part in a research project as a subject of study. This term implies that the person takes an active role in the research by performing actions or providing information.

Participation   Data gained by experiences that can perhaps be seen as an intensified form of observations (e.g. the experience of learning to drive a car tells you different things above cars and traffic than just watching).

Phenomenology   A philosophy or method of inquiry based on the premise that reality consists of objects and events as they are perceived or understood in human terms.

Pilot study   A pre-test of a questionnaire or other type of survey on a small number of cases in order to test the procedures and quality of responses.

Plagiarism   The taking and use of other people's thoughts or writing as your own. This is sometimes done by students who copy out chunks of text from publications or the Internet and include it in their writing without any acknowledgement to its source.

Population   A collective term used to describe the total quantity of cases of the type which is the subject of the study. It can consist of objects, people and even events.

Positivism   The application of the natural sciences to the study of social reality. An objective approach that can test theories and establish scientific laws. It aims to establish causes and effects.

Postmodernism   A term applied to a wide-ranging set of developments in critical theory, philosophy, architecture, art, literature, and culture, which are generally characterized as either emerging from, in reaction to, or superseding, modernism. In sociology, postmodernism is described as being the result of economic, cultural and demographic changes (related terms in this context include 'post-industrial society' and 'late capitalism'). It is attributed to (1) factors that have emerged from the service economy, (2) the importance of the mass media, and (3) the rise of an increasingly interdependent world economy.

Post-structuralism   Any of various theories or methods of analysis, including deconstruction and some psychoanalytic theories that deny the validity of structuralism's method of binary opposition and maintain that meanings and intellectual categories are shifting and unstable.

Prediction studies   These aim to foretell the outcome of a phenomenon on the basis of previous experience – one of the common objectives of research.

Primary data Data gained by direct, detached observation or measurement of phenomena in the real world, undisturbed by any intermediary interpreter.

Probability sampling   Sampling based on random selection. These techniques give the most reliable representation of the whole population from which predictions can be made about the population.

Problem area   An issue within a general body of knowledge or subject from which a research project might be selected.

Proportional stratified sampling   A sampling method used when cases in a population fall into distinctly different categories (strata) of a known proportion of that population.

Proposition   A theoretical statement that indicates the clear direction and scope of a research project.

Purposive sampling   A sampling method where the researcher selects what he/she thinks is a 'typical' sample based on specialist knowledge on selection criteria.

Qualitative data   Data that cannot be accurately measured and counted, and are generally expressed in words rather than numbers. These kinds of data are therefore descriptive in character, and rarely go beyond the nominal and ordinal levels of measurement.

Qualitative research   Relies heavily on language for the interpretation of its meaning, so data collection methods tend to involve close human involvement and a creative process of theory development rather than testing.

Quantification (of concepts)   Measurement techniques used in association with operational definitions.

Quantitative data   Data that can be measured, more or less exactly. Measurement implies some form of magnitude, usually expressed in numbers. Mathematical procedures can be applied to analyse the data. These might be extremely simple, such as counts or percentages, or more sophisticated, such as statistical tests or mathematical models.

Quantitative research   Relies on collecting data that is numerically based and amenable to such analytical methods as statistical correlations, often in relation to hypothesis testing.

Quota sampling   An attempt to balance the sample by selecting responses from equal numbers of different respondents. This is an unregulated form of sampling as there is no knowledge of whether the respondents are typical of their class.

Random assignment   Random sampling methods used to select the experimental units (the things that are being experimented on, e.g. materials, components, persons, groups, etc.) in order to combat the problem of unknown variables. This process neutralizes the particular effects of individual variables and allows the result of the experiment to be generalized.

Ratio (level of measurement)   A scale with equal units of measurement and containing a true zero equal to nought, that is the total absence of the quantity being measured.

Rationalism   Knowledge gained by reasoning (using deductive reasoning).

Realism (particularly social realism)   This maintains that structures do underpin social events and discourses, but as these are only indirectly observable they must be expressed in theoretical terms and are thus likely to be provisional in nature. This does not prevent them being used in action to change society.

Reasoning   A method of coming to conclusions by the use of logical argument.

Regression A statistical technique for using the values of one variable to predict the value of another, based on information about their relationship.

Relational studies An investigation of possible relationships between phenomena to establish if a correlation exists and, if so, its extent. The information about relationships between concepts form the bedrock of scientific knowledge, and explain, predict and provide us with a sense of understanding of our surroundings.

Relativism The stance that implies that judgement is principally dependent on the values of the individuals or society and the perspectives from which they make their judgements. No universal criteria can be 'rationally' applied, and an understanding of decisions made by individuals or organizations can only be gained through knowledge of the historical, psychological and social backgrounds of the individuals.

Reliability The degree to which the results of research are repeatable. This is based on: stability – the degree to which a measure is stable over time; internal reliability – the degree to which the indicators that make up the scale or index are consistent; and inter-observer consistency – the degree to which there is consistency in the decisions of several 'observers' in their recording of observations or translation of data into categories.

Replicability Whether the research can be repeated and whether similar results are obtained. This is a check on the objectivity and lack of bias of the research findings. It requires a detailed account of the concepts used in the research, the measurements applied and methods employed.

Research question A theoretical question that indicates a clear direction and scope for a research project.

Research problem A general statement of an issue meriting research. It is usually used to help formulate a research project and is the basis on which specific research questions, hypotheses or statements are formed.

Sample The small part of a whole (population) selected to show what the whole is like. There are two main types of sampling procedure – random and non-random.

Sampling error The differences between the random sample and the population from which it has been selected.

Sampling frame A complete list of cases in a population.

Scientific method The foundation of modern scientific inquiry. It is based on observation and testing of the soundness of conclusions, commonly by using the hypothetico-deductive method. The four-step method is: (1) identification of a problem, (2) formulation of a hypothesis, (3) practical or theoretical testing of the hypothesis, and (4) rejection or adjustment of the hypothesis if it is falsified.

Secondary data Data that have been subject to interpretation by others, usually in the form of publications.

Semiotics The 'science of signs'. This approach is used to examine other media (e.g. visual communication and design) as well as written texts. It attempts to gain a deep understanding of meanings by the interpretation of single elements of a subject rather than to generalize through a quantitative assessment of components.

Semi-structured interview   One that contains structured and unstructured sections with standardized and open-format questions.

Sense of understanding   A complete explanation of a phenomenon provided by a wider study of the processes that surround, influence and cause it to happen.

Simple random sampling   A sampling method used to select cases at random from a uniform population.

Simple stratified sampling   A sampling method that recognizes the different strata in a population in order to select a representative sample.

Snowball sampling   A sampling method where the researcher contacts a small number of members of a target population and gets them to introduce him/her to others.

Stability   The degree to which a measure is stable over time.

Standard deviation   The amount of variability within the population expressed as the square root of the variance.

Standardized tests   Devised by social scientists and psychologists to establish people's abilities, attitudes, aptitudes, opinions, etc. The objective of the tests is usually to measure in some way the abilities of the subjects according to a standardized scale so that easy comparisons can be made.

Statement   An assertion based on a combination of concepts.

Statistical inference   The process of using a test of statistical significance to generalize from a sample to a population.

Statistical significance   A measure of how much statistical results are simply occasioned by chance or how truly representative they are of a population. An example of a test is the chi-square test.

Structuralism   A method of analysing phenomena, as in anthropology, linguistics, psychology or literature. It is chiefly characterized by contrasting the elemental structures of the phenomena in a system of binary opposition.

Structured interview   Interviews that use standardized questions read out by the interviewer according to an interview schedule. Answers may be closed-format.

Subject   The participant in a research project. The term implies a passive role in the project, that is, things are done to the subject in the form of a test or an experiment.

Sub-problem   A component of a main problem, usually expressed in less abstract terms to indicate an avenue of investigation.

Symbol   A sign used to communicate concepts in the form of natural or artificial language.

Symbolic interactionism   A sociological perspective that examines how individuals and groups interact, focusing on the creation of personal identity through interaction with others. Of particular interest is the relationship between individual action and group pressures. This perspective examines the idea that subjective meanings are socially constructed, and that these subjective meanings interrelate with objective actions.

Systematic sampling   A sampling method that selects samples using a numerical method, for example the selection of every tenth name on a list.

Systematic matching sampling   A sampling method that is used when two groups of very different size are compared by selecting a number from the larger group to match the number and characteristics of the smaller one.

Theory   A system of ideas based on interrelated concepts, definitions and propositions with the purpose of explaining or predicting phenomena.

Theoretical sampling   The selection of a sample of the population that the researcher thinks knows most about the subject. This approach is common in qualitative research where statistical inference is not required.

Univariate analysis   Analyses the qualities of one variable at a time.

Unstructured interview   A flexible format interview, usually based on a question guide but where the format remains the choice of the interviewer, who can allow the interview to 'ramble' in order to get insights into the attitudes of the interviewee. No closed-format questions are used.

Validity of argument   The property of an argument to draw conclusions from premises correctly according to the rules of logic.

Validity of research   The degree to which the research findings are true.

Value   The actual unit or method of measurement of a variable. These are data in their most concrete form.

Variable   The component of an indicator which can be measured.

Visual ethnography   Observation used for recording the nature or condition of objects or events visually, for example through photography, film or sketching.

Alldred, P. and Gillies, V. (2002) 'Eliciting research accounts: re/producing modern subjects?', in M. Mauthner, M. Birch, J. Jessop and T. Miller (eds), *Ethics in Qualitative Research*. London: Sage. Chapter 8, pp. 148–65.

Barr Greenfield, T. (1975) 'Theory about organisations: a new perspective and its implications for schools', in M.G. Hughes (ed.), *Administering Education: International Challenge*. London: Athlone Press.

Bernard, H.R. (2000) *Social Research Methods: Qualitative and Quantitative Approaches*. Thousand Oaks, CA: Sage.

Booth, W.C., Colomb, G.G. and William, J.M. (1995) *The Craft of Research*. Chicago: University of Chicago Press.

Bromley, D.B. (1986) *The Case-Study Method in Psychology and Related Disciplines*. Chichester: Wiley.

Bryman, A. (2004) *Social Research Methods* (2nd edn). Oxford: Oxford University Press.

Campbell, D.T. and Stanley, J.C. (1963) *'Experimental and Quasi-Experimental Designs for Research on Teaching*. Chicago: Rand McNally.

Campbell, D.T. and Stanley, J.C. (1966) *Experimental and Quasi-Experimental Designs for Research*. Boston: Houghton Mifflin.

Cohen, L. and Manion, L. (1994) *Research Methods in Education*. London: Routledge.

Dixon, B.R. (1987) *A Handbook of Social Science Research*. New York: Oxford University Press.

Duncombe, J. and Jessop, J. (2002) '"Doing rapport" and the ethics of "faking friendship"', in M. Mauthner, M. Birch, J. Jessop and T. Miller (eds), *Ethics in Qualitative Research*. London: Sage. Chapter 6, pp. 107–22.

Field, A. (2000) *Discovering Statistics Using SPSS for Windows: Advanced Techniques for the Beginner*. London: Sage.

Forster, N. (1994) 'The analysis of company documentation', in C. Cassell and G. Symon (eds), *Qualitative Methods of Organizational Research: A Practical Guide*. London: Sage. pp. 147–66.

Foucault, M. (1972) *The Archaeology of Knowledge*. London: Tavistock.

Glaser, B. and Strauss, A. (1967) *The Discovery of Grounded Theory: Strategies for Qualitative Research*. Chicago: Aldine.

Gold, R. (1958) 'Roles in sociological fieldwork', *Social Forces*, 36: 217–23.

Guba, E. and Lincoln, Y. (1989) *Fourth Generation Evaluation*. Newbury Park, CA: Sage.

Hacking, I. (ed.) (1981) *Scientific Revolutions*. Oxford: Oxford University Press.

Harré, R. (1972) *The Philosophies of Science*. Oxford: Oxford University Press.

Hughes, J.A. and Sharrock, W.W. (1997) *The Philosophy of Social Research* (3rd edn). Harlow: Longman.

Kerlinger, F. (1970) *Foundations of Behavioral Research*. New York: Holt, Rinehort & Winston.

Kvale, S. (1996) *Interviews: An Introduction to Qualitative Research Interviewing*. Thousand Oaks, CA: Sage.

Lazarfeld, P., Pasanella, A. and Rosenberg, M. (eds) (1972) *Continuities in the Language of Social Research*. New York: Free Press.

Leedy, P.D. (1989) *Practical Research: Planning and Design* (4th edn). London: Collier Macmillan.

Lofland, J. (1971) *Analysing Social Settings: A Guide to Qualitative Observation and Analysis*. Belmont, CA: Wadsworth.

Mangione, T. (1995) *Mail Surveys: Improving the Quality*. Thousand Oaks, CA: Sage.

Marsh, C. (1982) *The Survey Method: The Contribution of Surveys to Sociological Explanation*. London: Allen and Unwin.

Miles, M.B. and Huberman, A.M. (1994) *Qualitative Data Analysis: An Expanded Sourcebook*. London: Sage.

Miller, T. and Bell L. (2002) 'Consenting to what? Issues of access, gatekeeping and "informed" consent', in M. Mauthner, M. Birch, J. Jessop and T. Miller (eds), *Ethics in Qualitative Research*. London: Sage. Chapter 3, pp. 53–69.

Open University (1993) *An Equal Opportunities Guide to Language and Image*. Milton Keynes: Open University.

Phillips, N. and Brown, J. (1993) 'Analyzing communications in and around organizations: a critical hermeneutic approach', *Academy of Management Journal*, 36: 1547–76.

Preece, R. (1994) *Starting Research: An Introduction to Academic Research and Dissertation Writing*. London: Pinter.

Quine, W.V.O. (1969) *Ontological Relativity and Other Essays*. New York: Columbia University Press.

Reynolds, P.D. (1977) *A Primer in Theory Construction*. Indianapolis, IN: Bobbs-Merrill.

Robson, C. (2002) *Real World Research: A Resource for Social Scientists and Practitioner-Researchers* (2nd edn). Oxford: Blackwell.

Seale, C. (ed.) (1998) *Researching Society and Culture*. London: Sage.

Seale, C. (ed.) (2004) *Researching Society and Culture* (2nd edn). London: Sage.

Seale, C. and Filmer, P. (1998) 'Doing social surveys', in C. Seale (ed.), *Researching Society and Culture*. London: Sage. Chapter 11, pp. 125–45.

Siegel, S. and Castellan, N. (1988) *Nonparametric Statistics for the Behavioral Sciences* (2nd edn). New York: McGraw-Hill.

Silverman, D. (1993) *Interpreting Qualitative Data: Methods for Analysing Qualitative Data*. London: Sage.

Silverman, D. (1998) 'Research and social theory', in C. Seale (ed.), *Researching Society and Culture*. London: Sage.

Slater, D. (1998) 'Analysing cultural objects: content analysis and semiotics', in C. Seale (ed.), *Researching Society and Culture*. London: Sage.

Swales, J. and Feak, C. (2000) *English in Today's Research World: A Writing Guide*. Michigan: University of Michigan Press.

van Dijk, T.A. (1994) 'Discourse and cognition in society', in C. Crowly and D. Michell (eds), *Communication Theory Today*. Cambridge: Polity Press. pp. 107–26.

Williams, M. and May, T. (1996) *Introduction to the Philosophy of Social Research*. London: UCL Press.

index

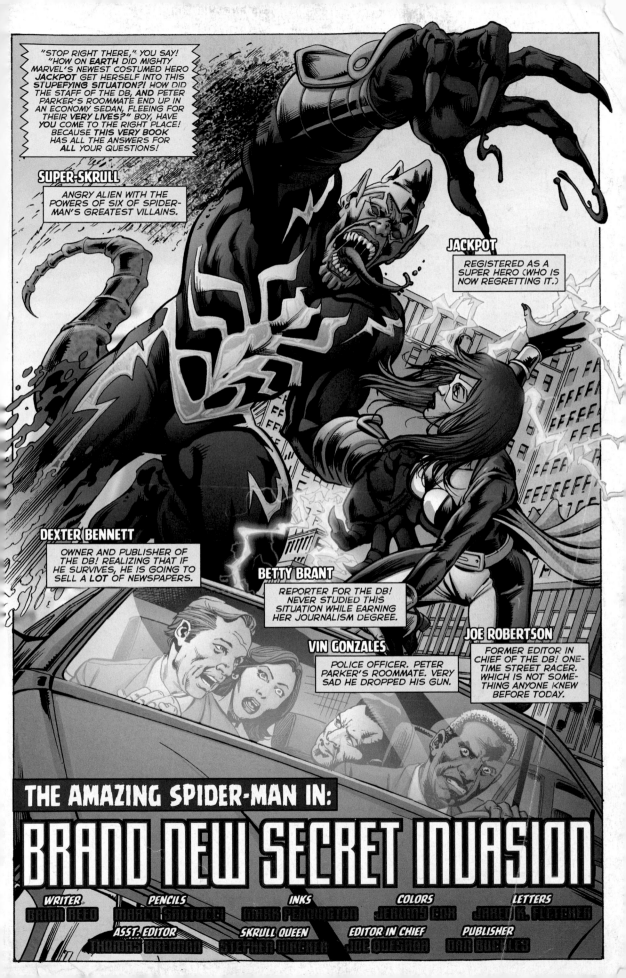

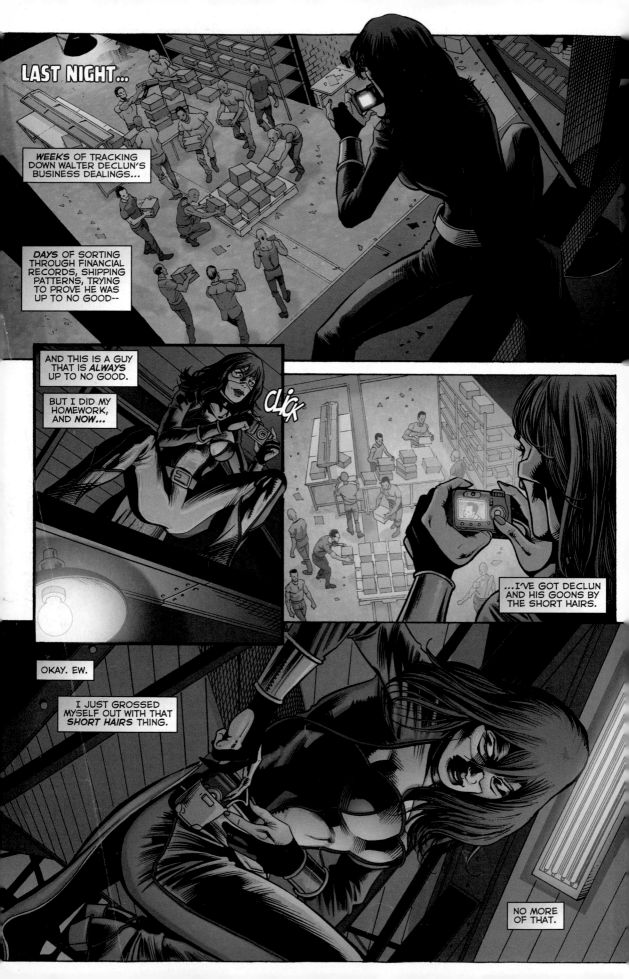

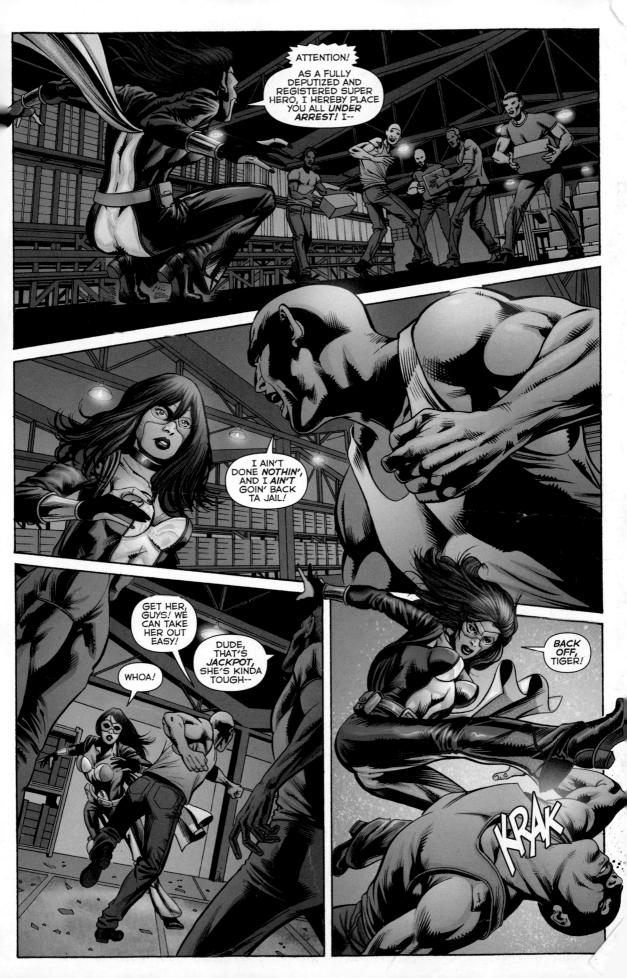

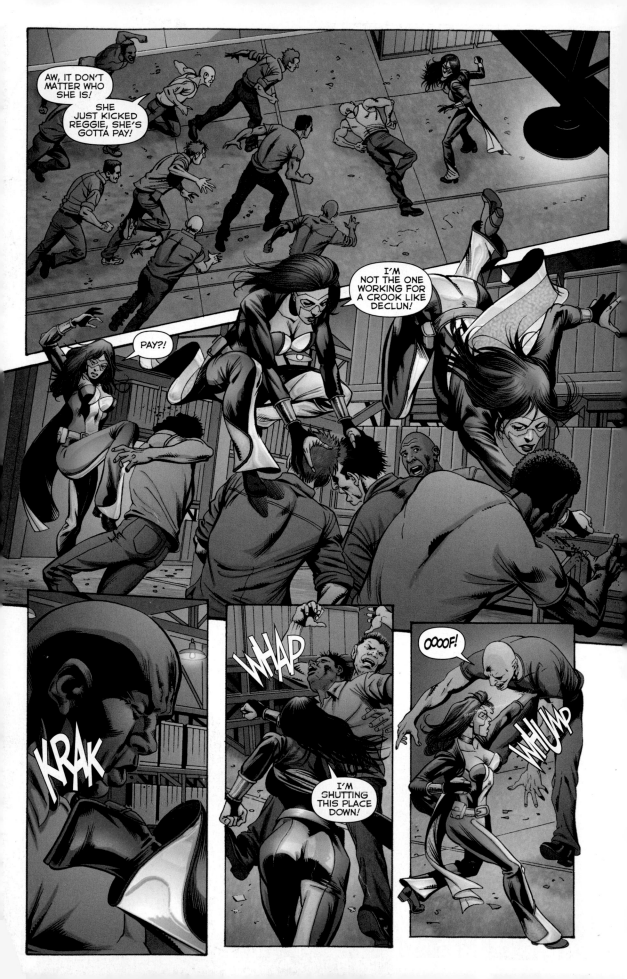

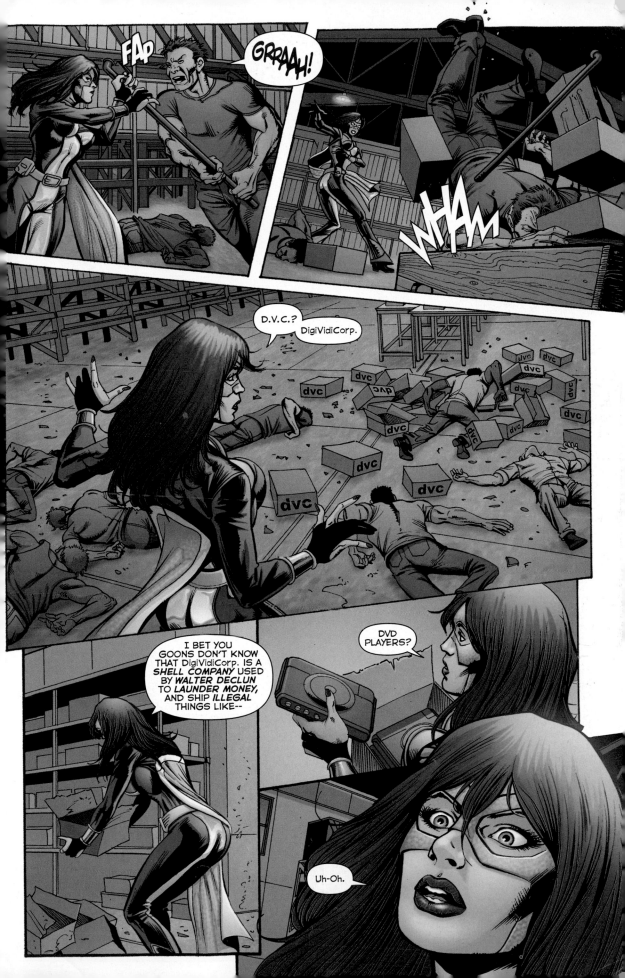

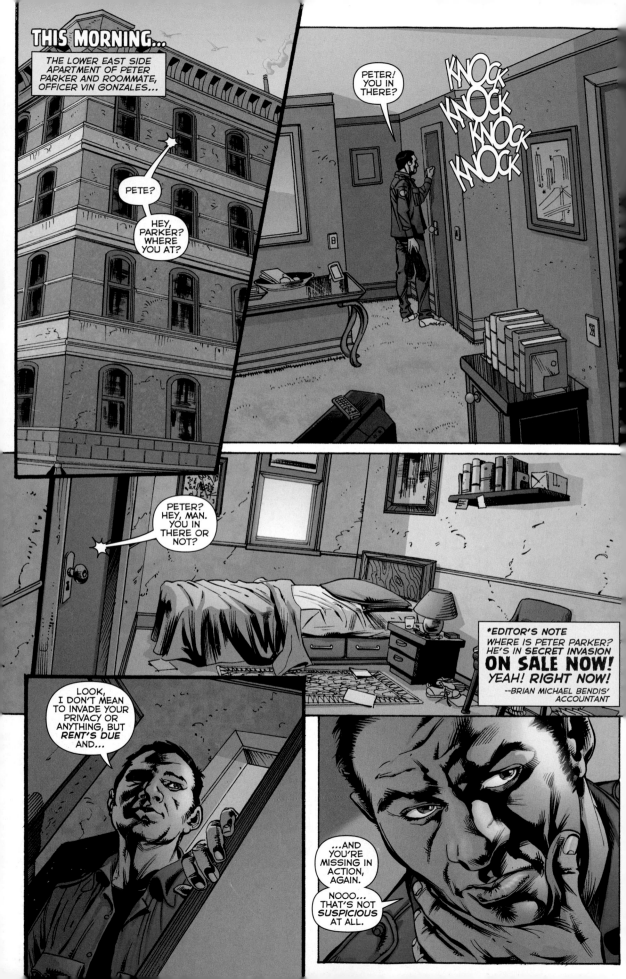

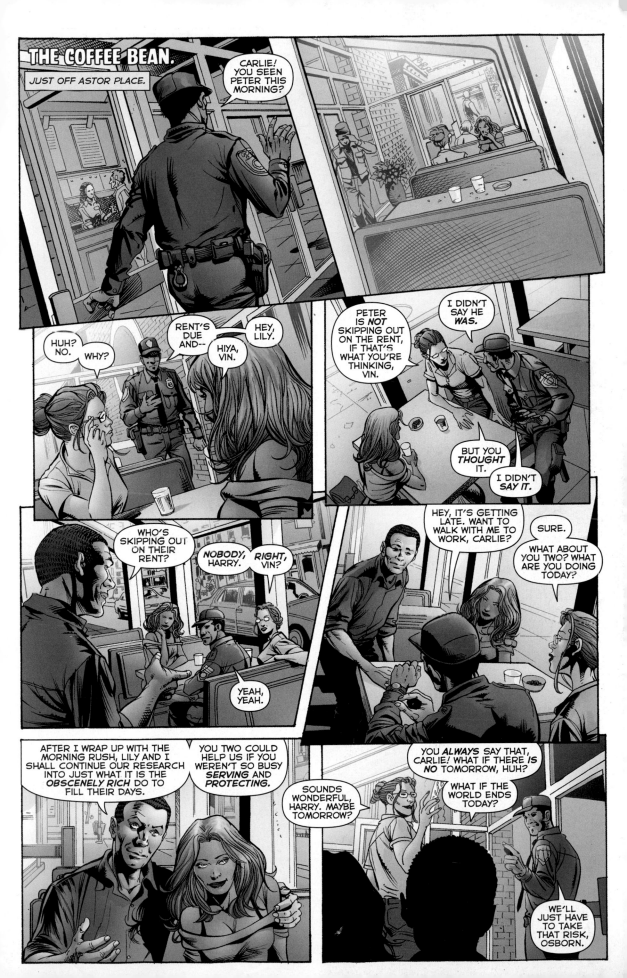

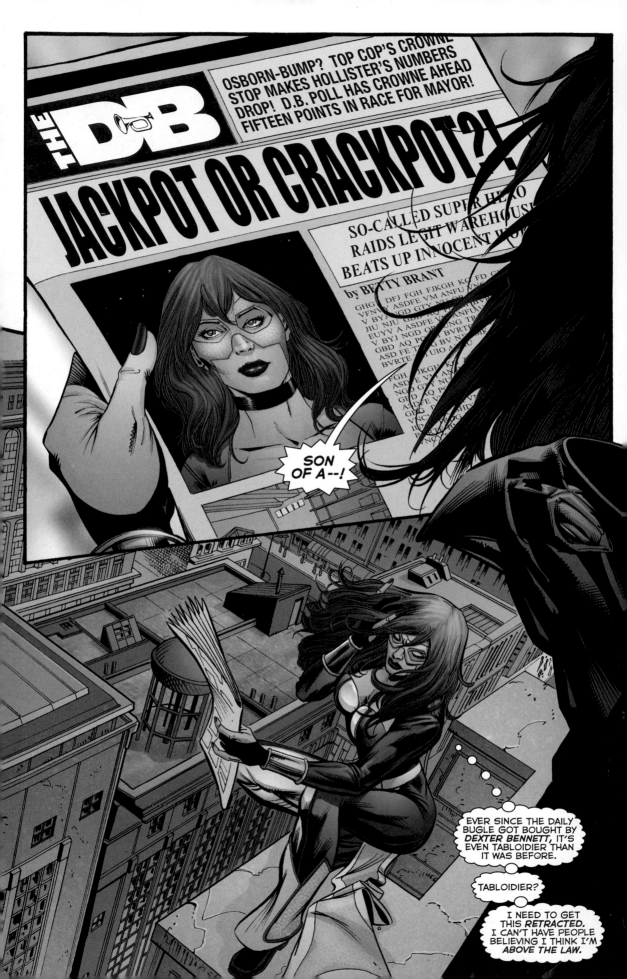

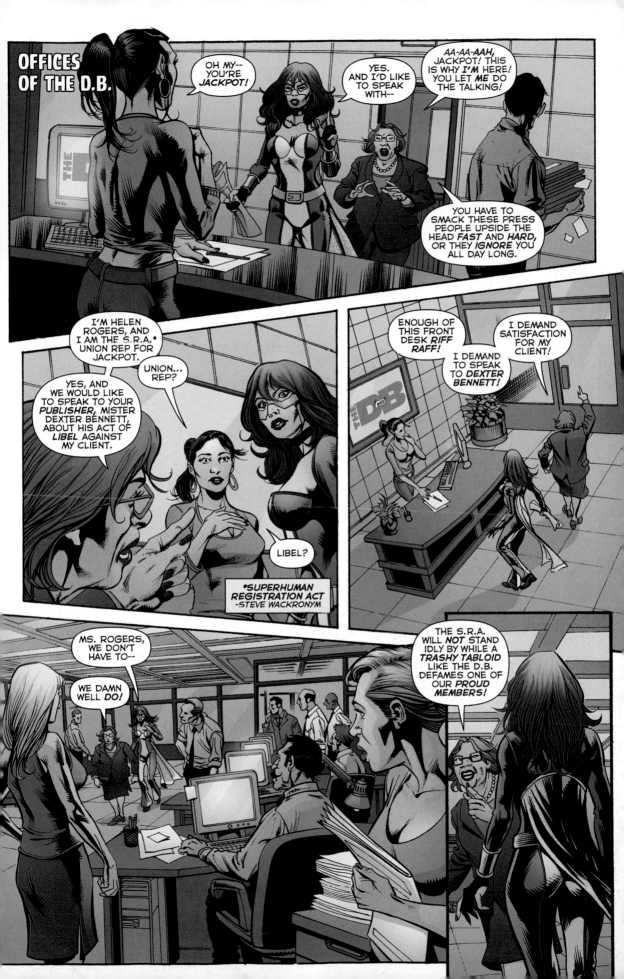

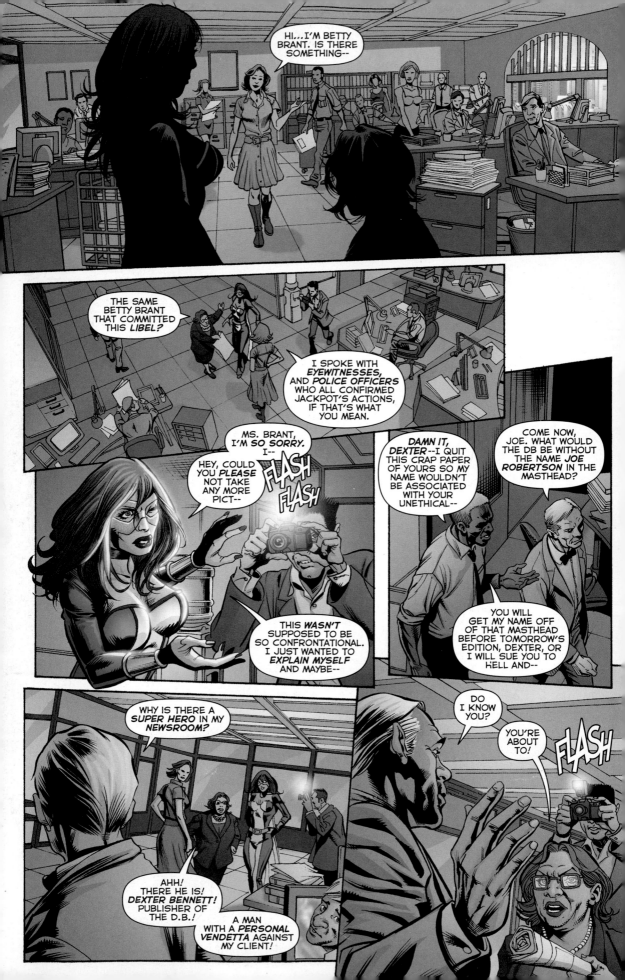

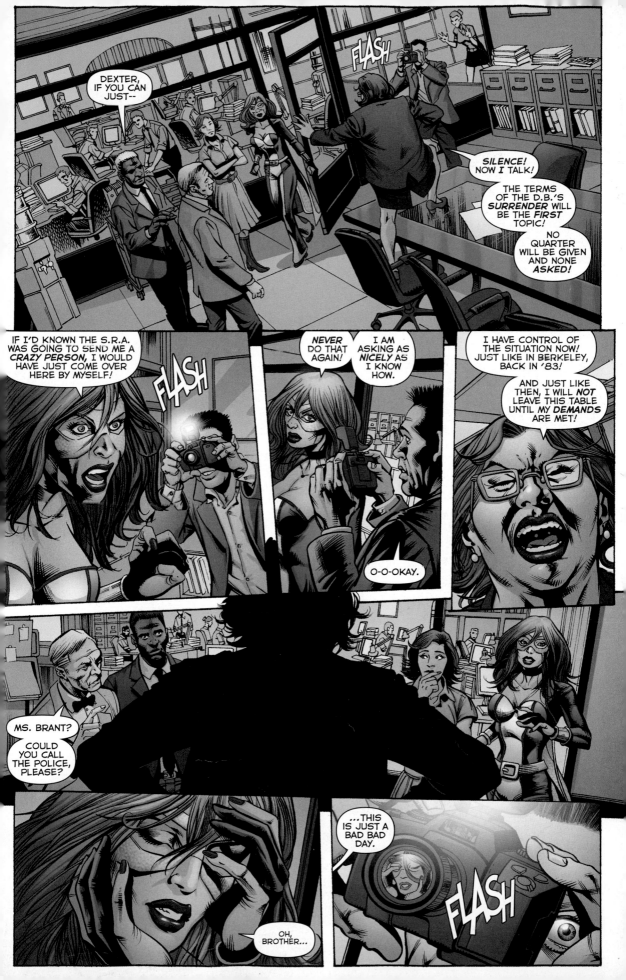

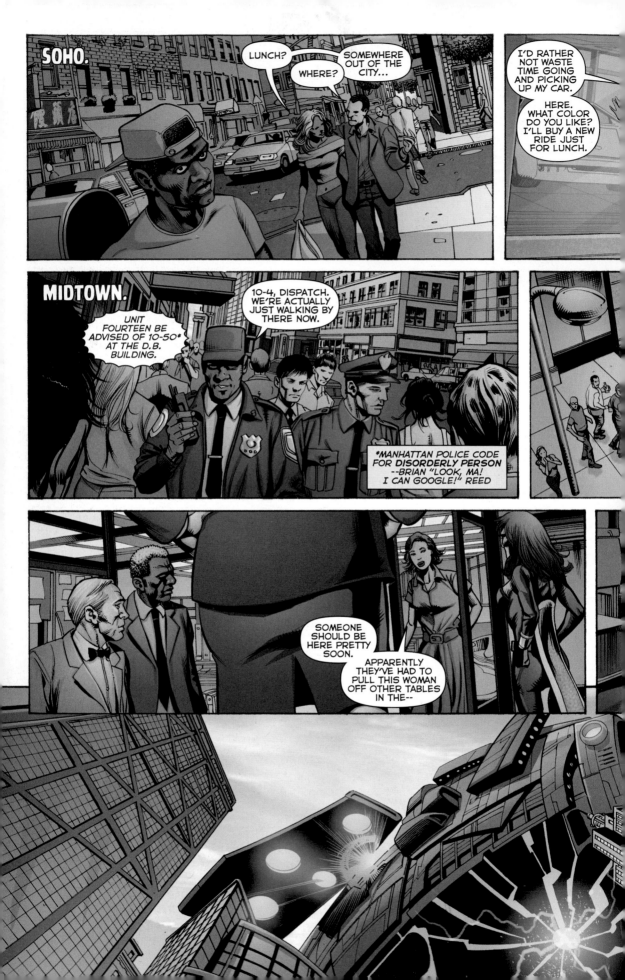

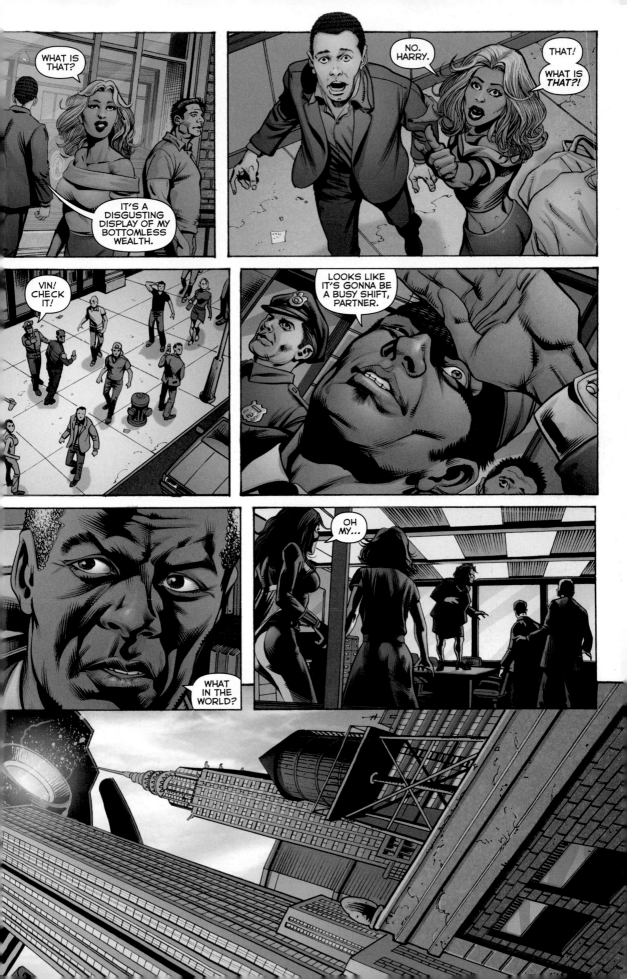

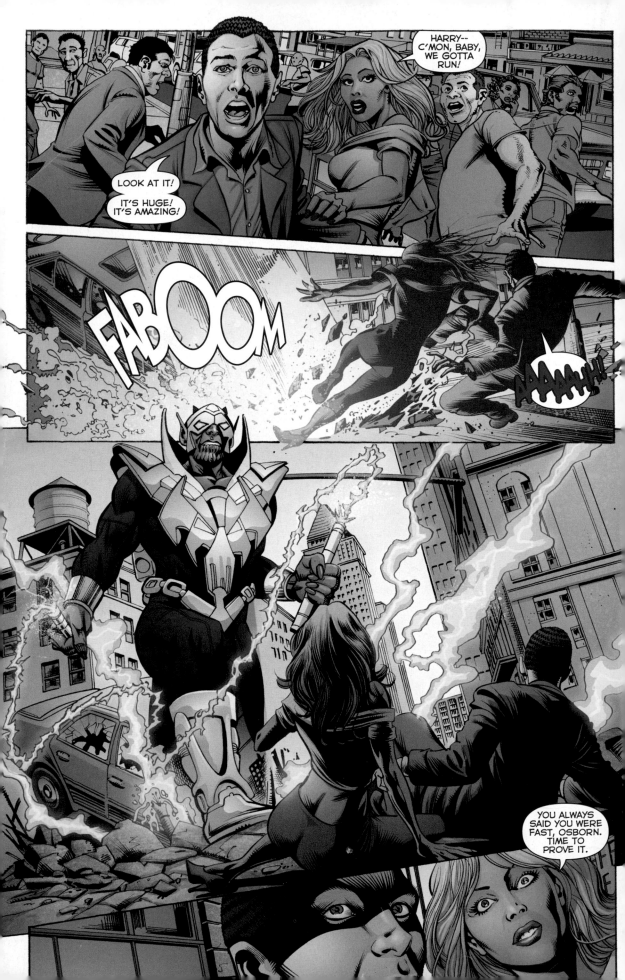

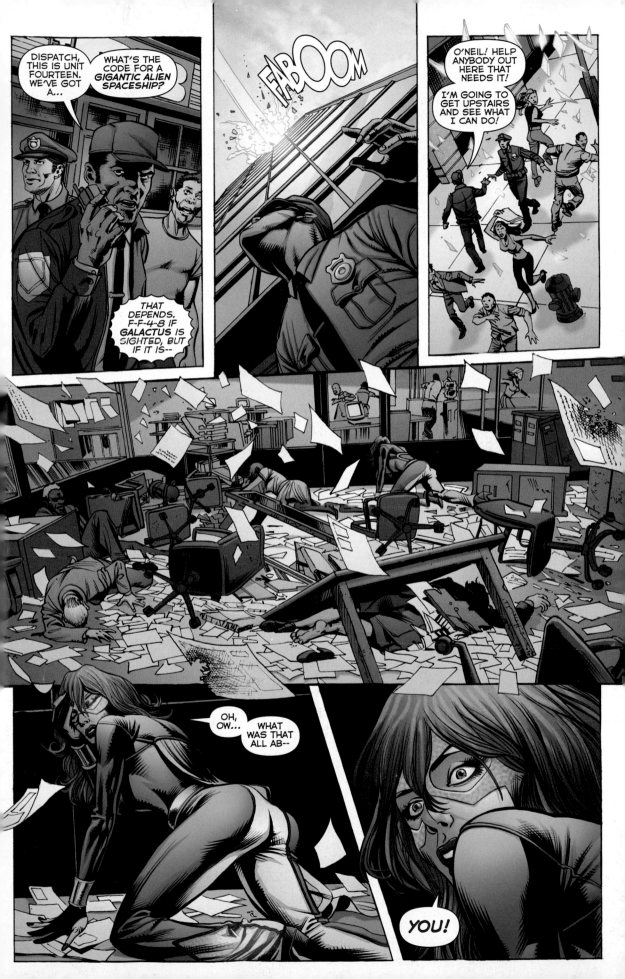

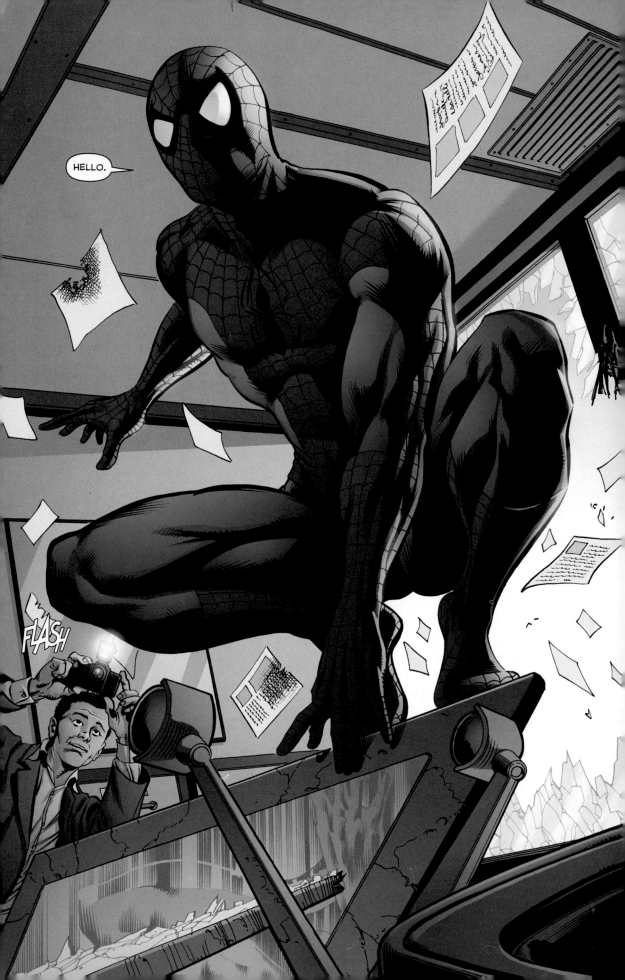

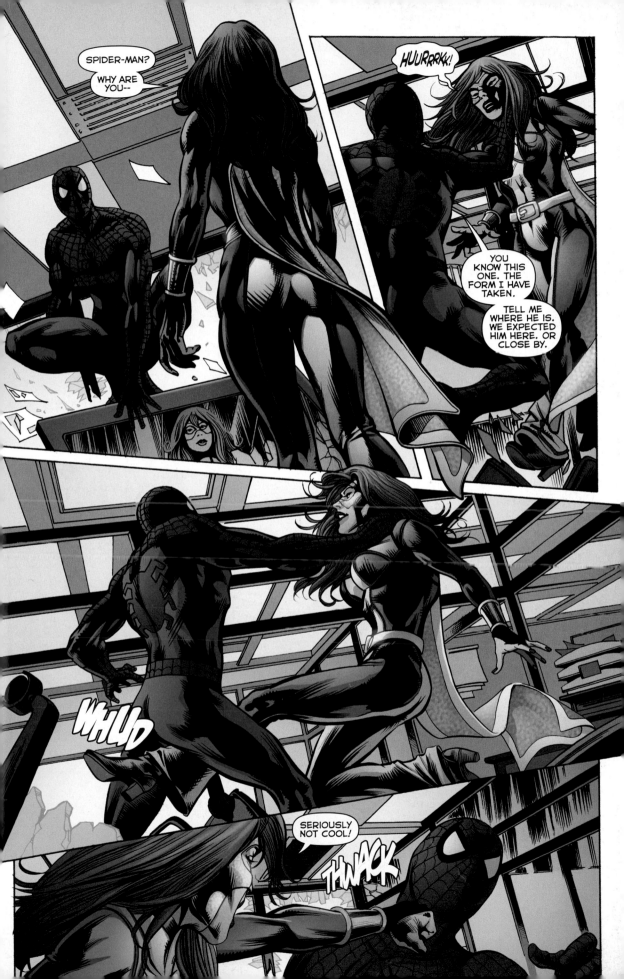

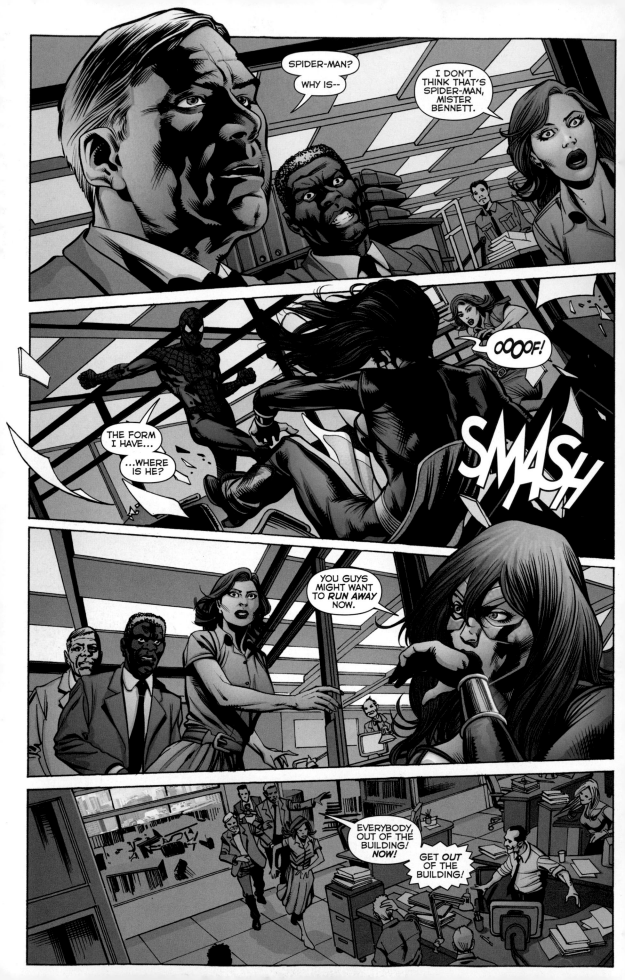

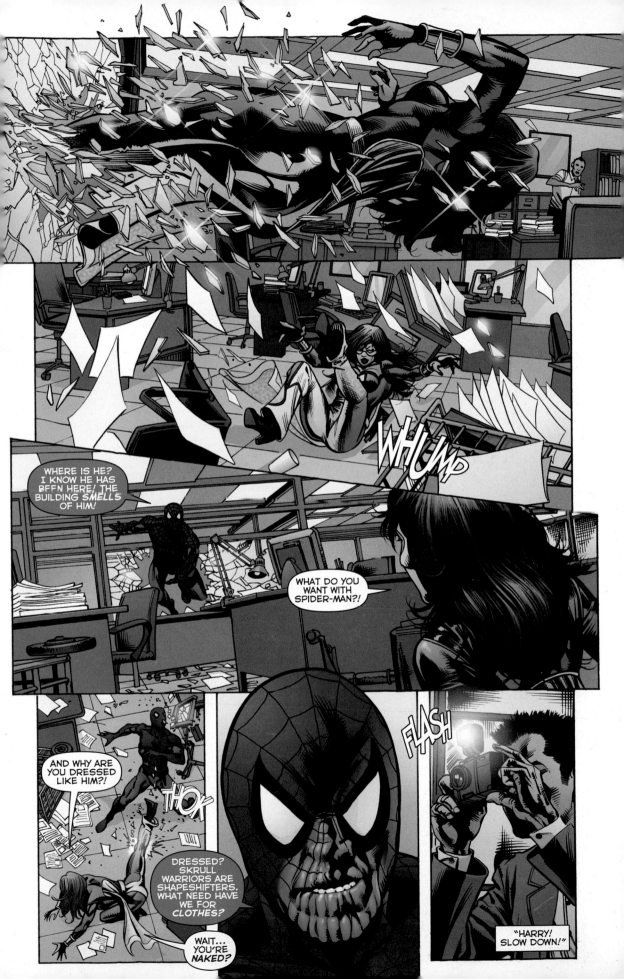

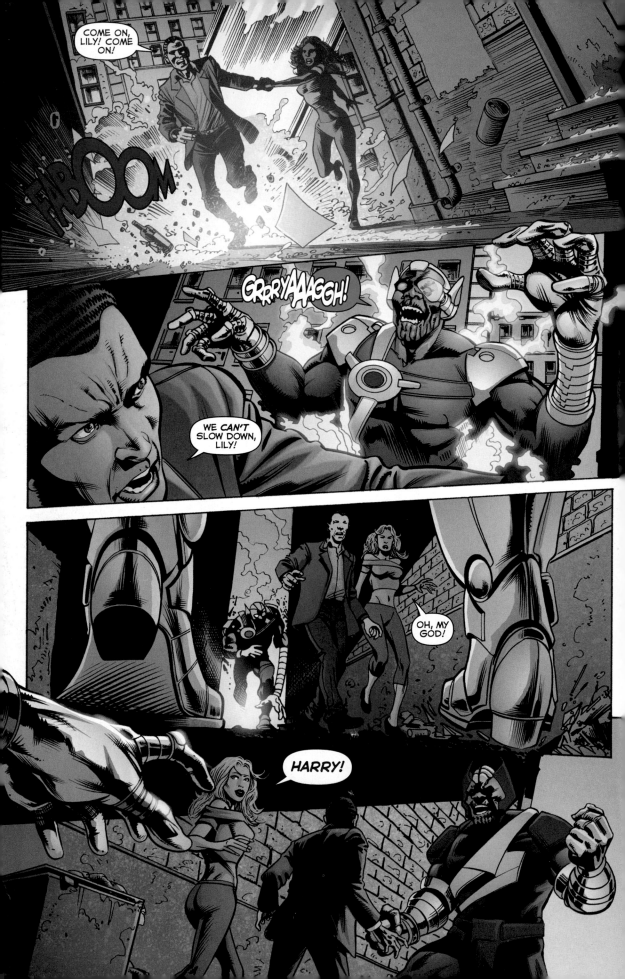

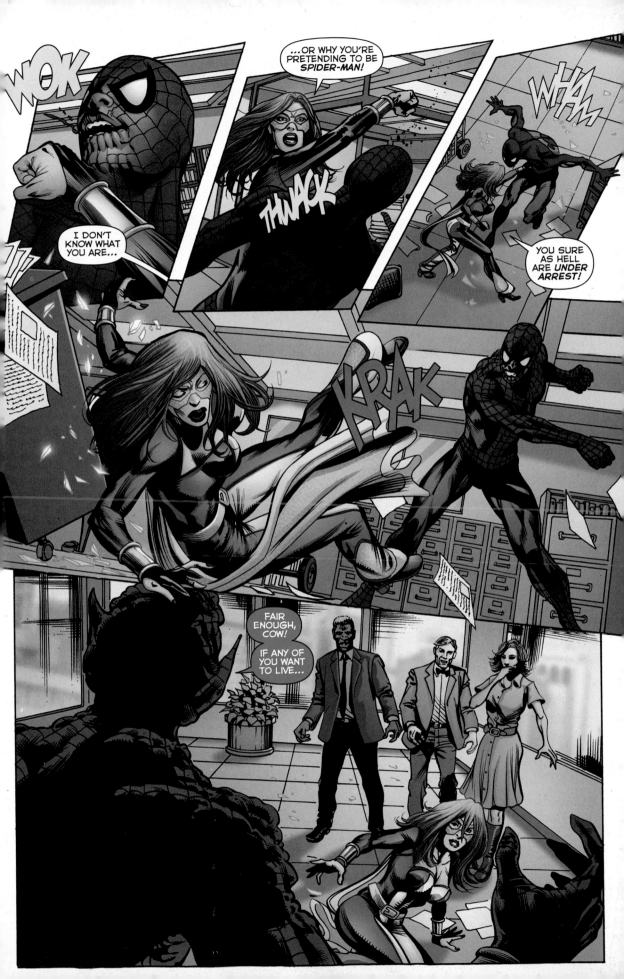

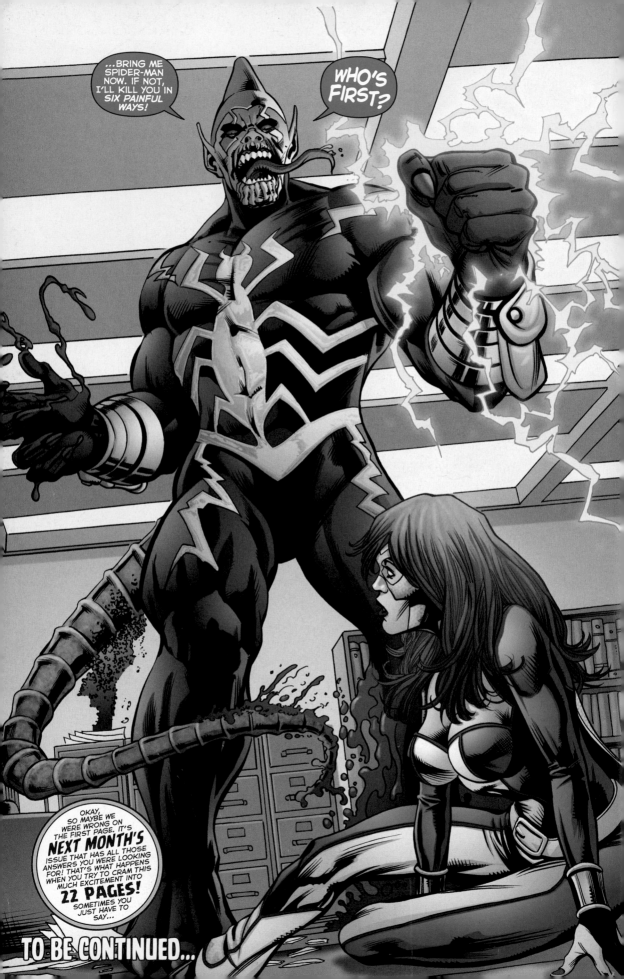

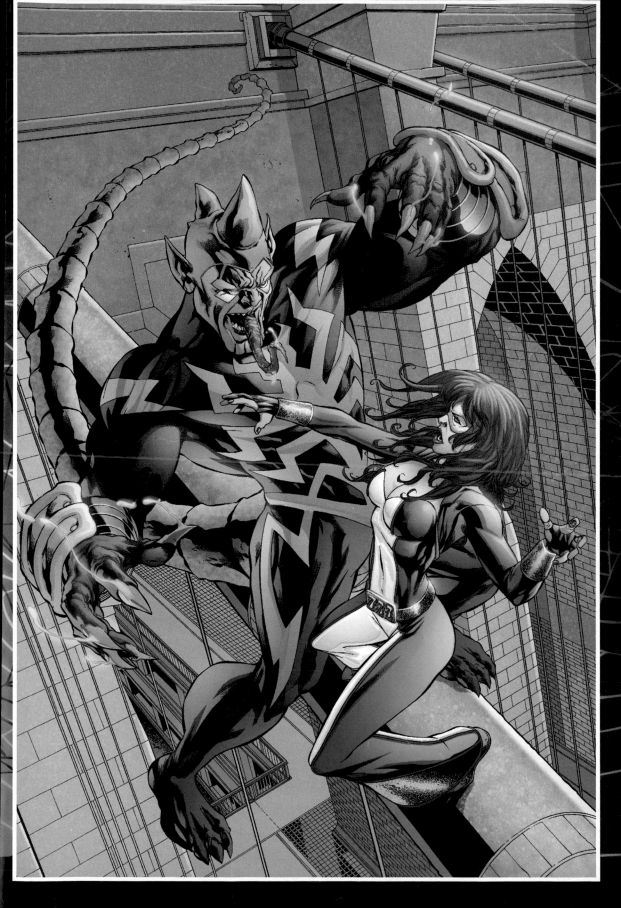

SECRET INVASION: THE AMAZING SPIDER-MAN #2

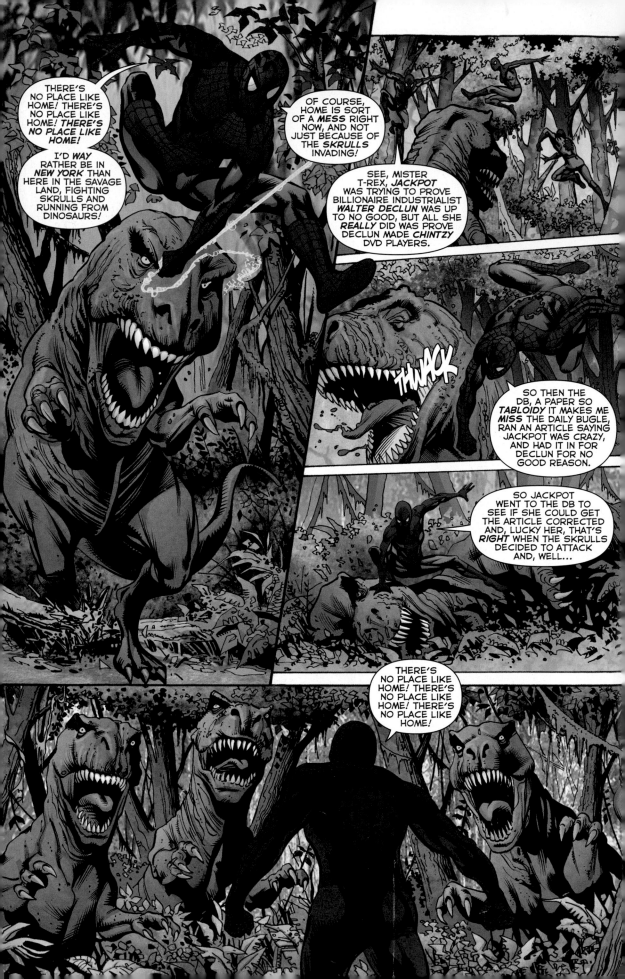

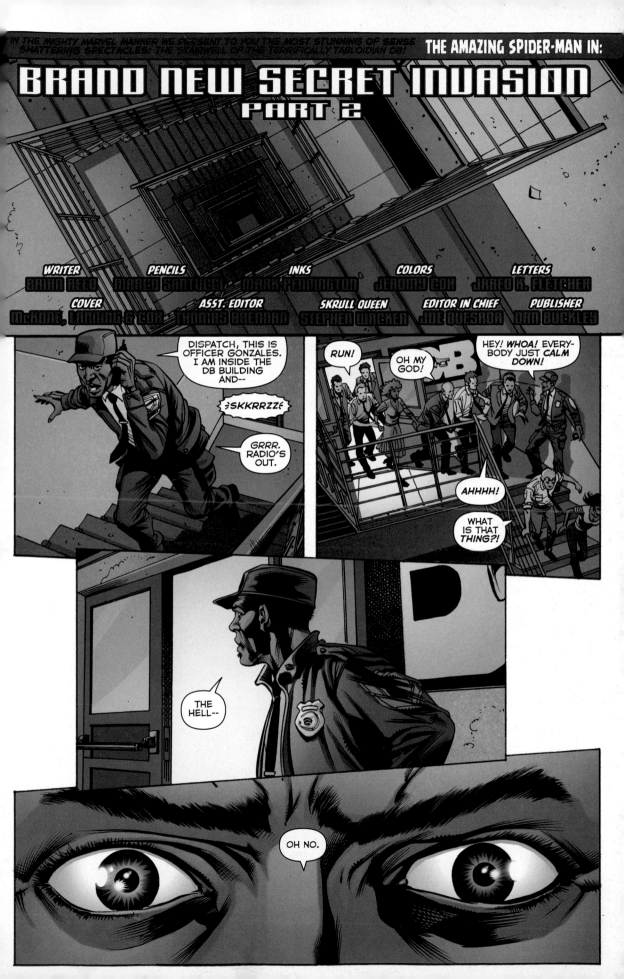

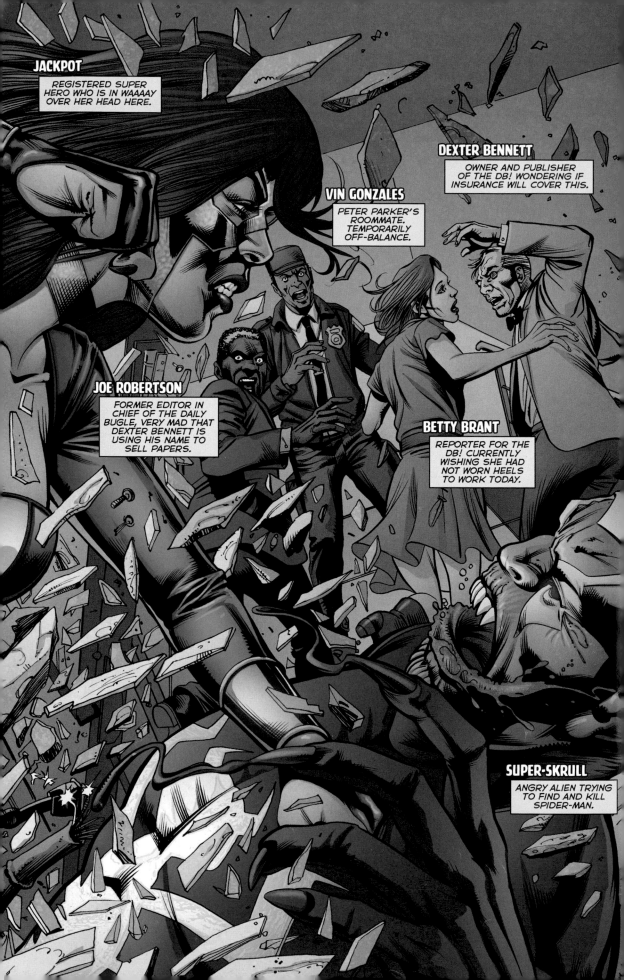

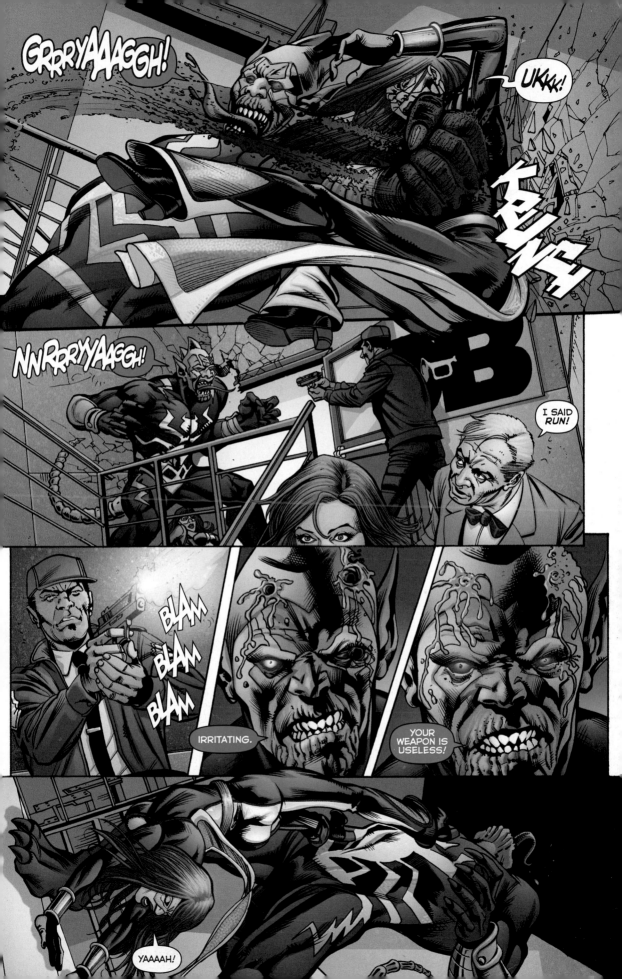

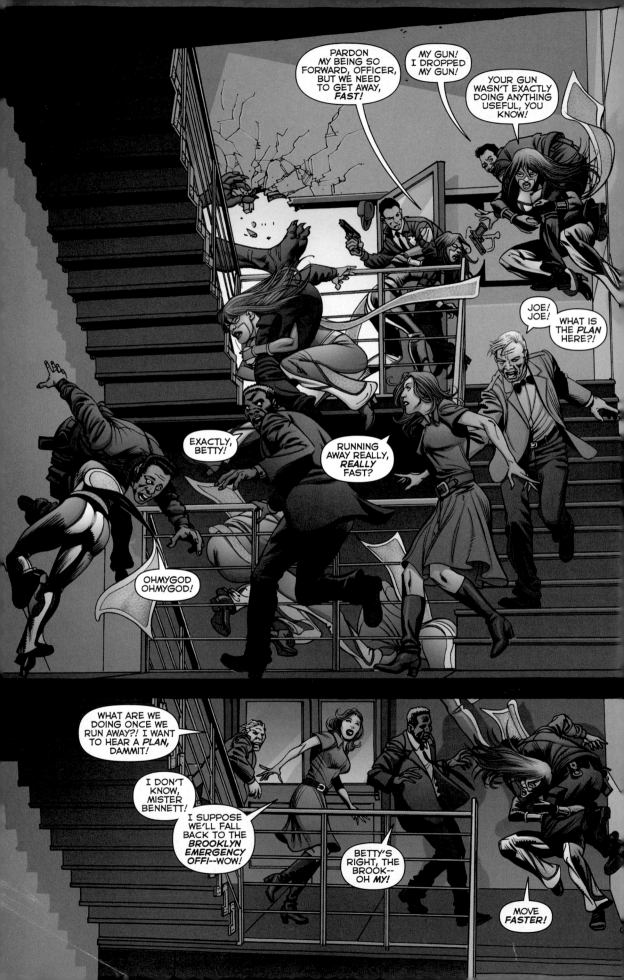

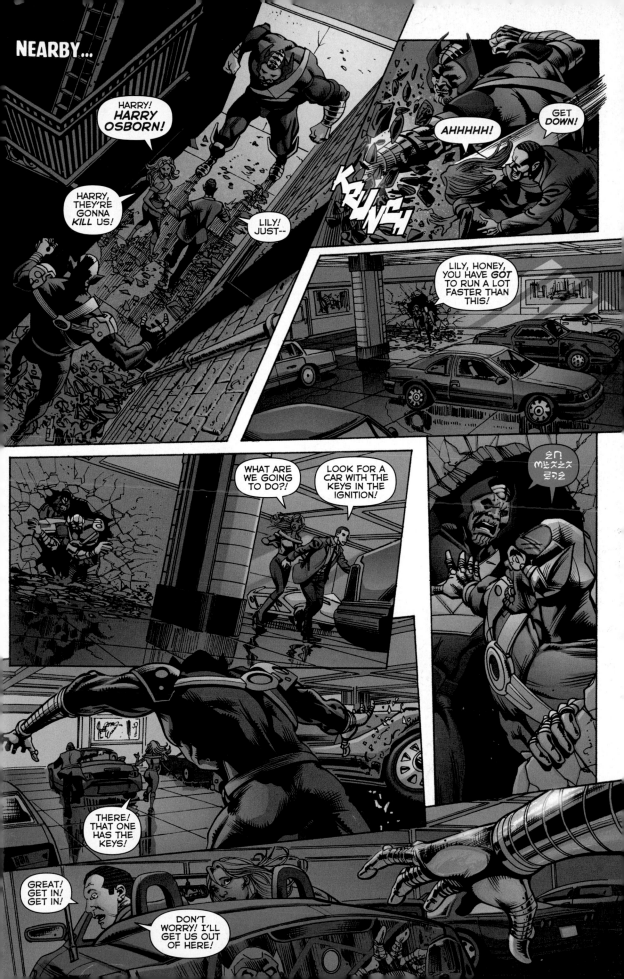

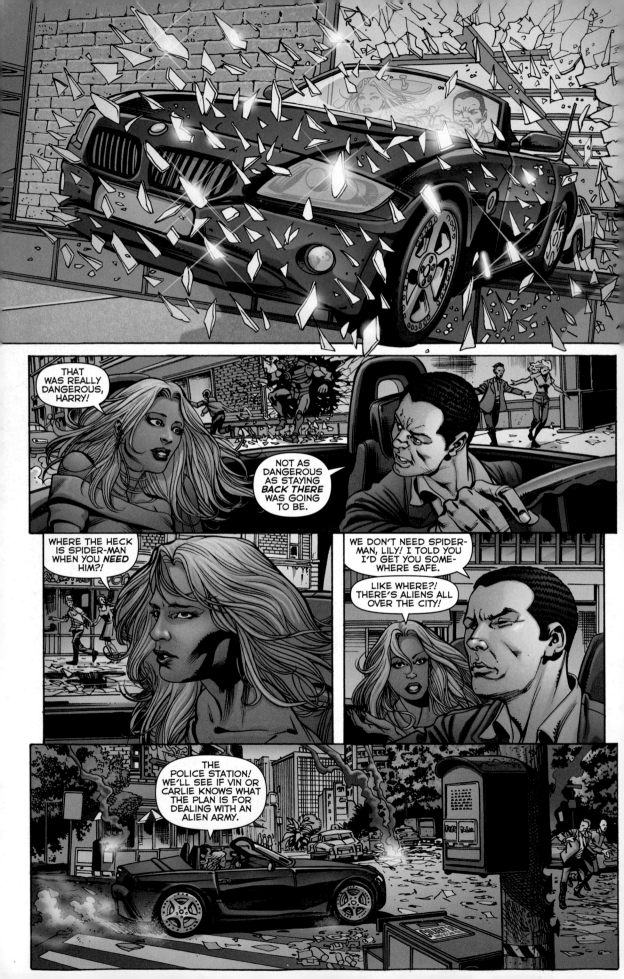

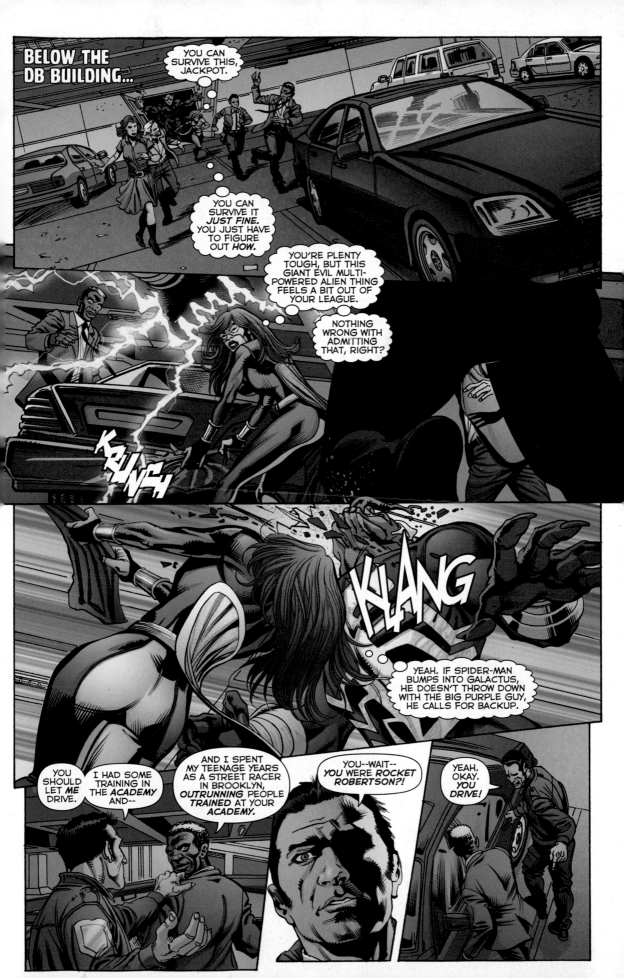

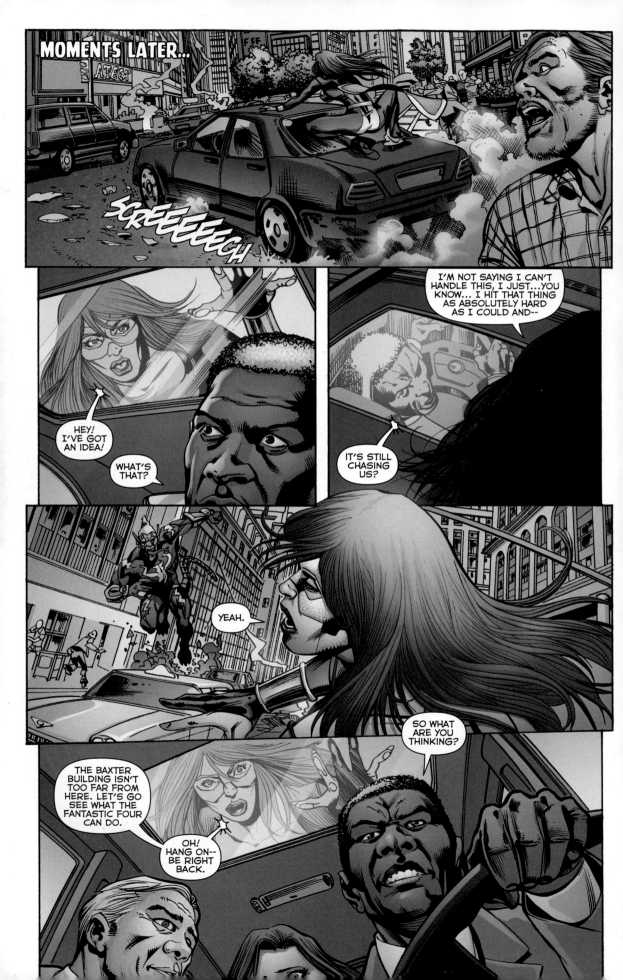

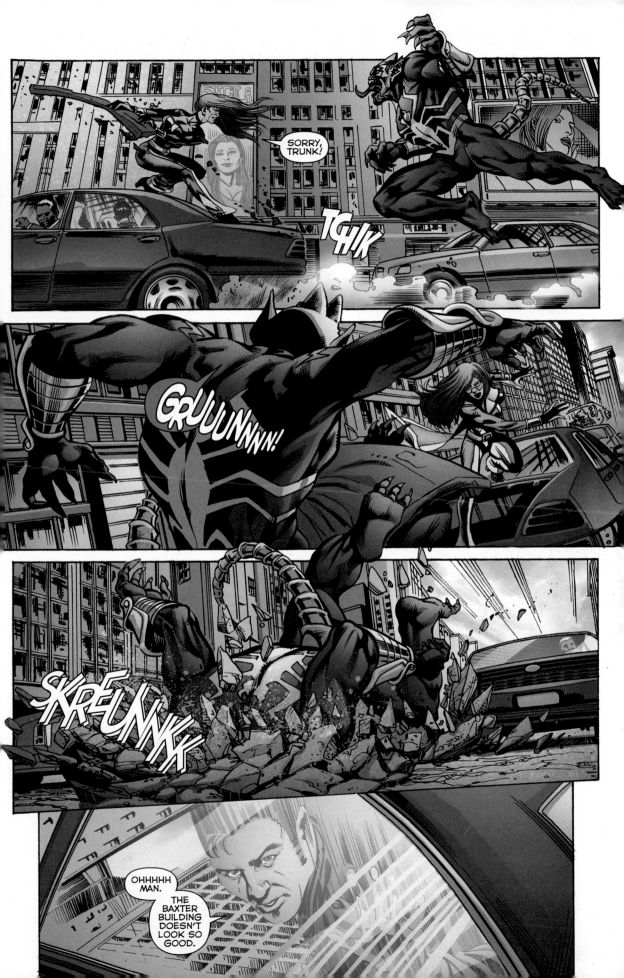

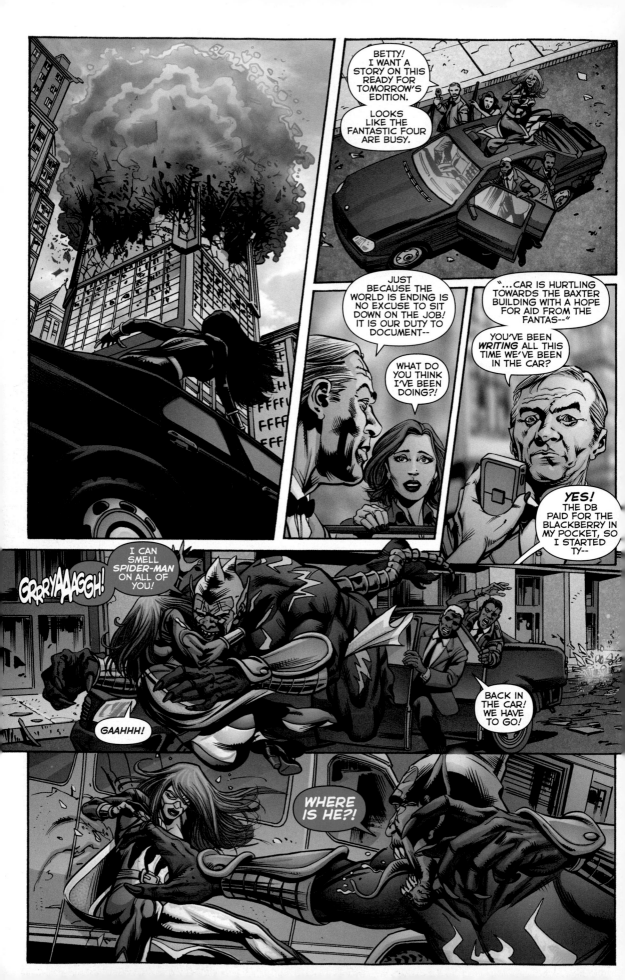

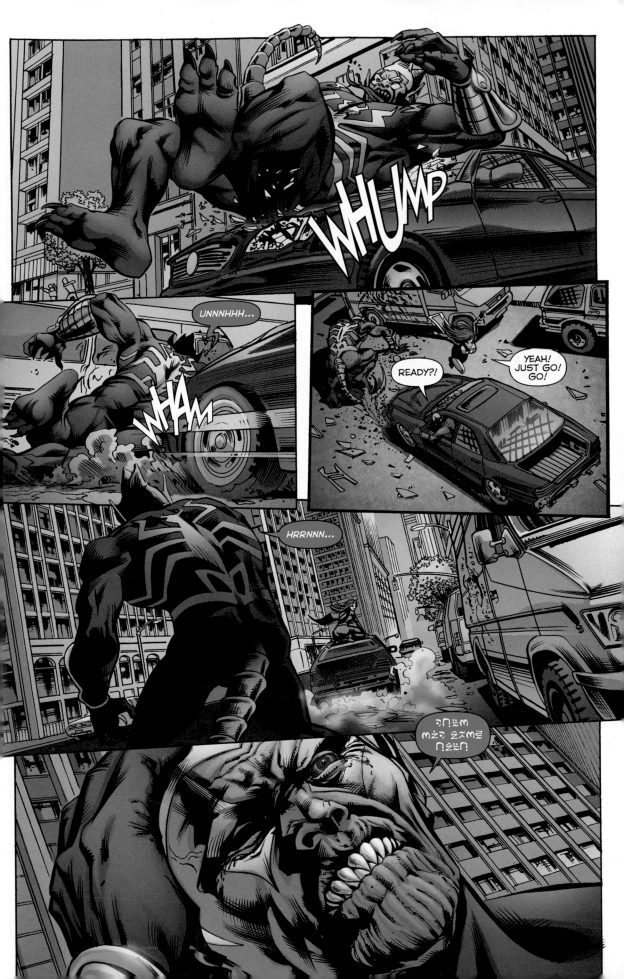

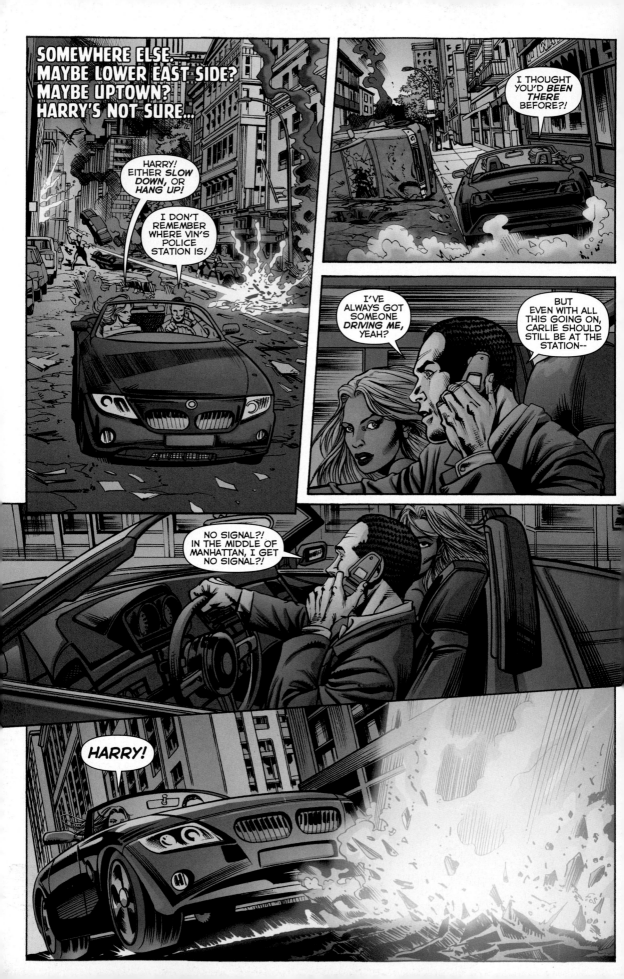

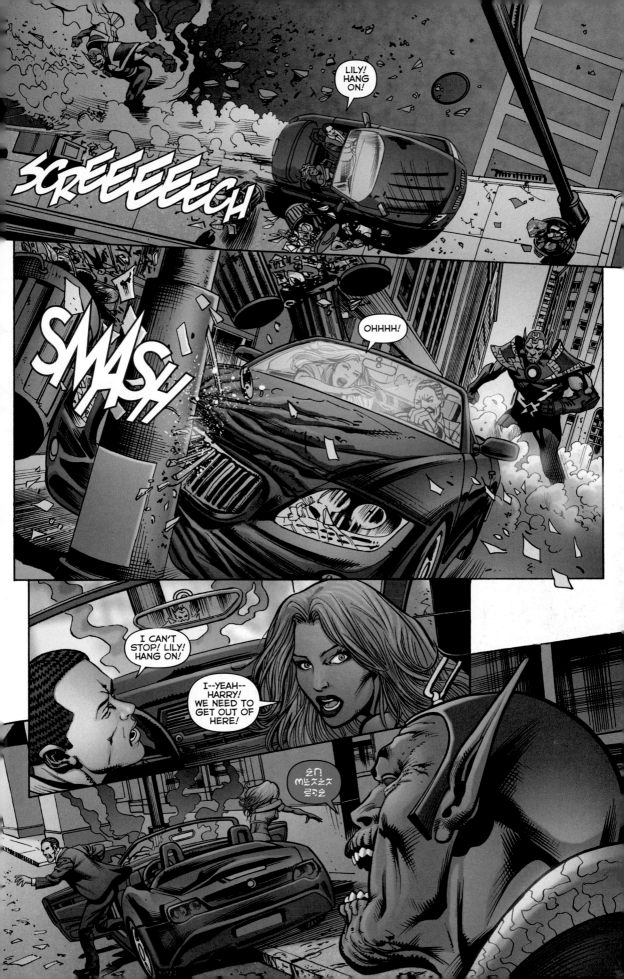

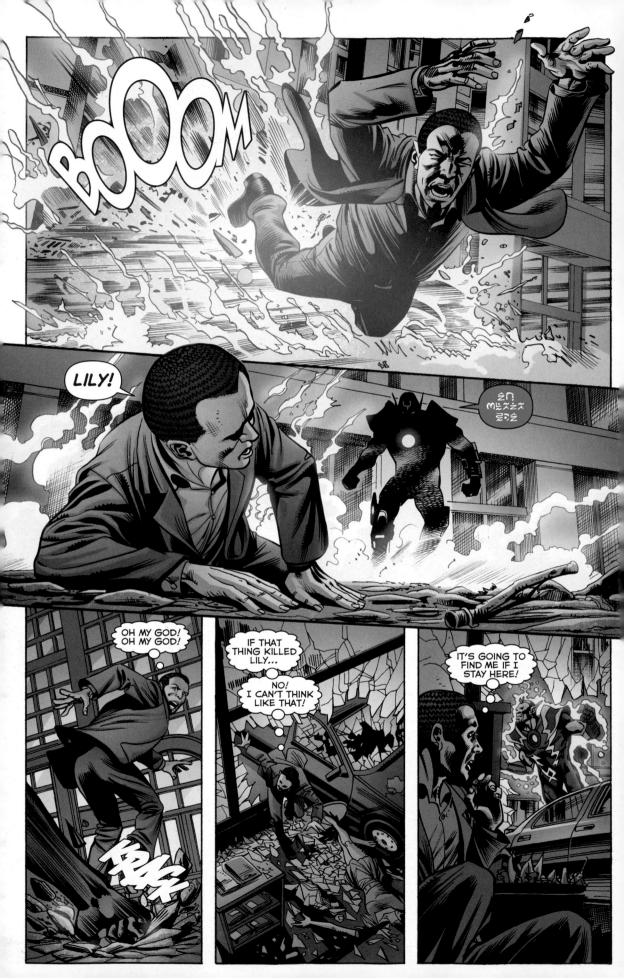

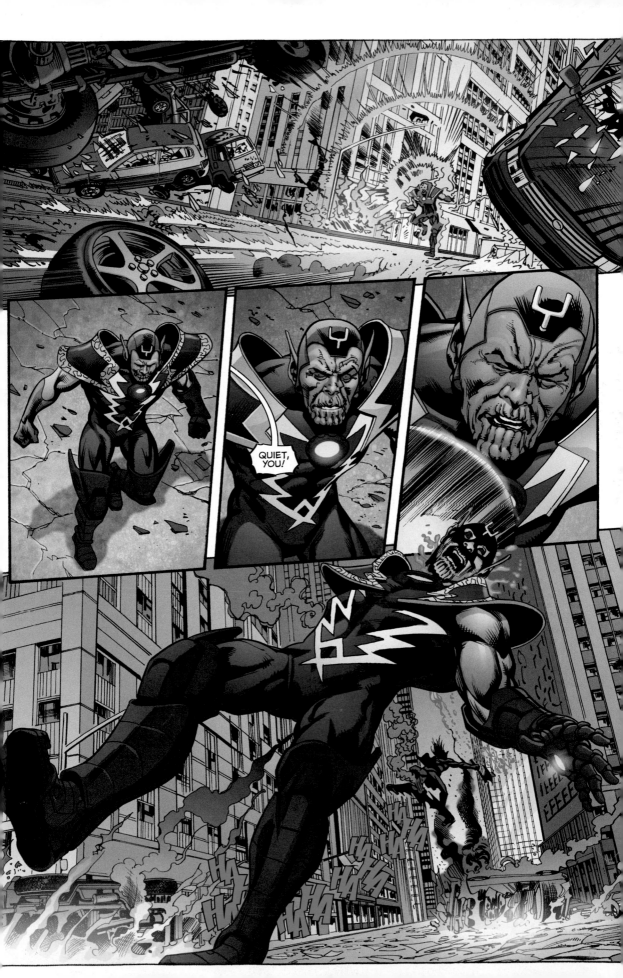

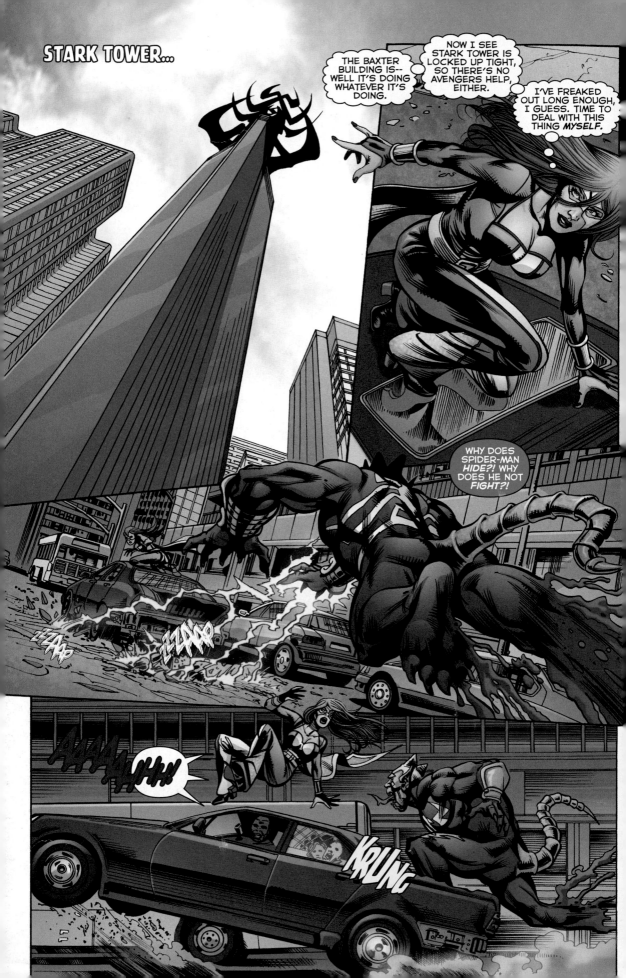

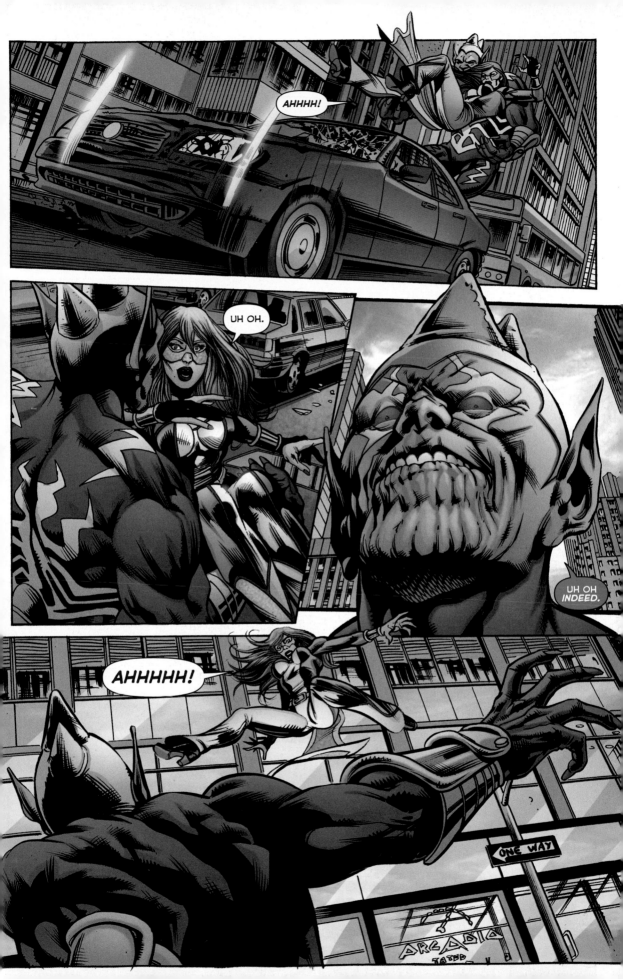

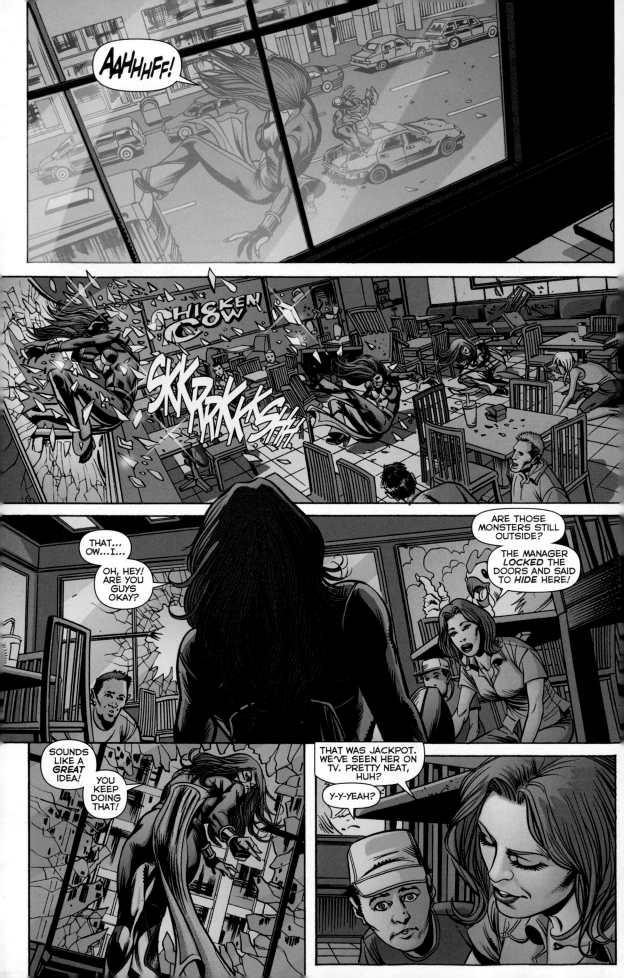

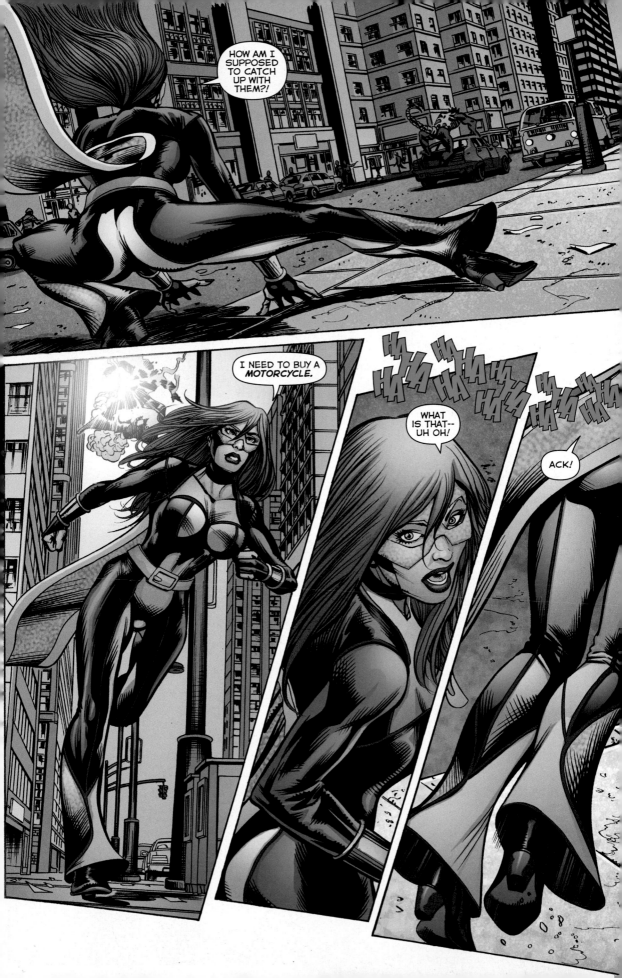

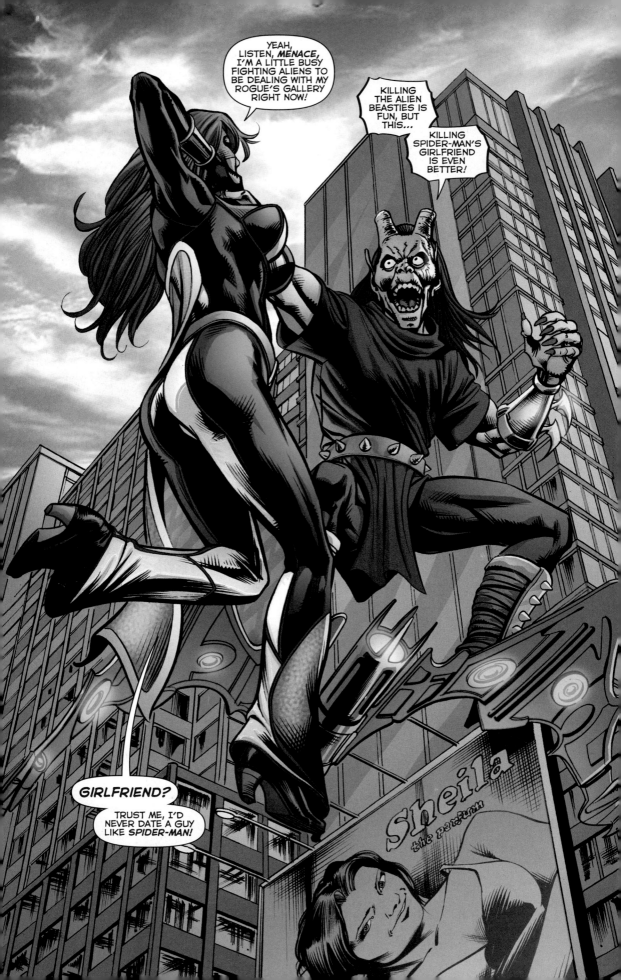

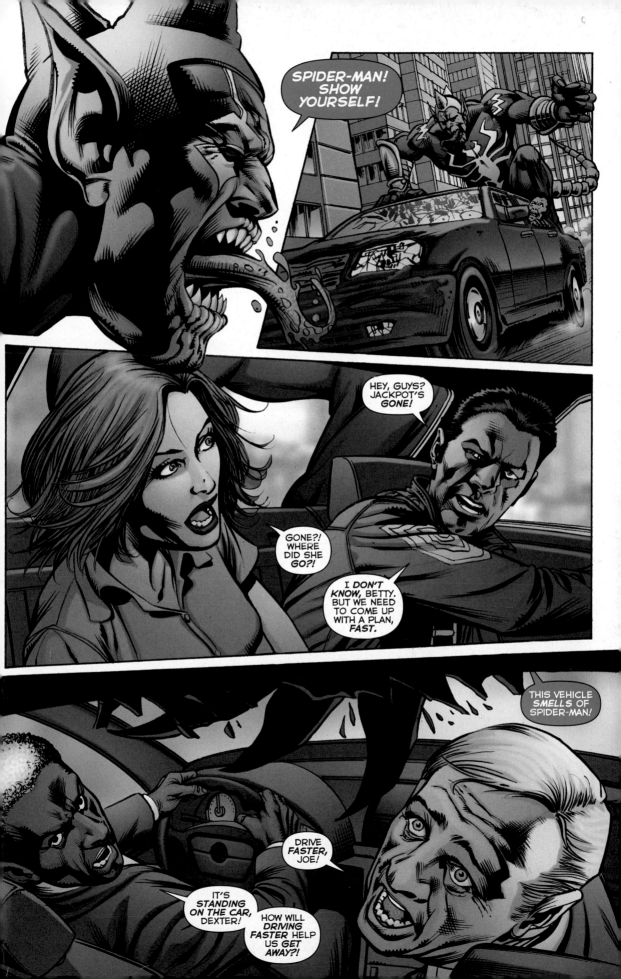

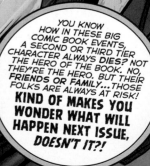

TO BE CONTINUED...

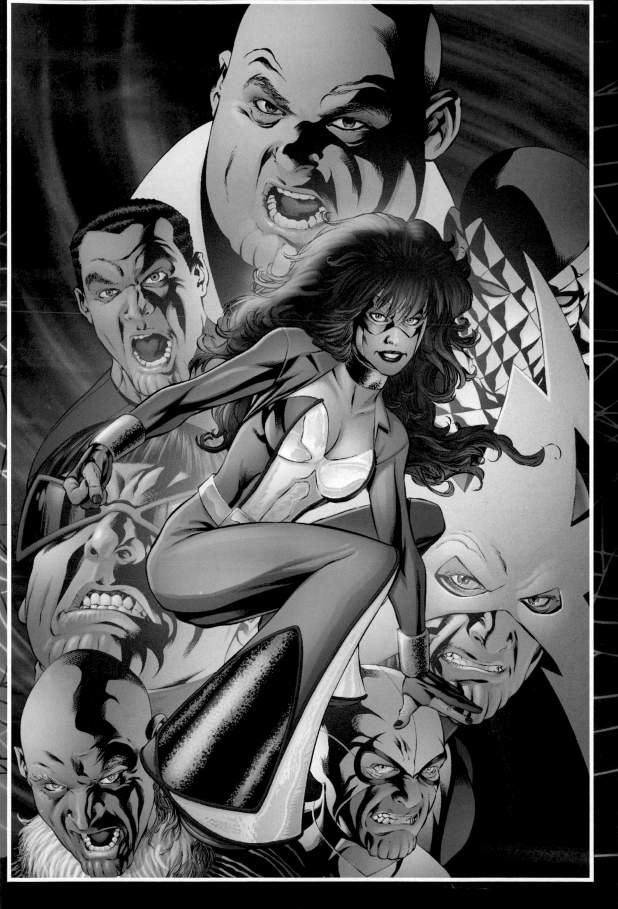

SECRET INVASION: THE AMAZING SPIDER-MAN #3

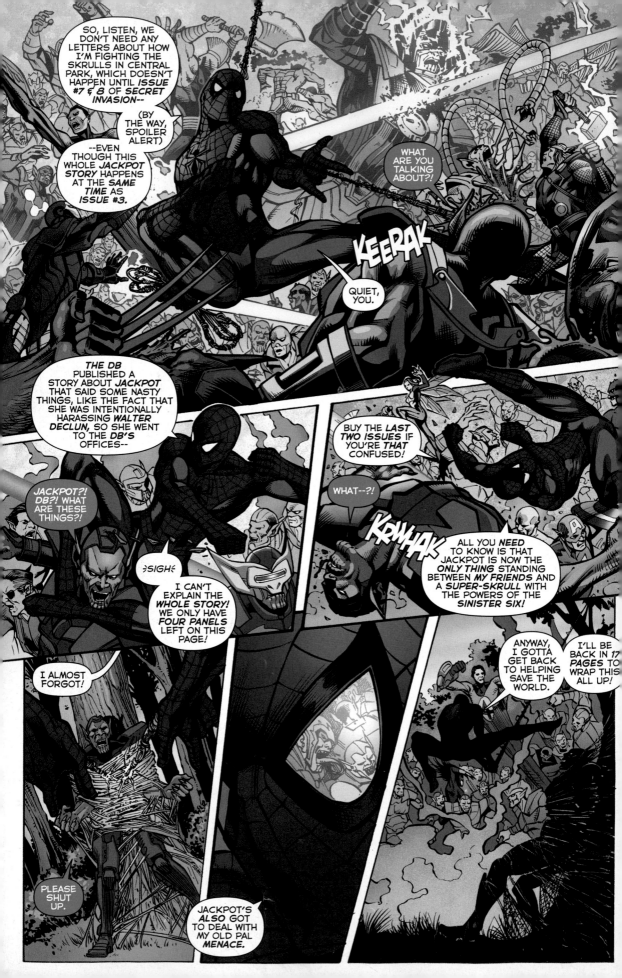

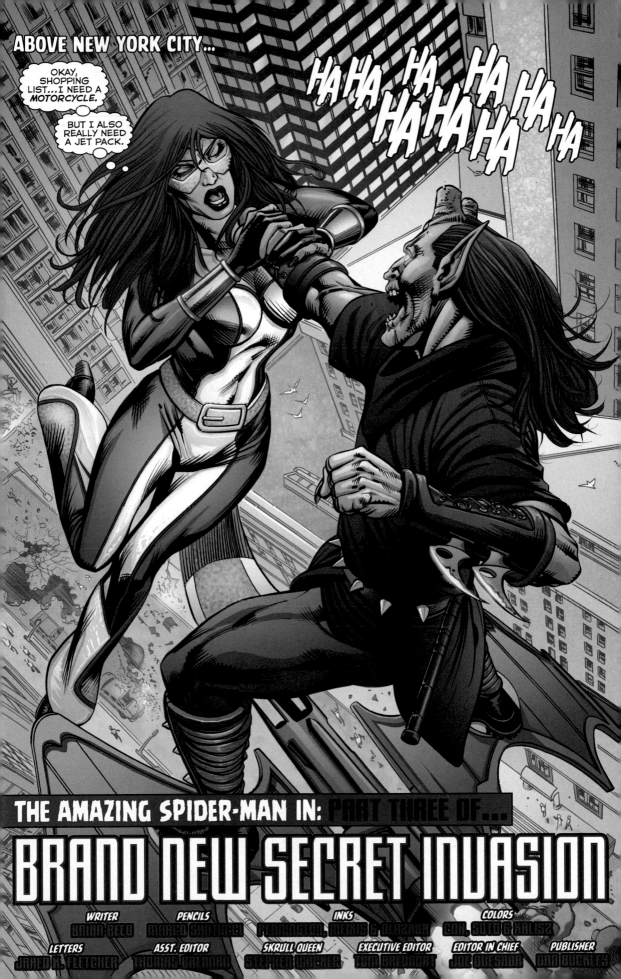

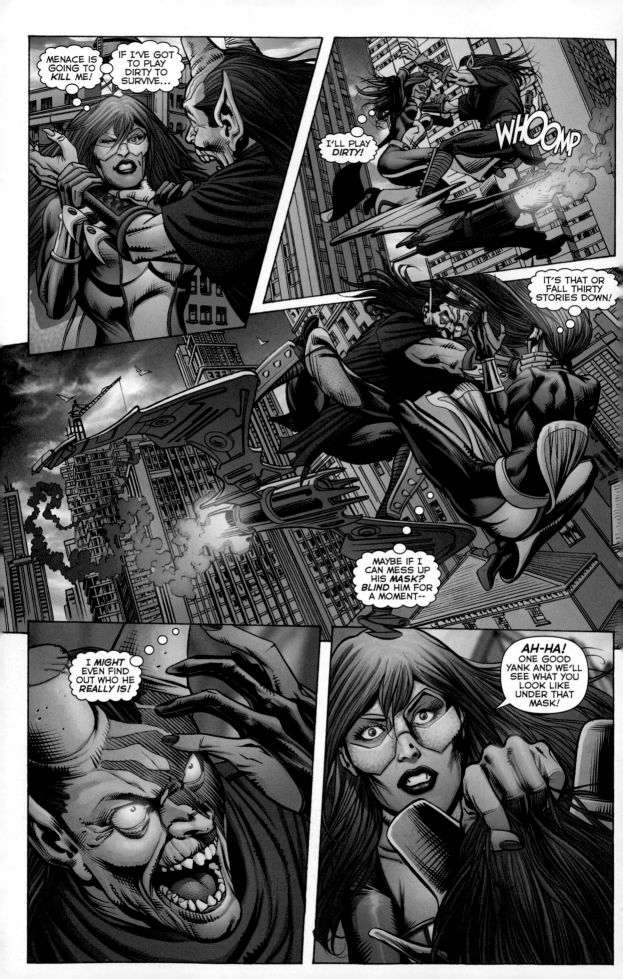

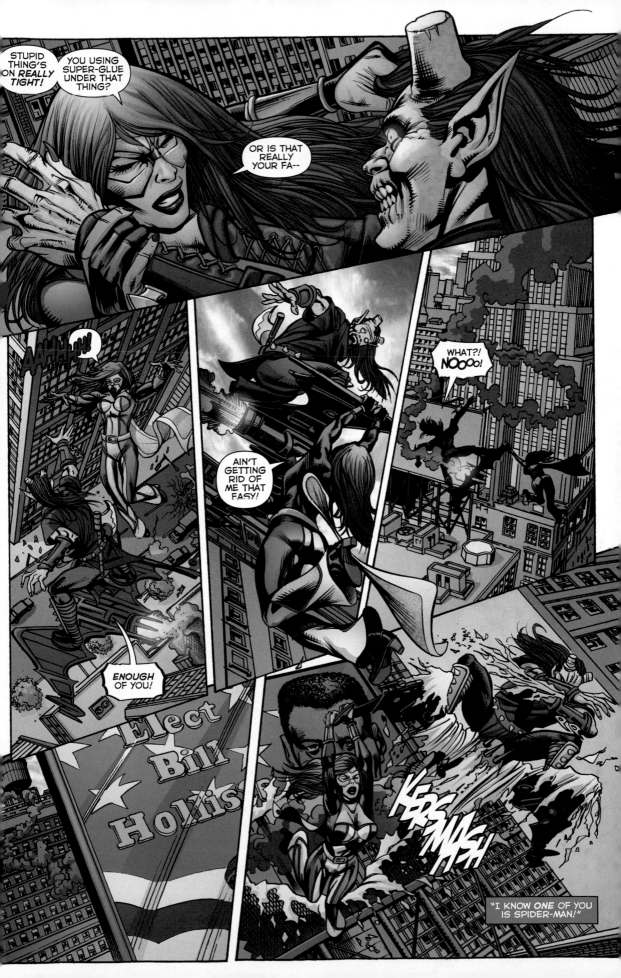

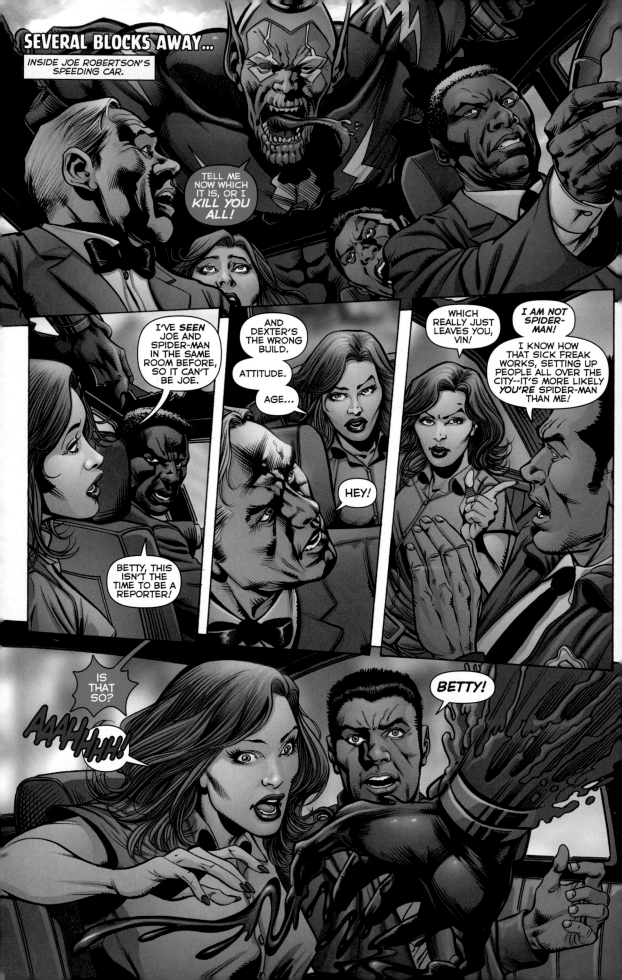

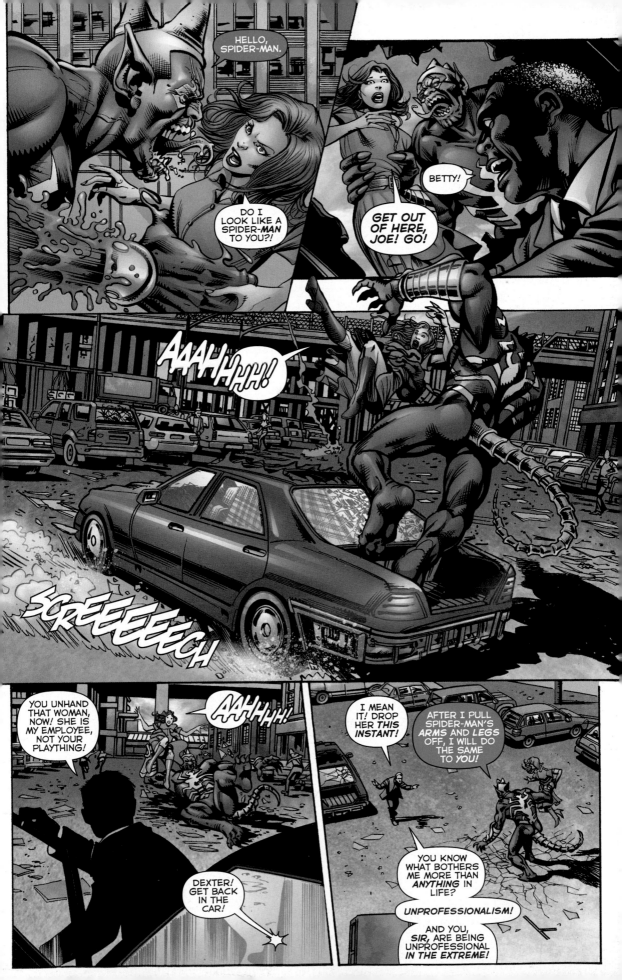

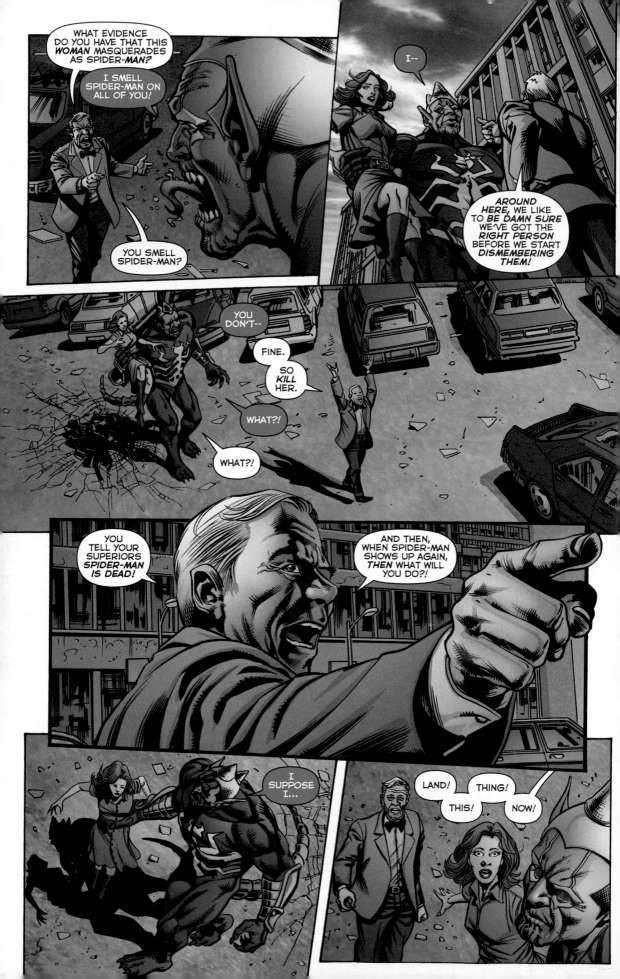

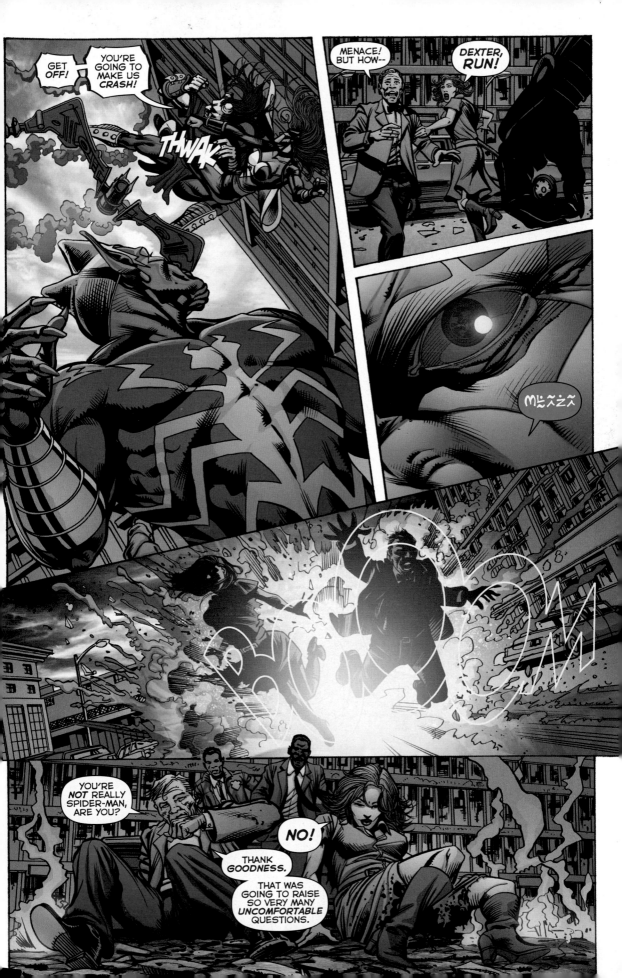

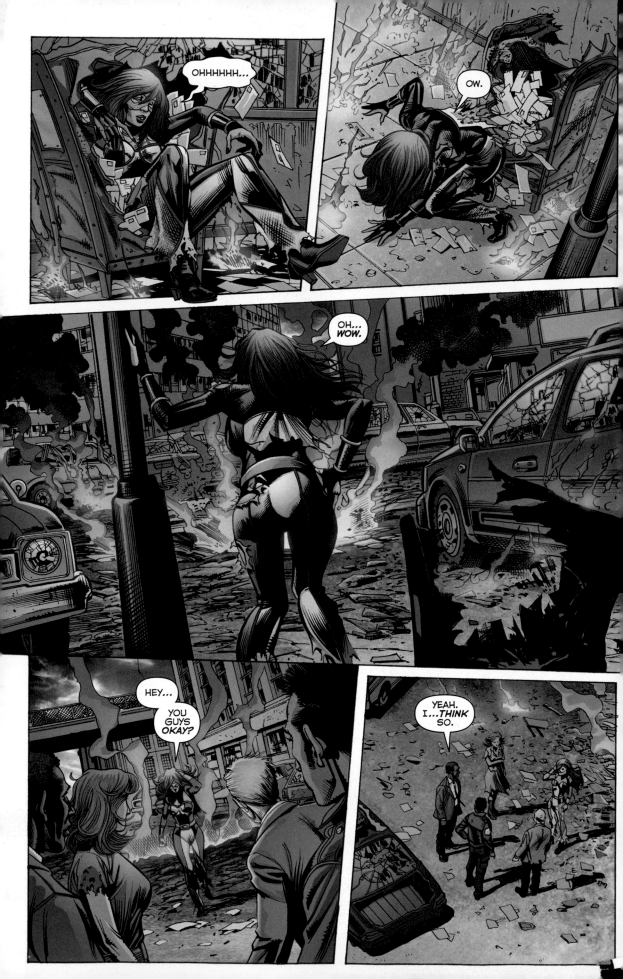

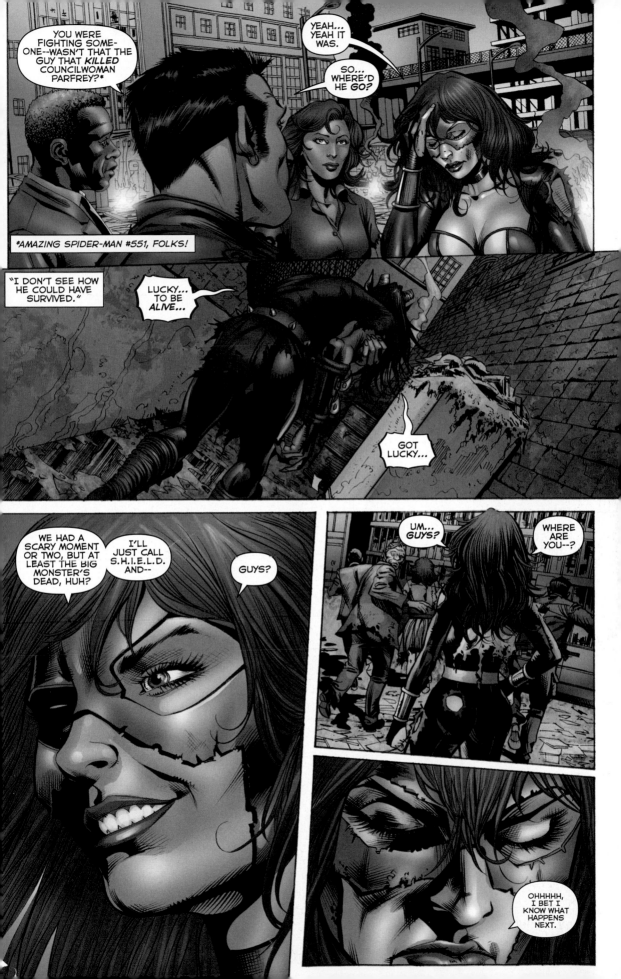

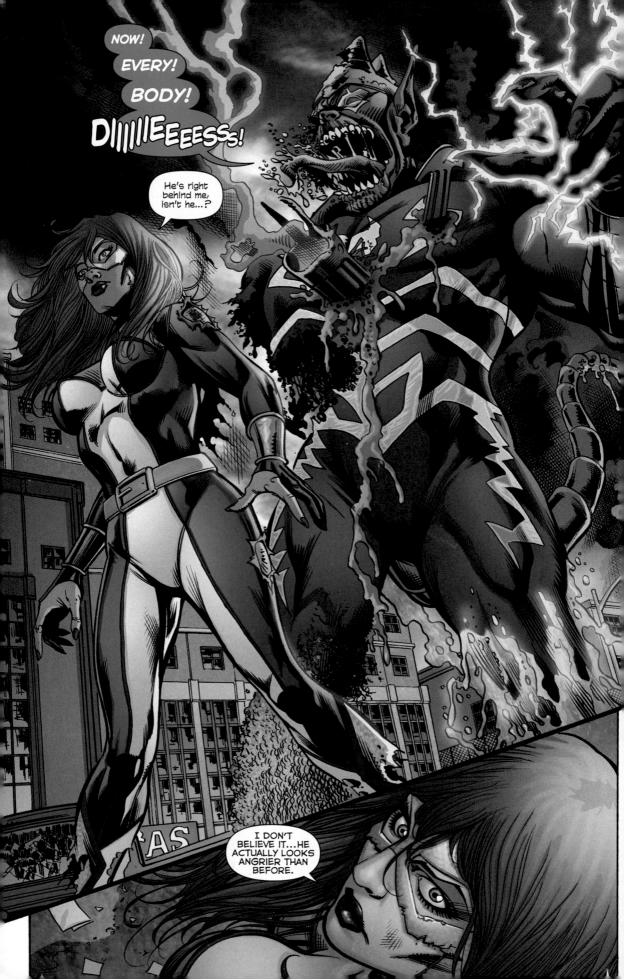

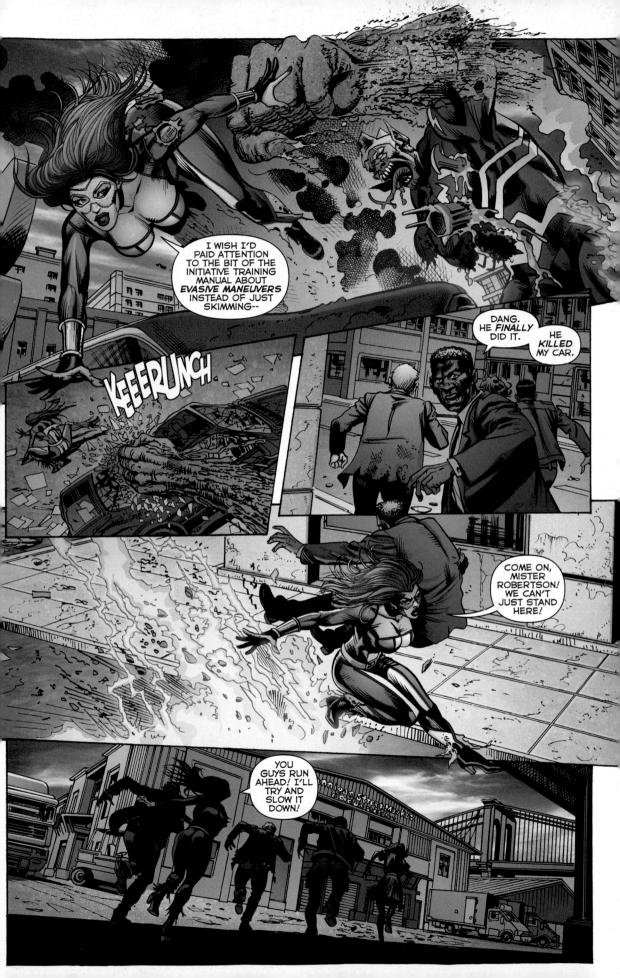

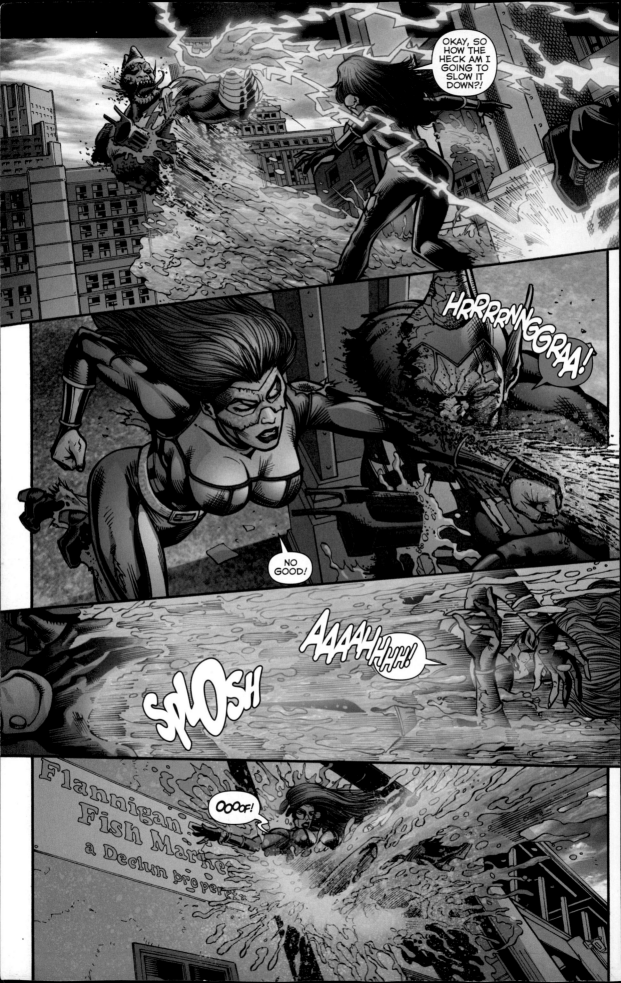

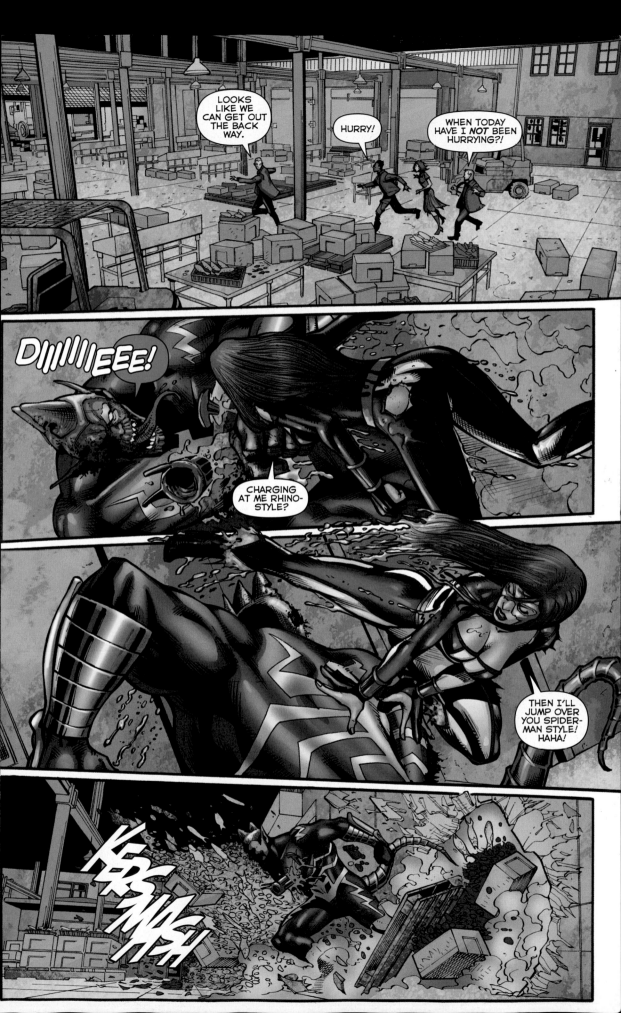

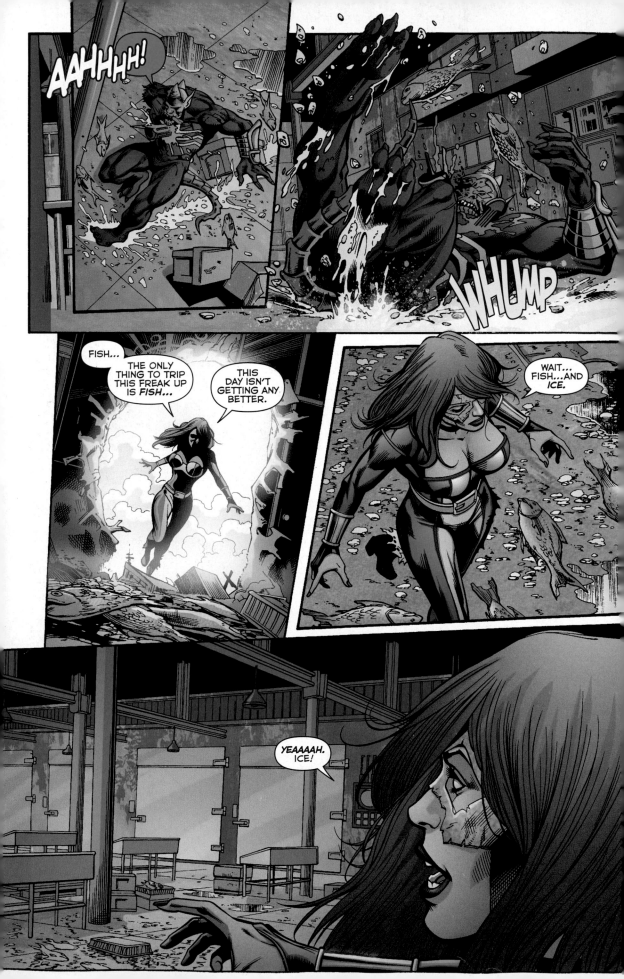

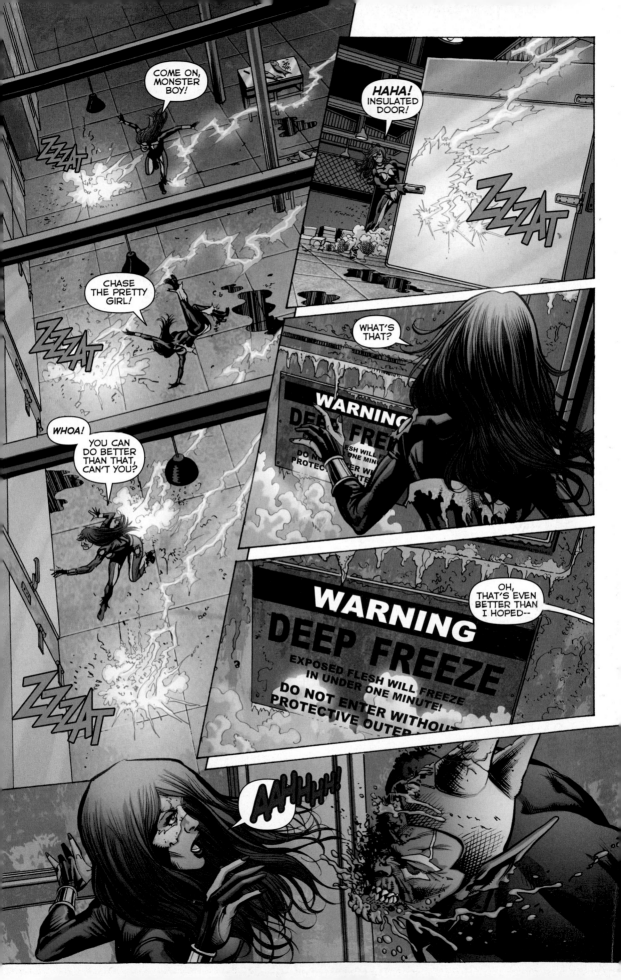

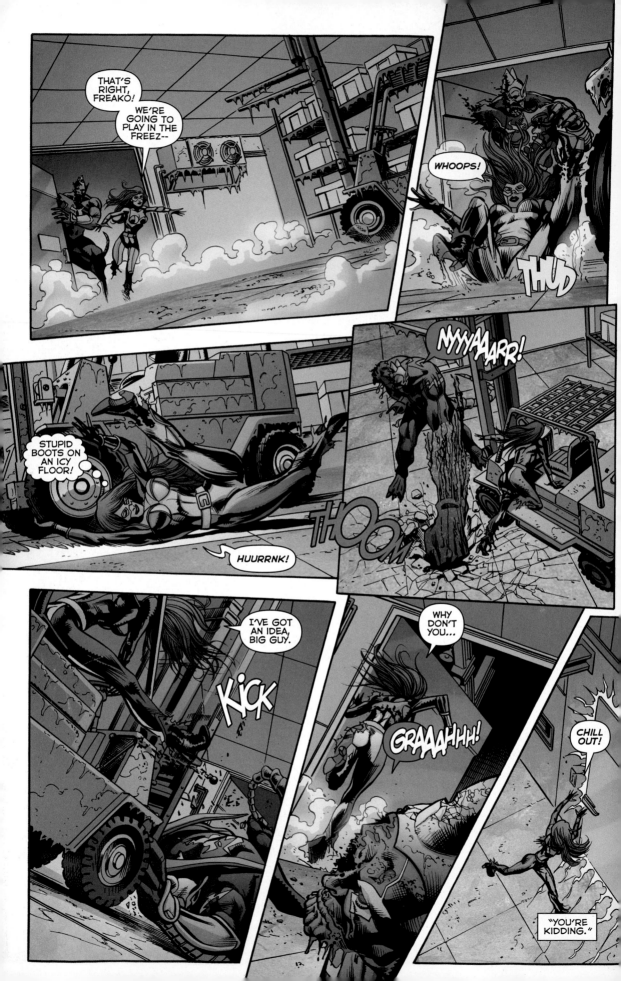

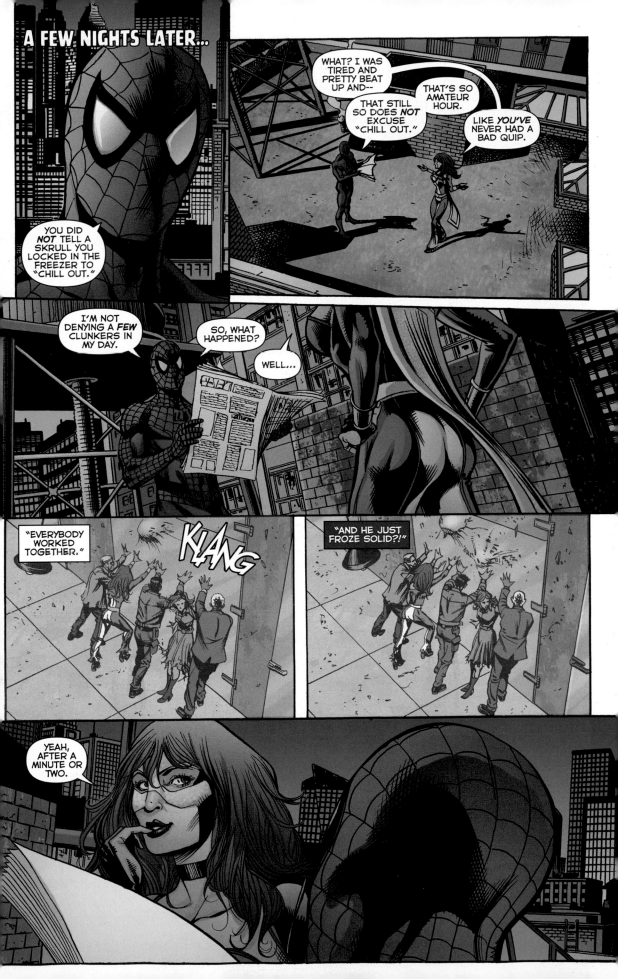

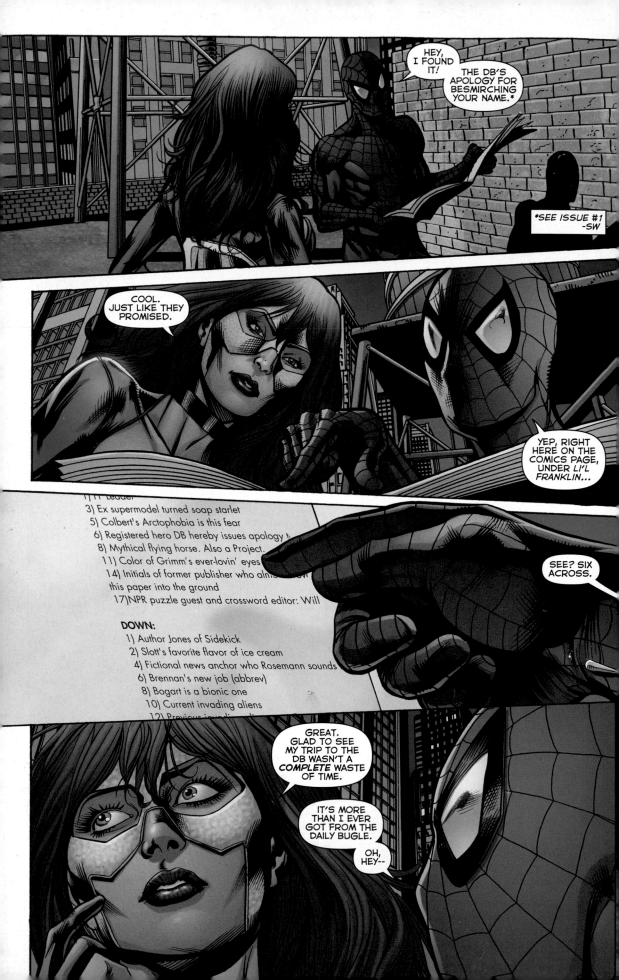

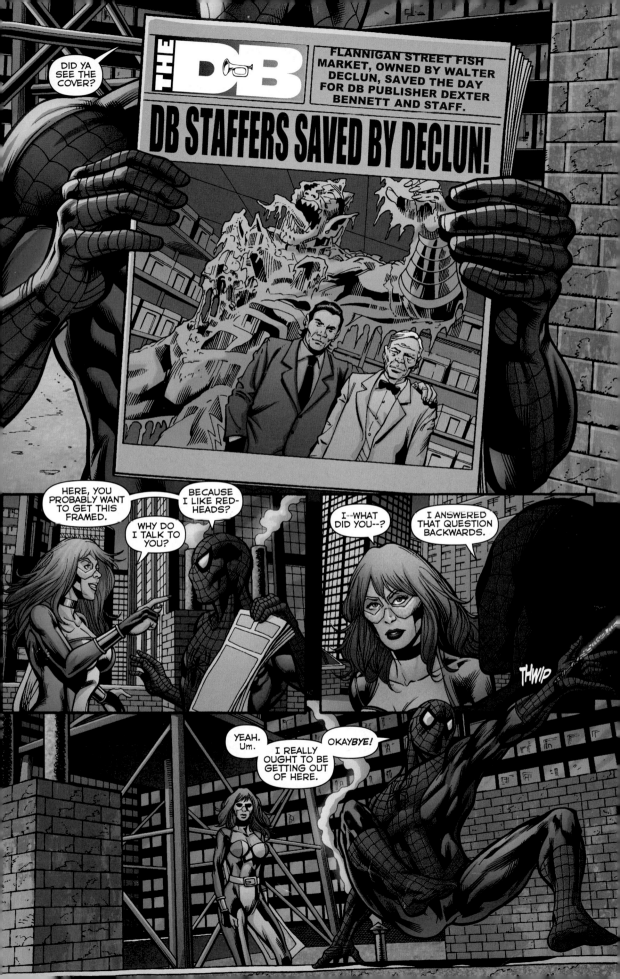

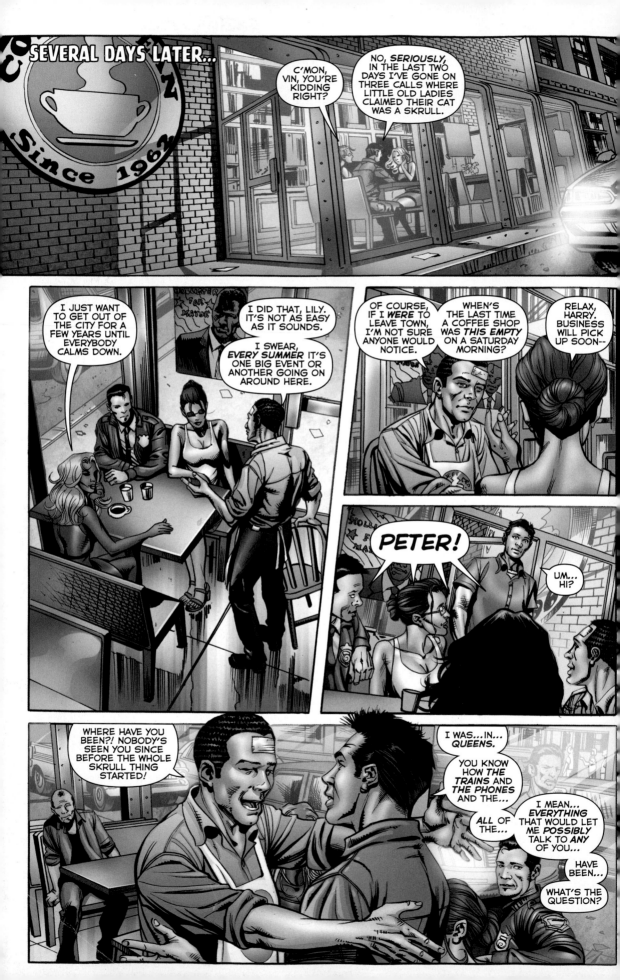

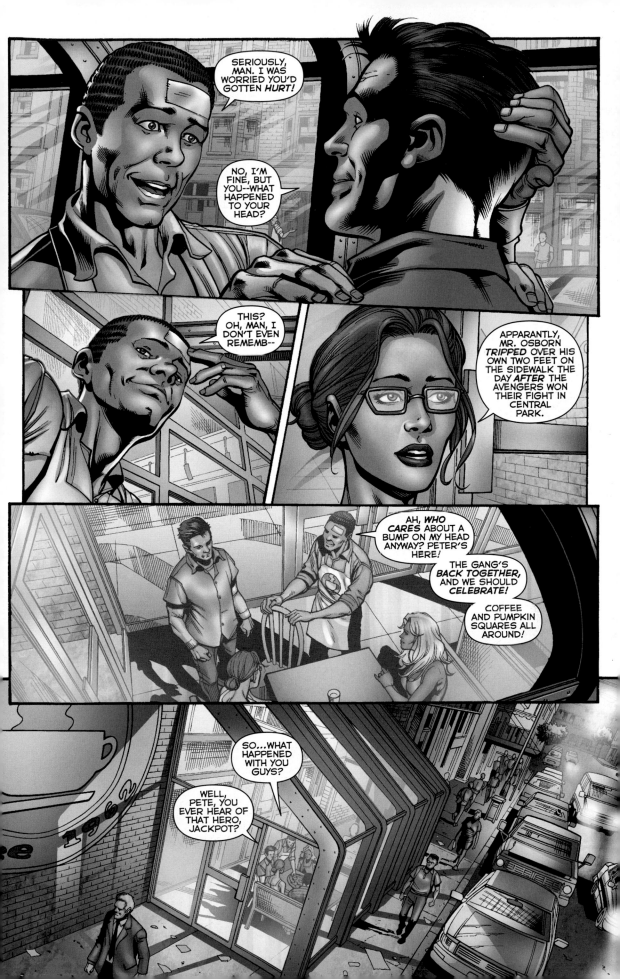

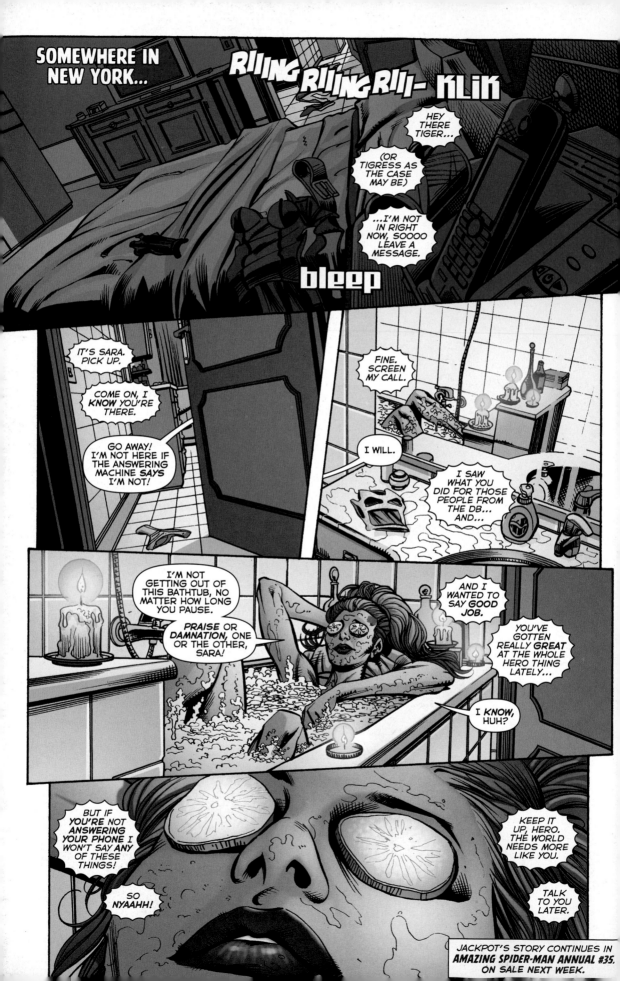

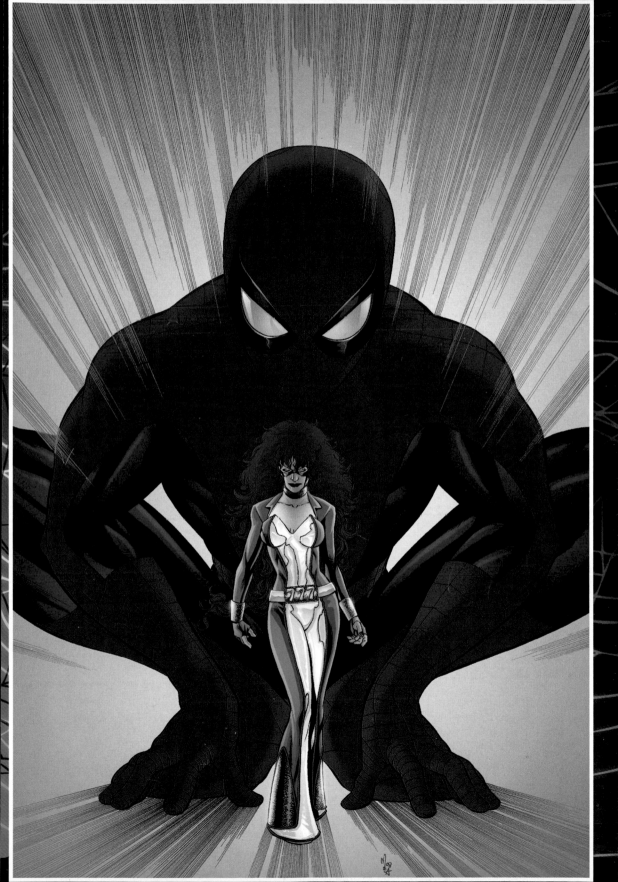

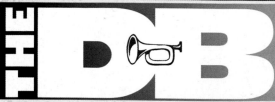

THE DB! SPECIAL EDITION!

OCTOBER 29, 2008 • WEDNESDAY

WHO IS JACKPOT?

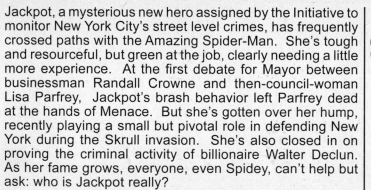

VISIT THE SPIDEY-BLOG! www.marvel.com/blogs/spider-office

Jackpot, a mysterious new hero assigned by the Initiative to monitor New York City's street level crimes, has frequently crossed paths with the Amazing Spider-Man. She's tough and resourceful, but green at the job, clearly needing a little more experience. At the first debate for Mayor between businessman Randall Crowne and then-council-woman Lisa Parfrey, Jackpot's brash behavior left Parfrey dead at the hands of Menace. But she's gotten over her hump, recently playing a small but pivotal role in defending New York during the Skrull invasion. She's also closed in on proving the criminal activity of billionaire Walter Declun. As her fame grows, everyone, even Spidey, can't help but ask: who is Jackpot really?

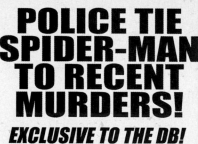

POLICE TIE SPIDER-MAN TO RECENT MURDERS!

EXCLUSIVE TO THE DB!

In off-the-record conversations with DB staffers, police have confirmed that Spider-Man is the key suspect in the string of recent murders that has shocked this city. Although police have been reluctant to discuss the specifics of the murders, so-called "Spider Tracers" have definitely been found on each victim, leaving no doubt as to the involvement of Spider-Man. Spider-Man is already wanted for violations of…

CONTINUED ON A2

WHO IS THE MYSTERIOUS VILLAIN KNOWN AS **BLINDSIDE**?! (A NEW SUPER-BADDIE CREATED AND CONCEIVED IN THE MIGHTY MARVEL MANNER!)

WHO IS THE MYSTERIOUS SUPER-HEROINE KNOWN AS **JACKPOT**?! (HINT: SHE'S NOT WHO YOU THINK SHE IS!)

AND *INTRODUCING...* THE MOST DANGEROUS MARVEL VILLAIN SINCE THE KINGPIN... **THE MOGUL!** (ACTUALLY IT'S A GUY NAMED WALTER DECLUN, BUT LEGAL NEEDED SOMETHING TO TRADEMARK! HE'S A NASTY PIECE OF WORK, THOUGH!)

the **AMAZING SPIDER-MAN** IN

A TALE OF TWO JACKPOTS

| MARC GUGGENHEIM WRITER | MIKE McKONE PENCILS | ANDY LANNING INKS | JEROMY COX W/SOTOCOLOR COLORS | VC'S CORY PETIT LETTERS | TOM BRENNAN ASST. EDITOR | STEPHEN WACKER EDITOR | TOM BREVOORT EXECUTIVE EDITOR | JOE QUESADA EDITOR IN CHIEF | DAN BUCKLEY PUBLISHER |

GALE, GUGGENHEIM, SLOTT & WELLS SPIDEY'S BRAINTRUST

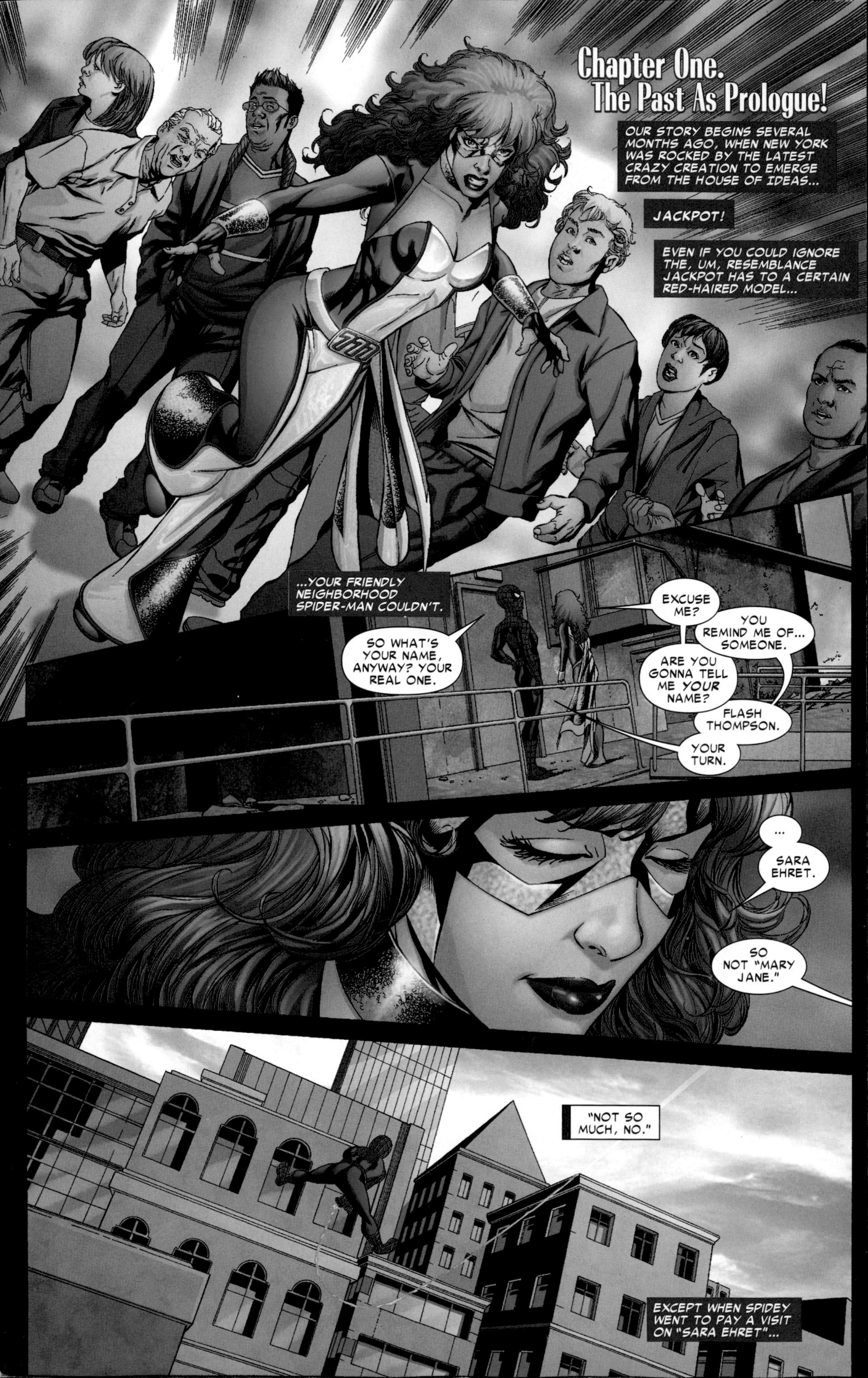
Chapter One. The Past As Prologue!
OUR STORY BEGINS SEVERAL MONTHS AGO, WHEN NEW YORK WAS ROCKED BY THE LATEST CRAZY CREATION TO EMERGE FROM THE HOUSE OF IDEAS...
JACKPOT!
EVEN IF YOU COULD IGNORE THE, UM, RESEMBLANCE JACKPOT HAS TO A CERTAIN RED-HAIRED MODEL...
...YOUR FRIENDLY NEIGHBORHOOD SPIDER-MAN COULDN'T.
SO WHAT'S YOUR NAME, ANYWAY? YOUR REAL ONE.
EXCUSE ME?
YOU REMIND ME OF... SOMEONE.
ARE YOU GONNA TELL ME YOUR NAME?
FLASH THOMPSON.
YOUR TURN.
...
SARA EHRET.
SO NOT "MARY JANE."
"NOT SO MUCH, NO."
EXCEPT WHEN SPIDEY WENT TO PAY A VISIT ON "SARA EHRET"...

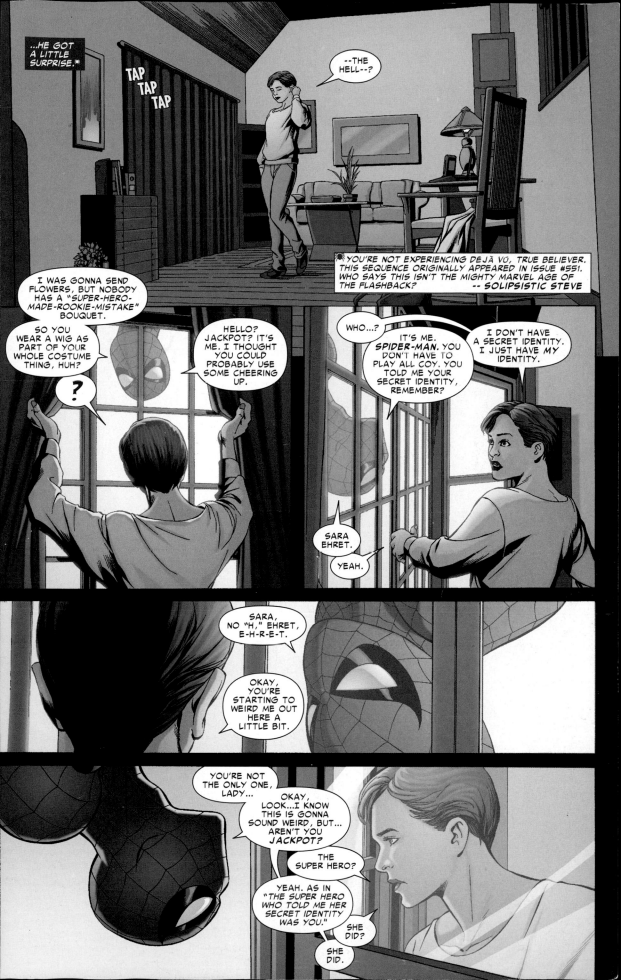

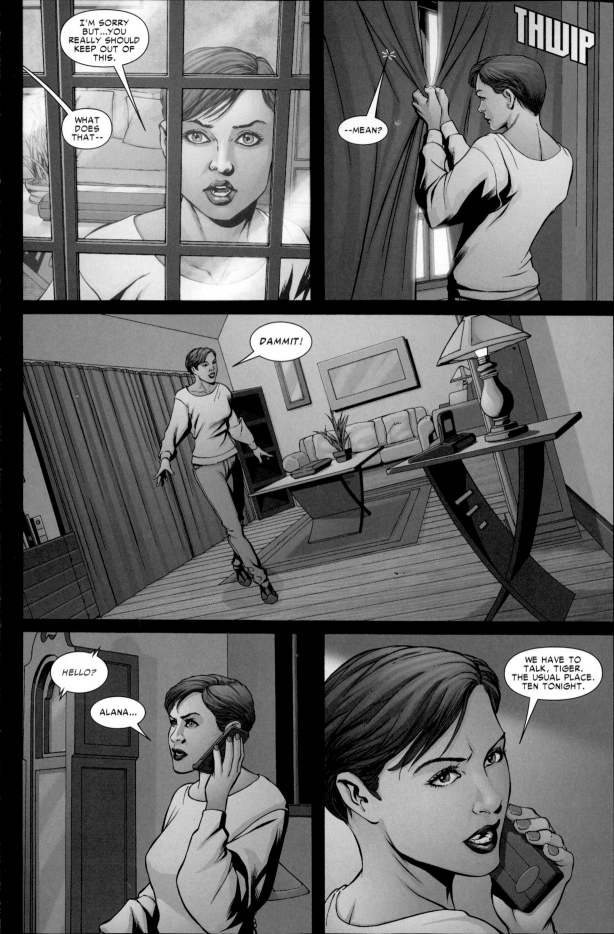

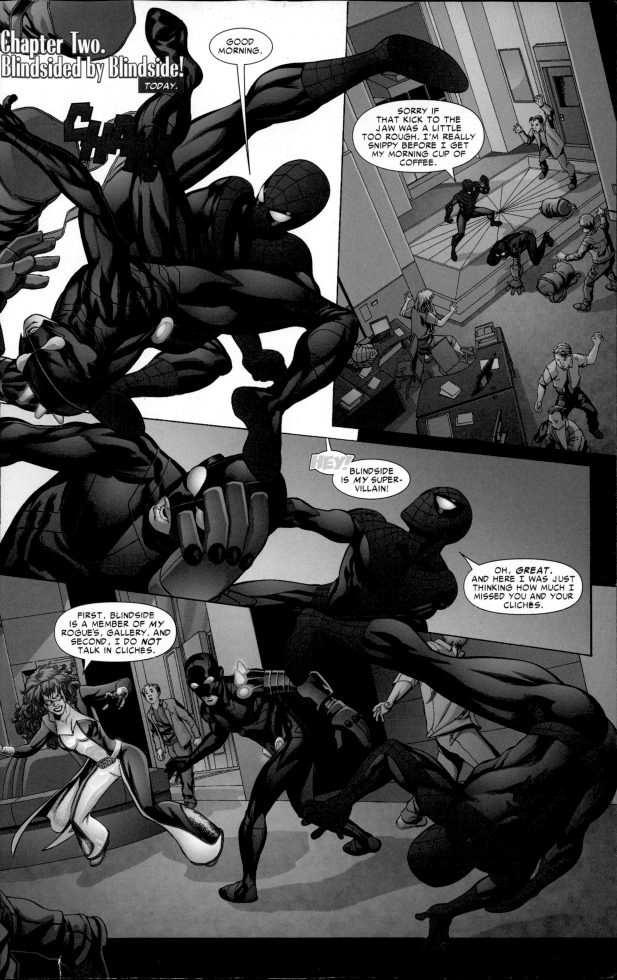

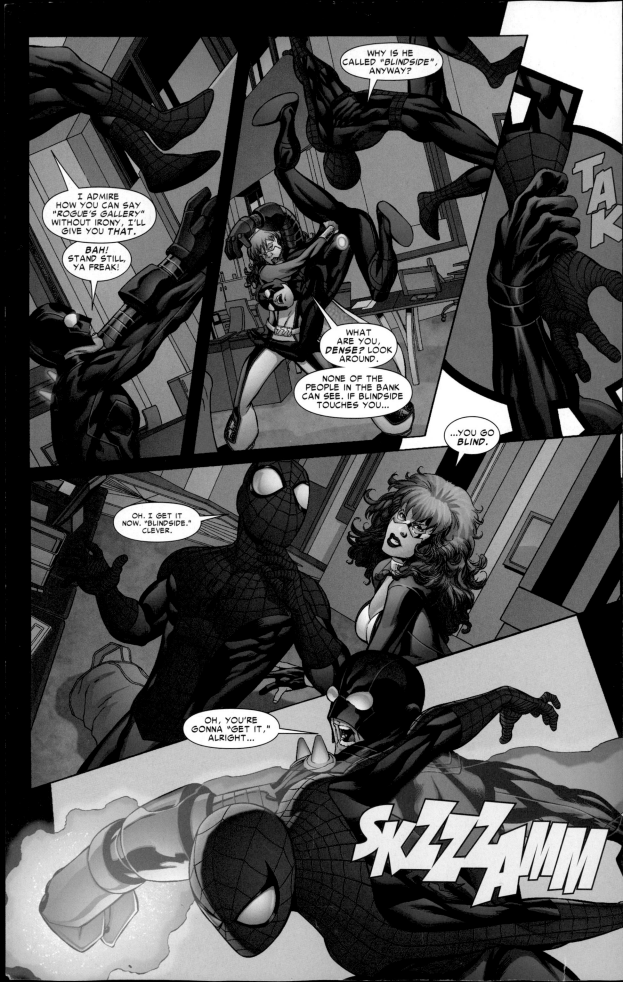

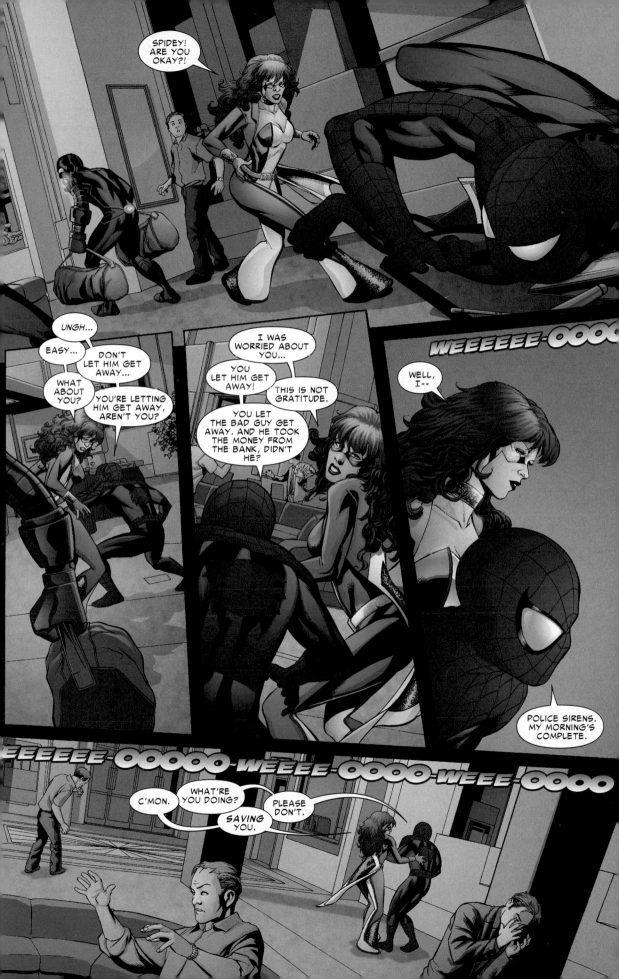

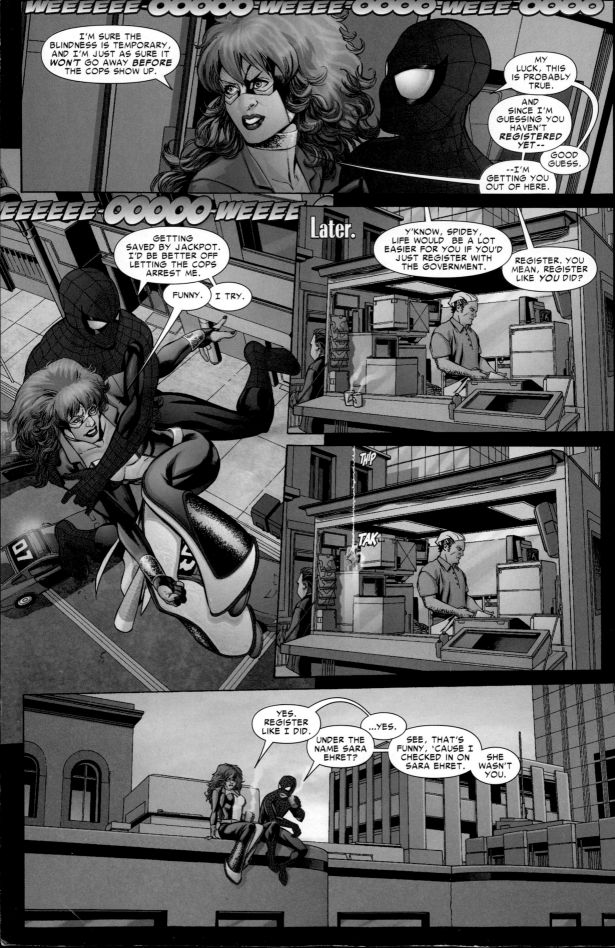

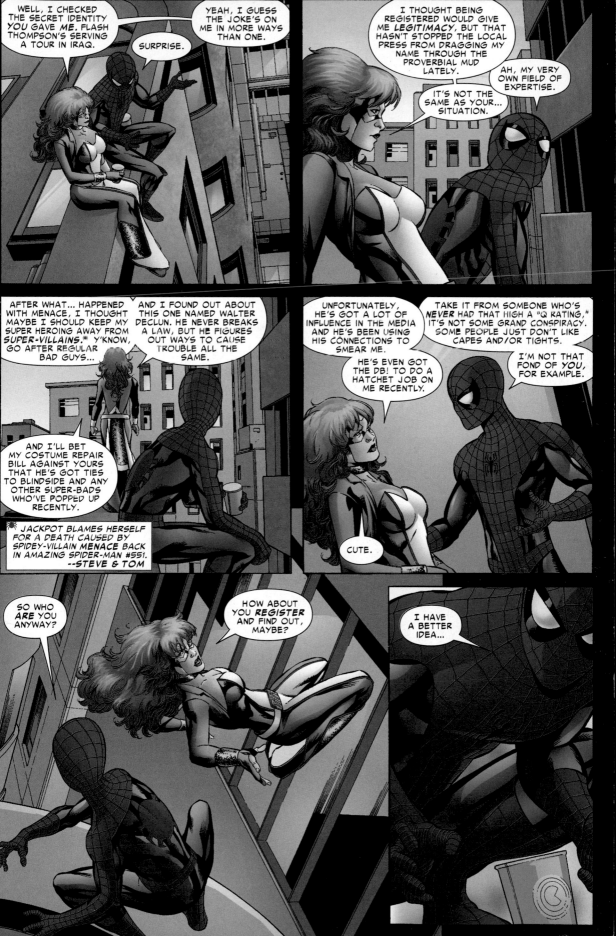

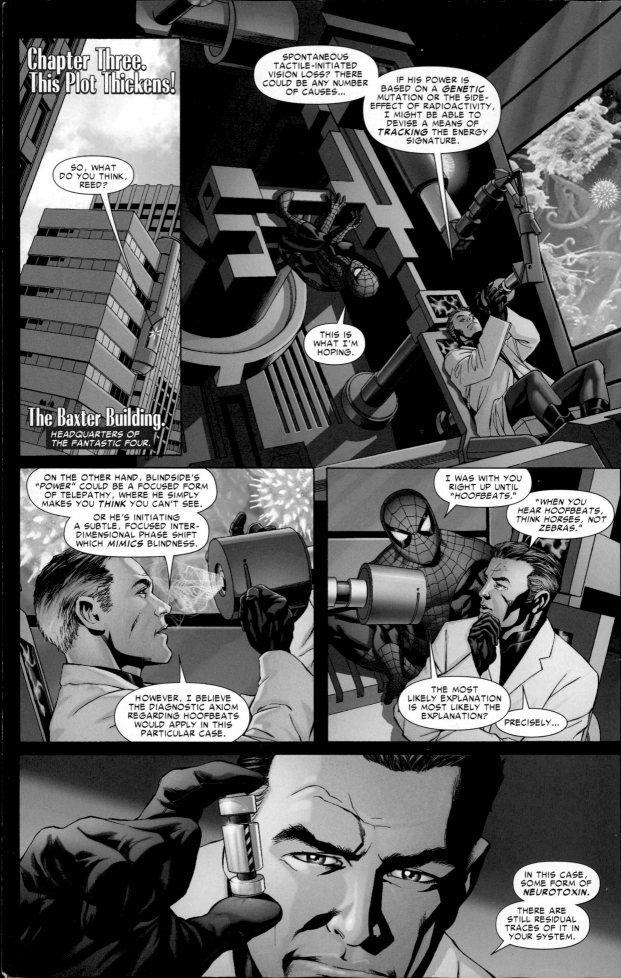

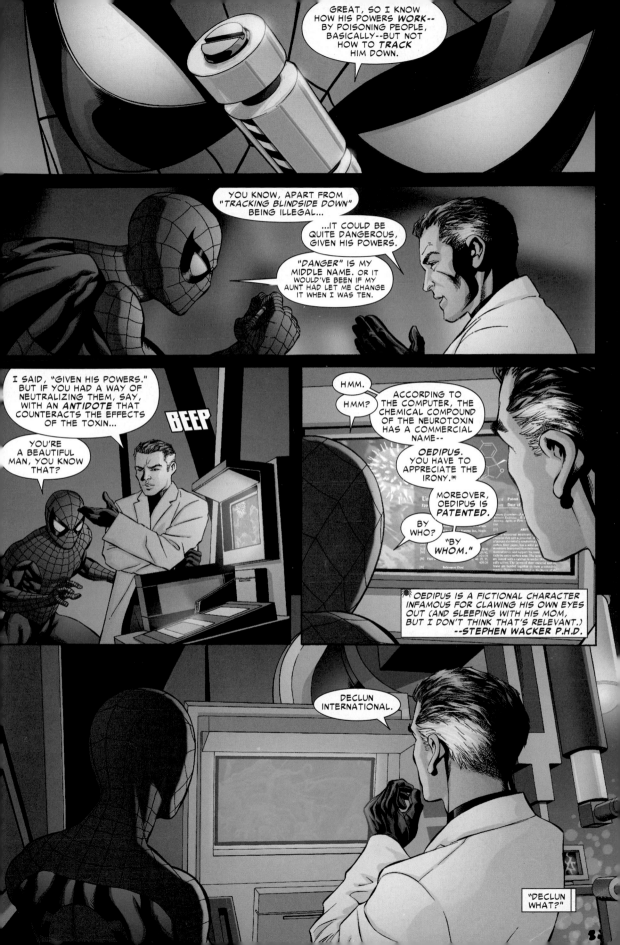

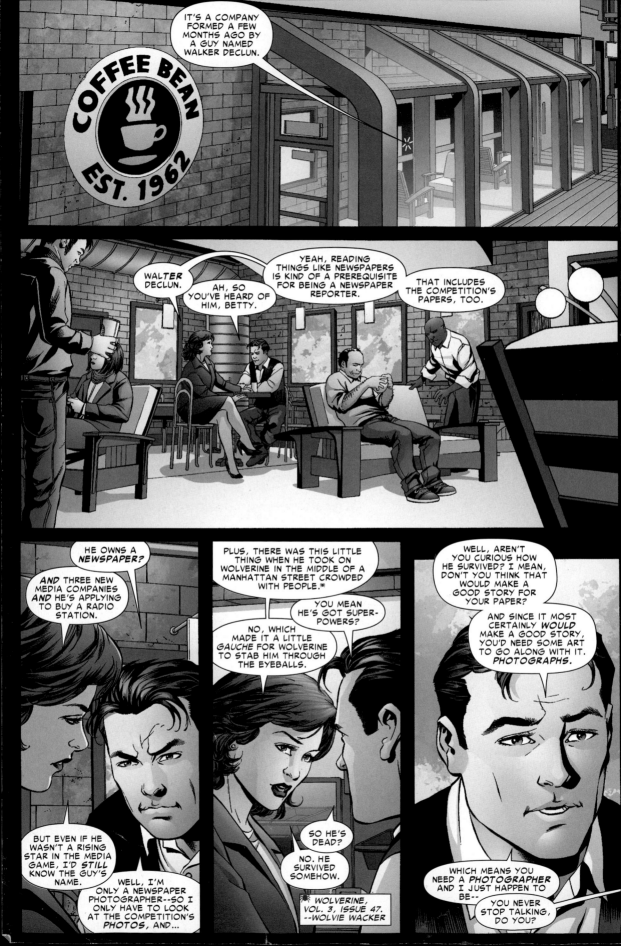

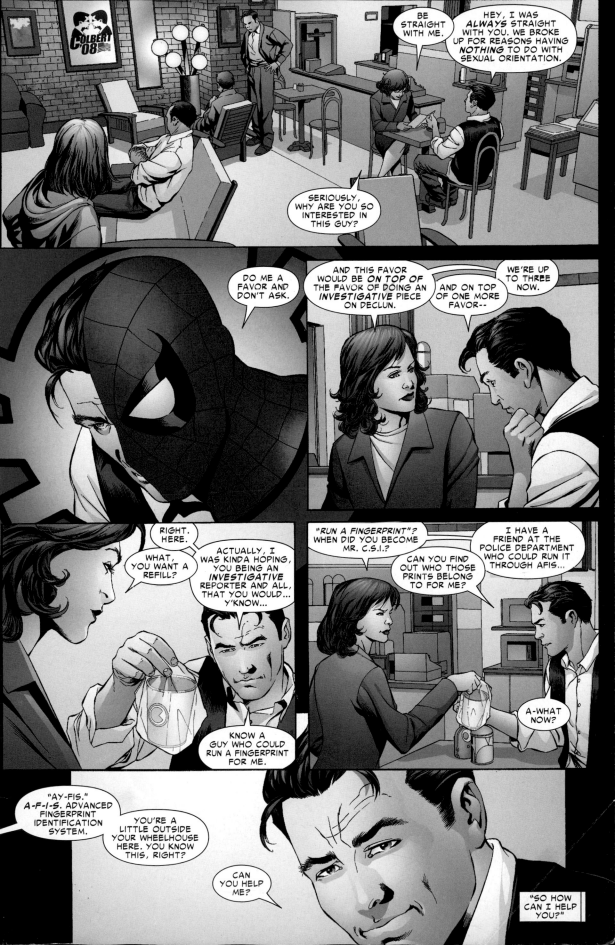

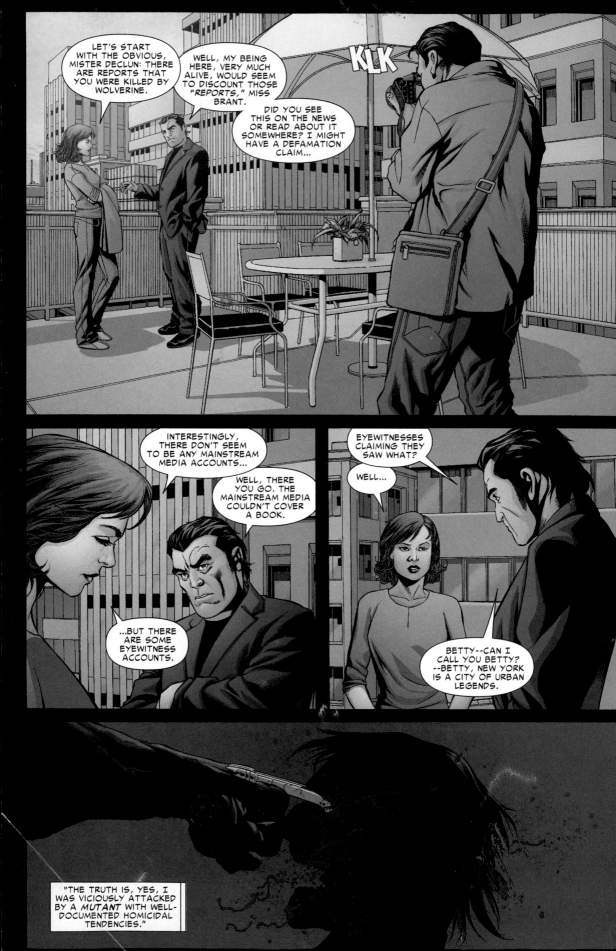

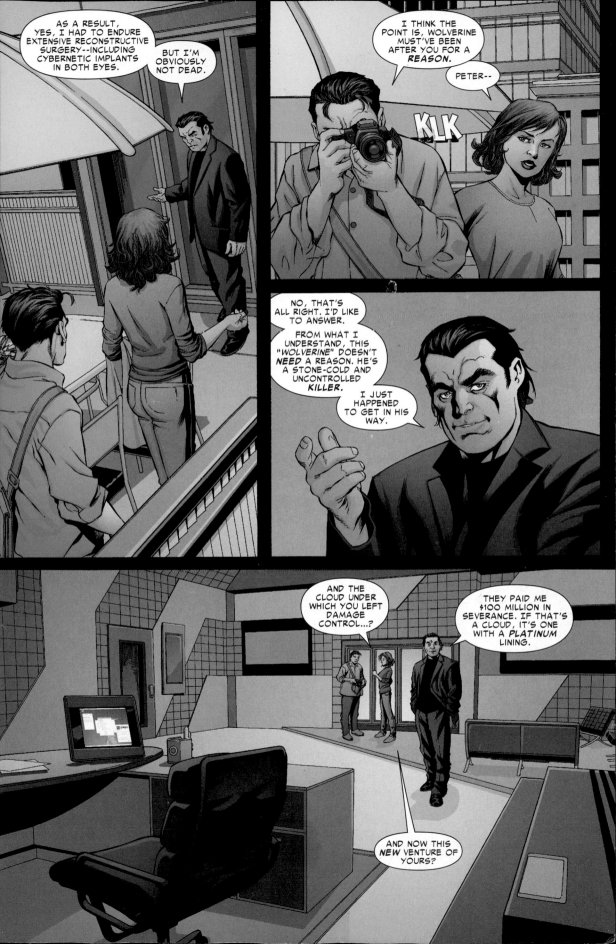

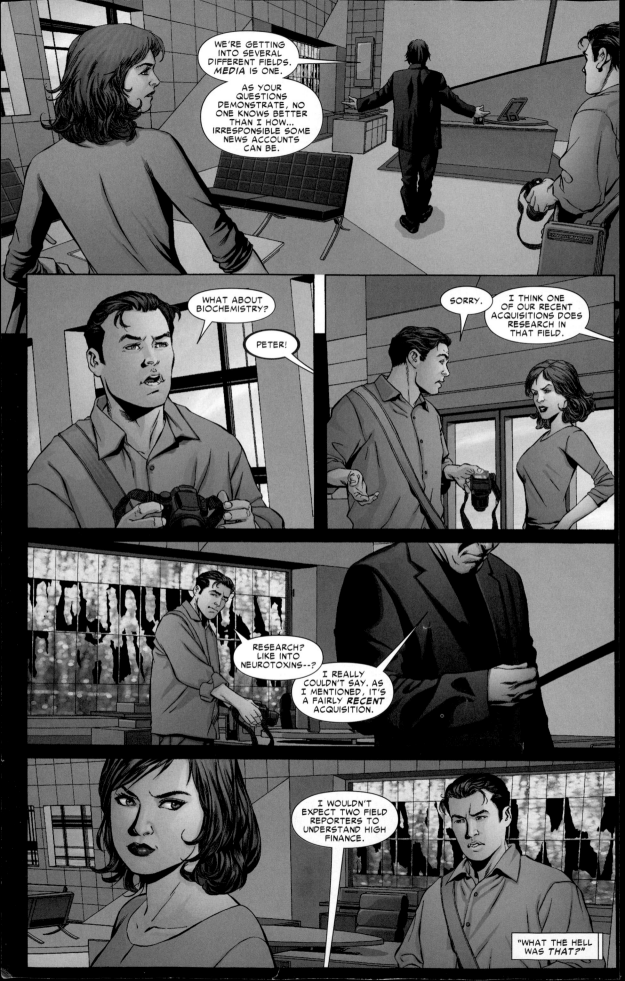

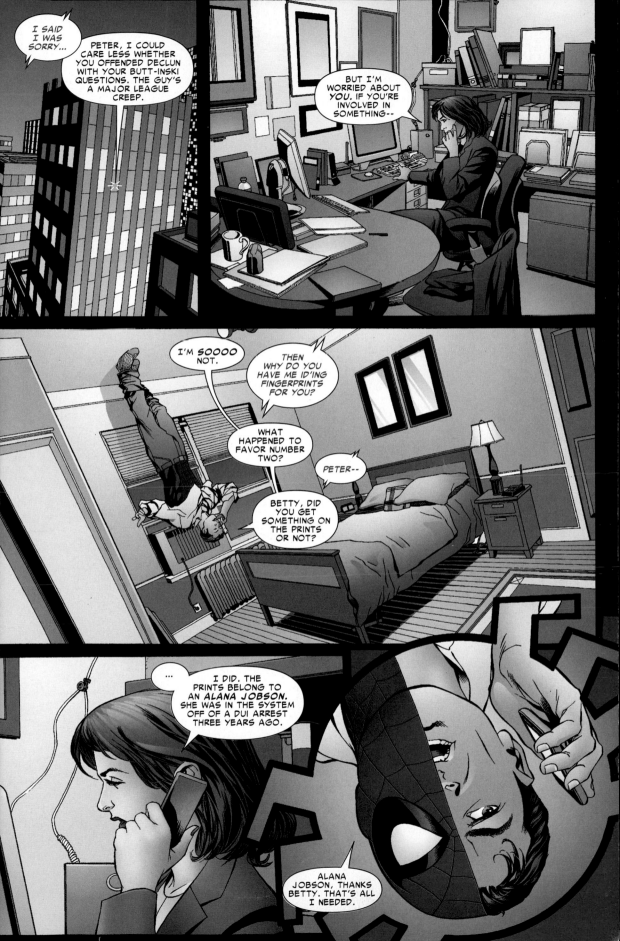

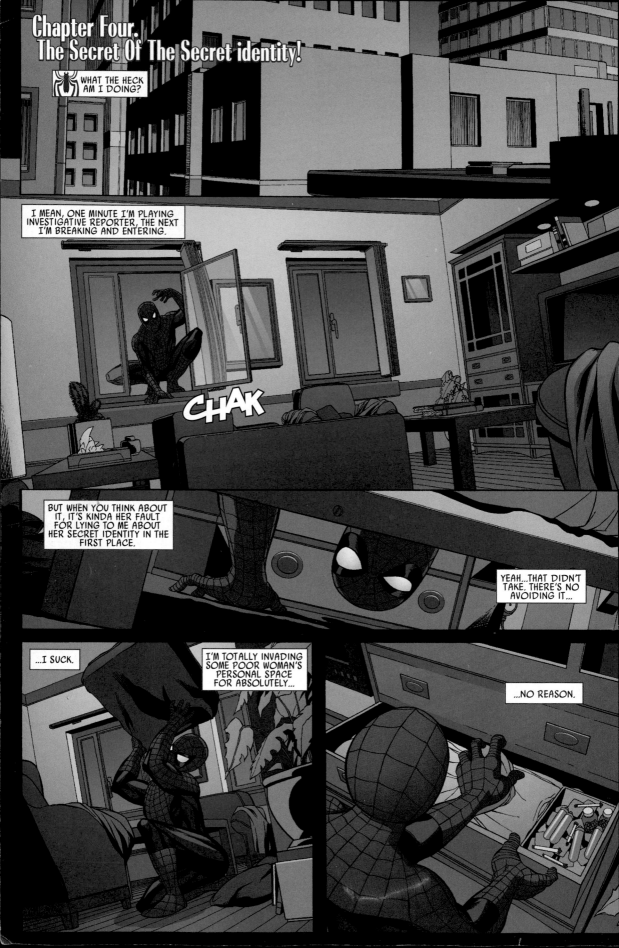

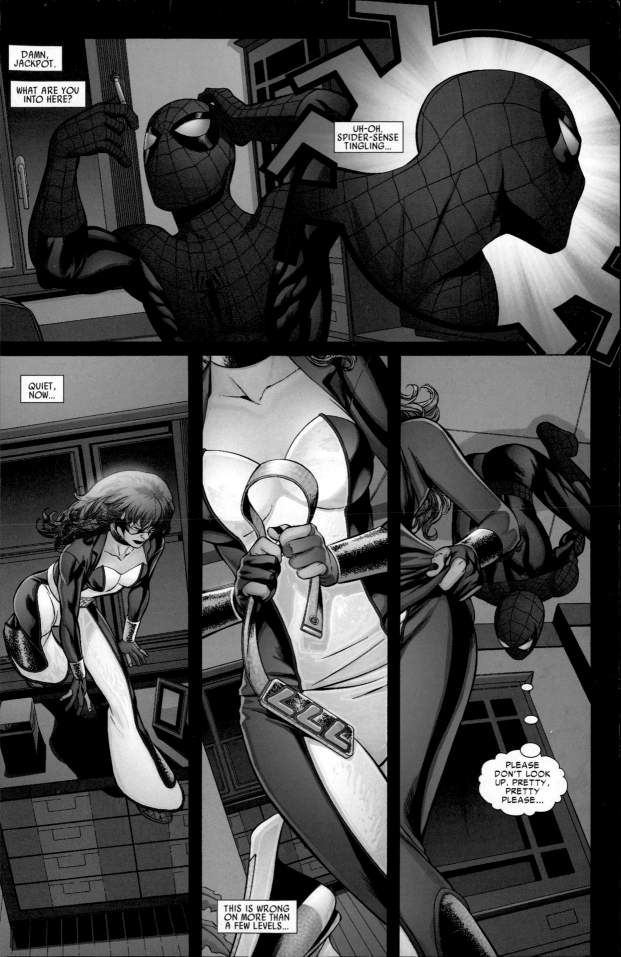

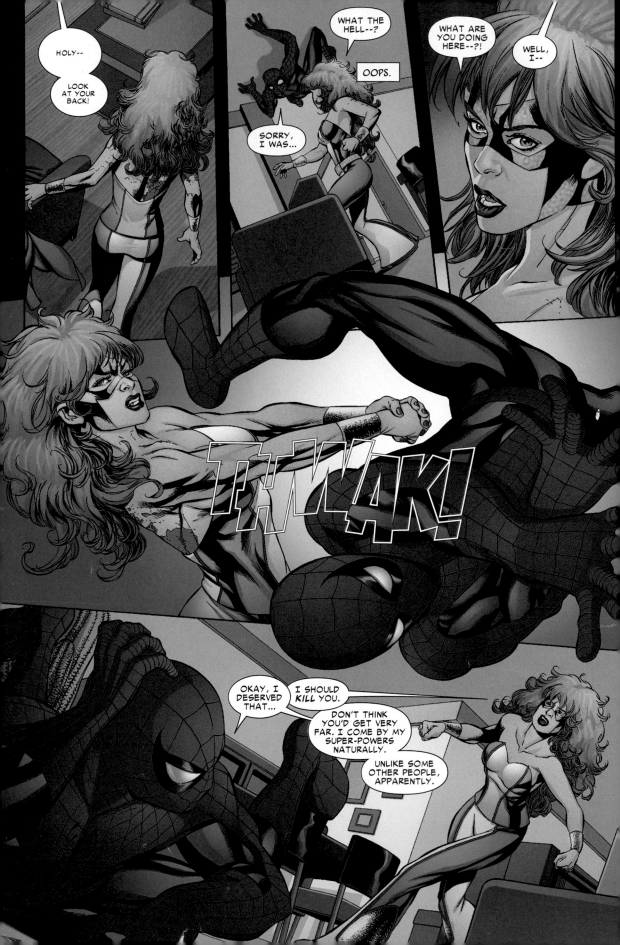

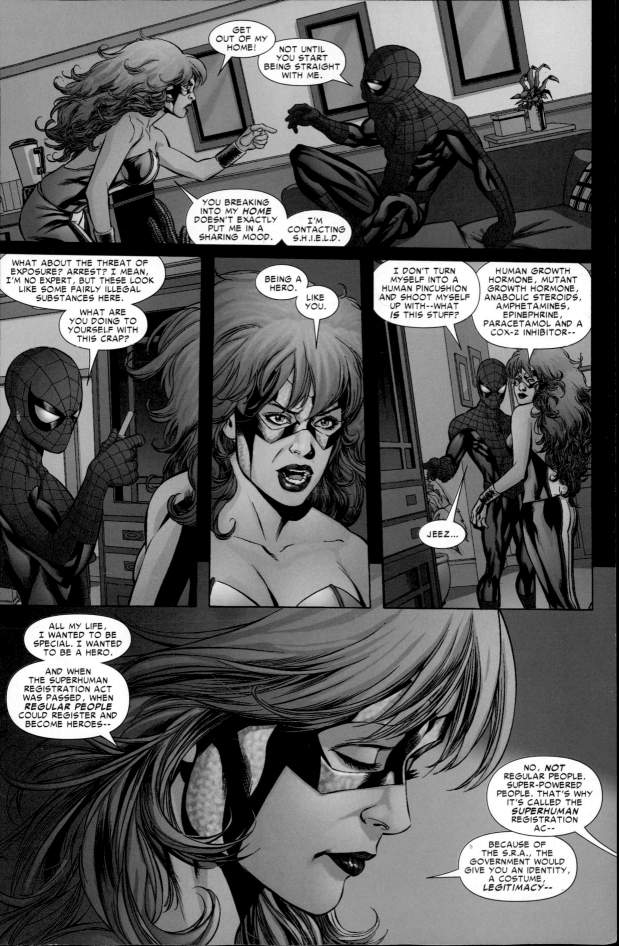

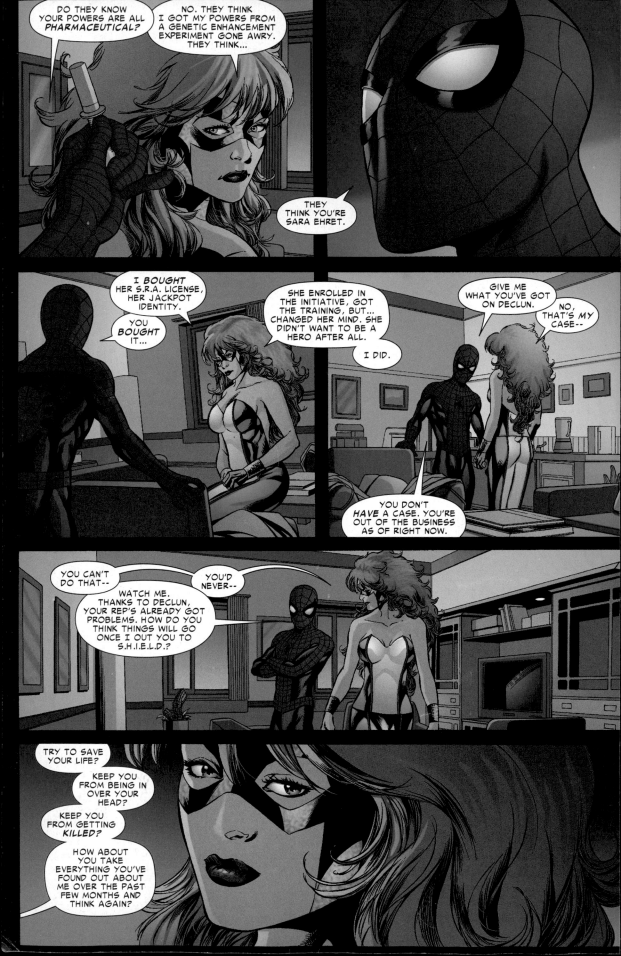

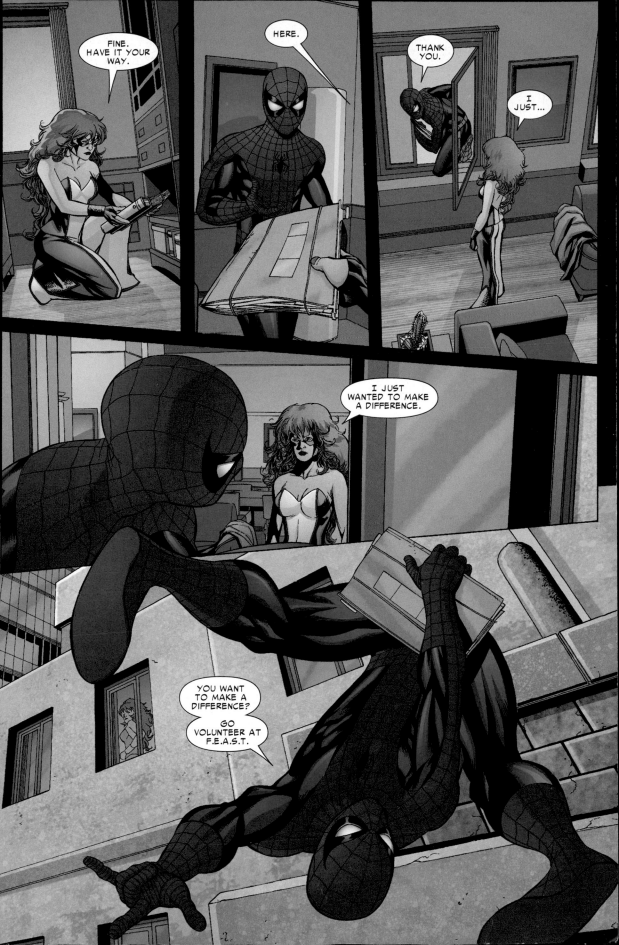

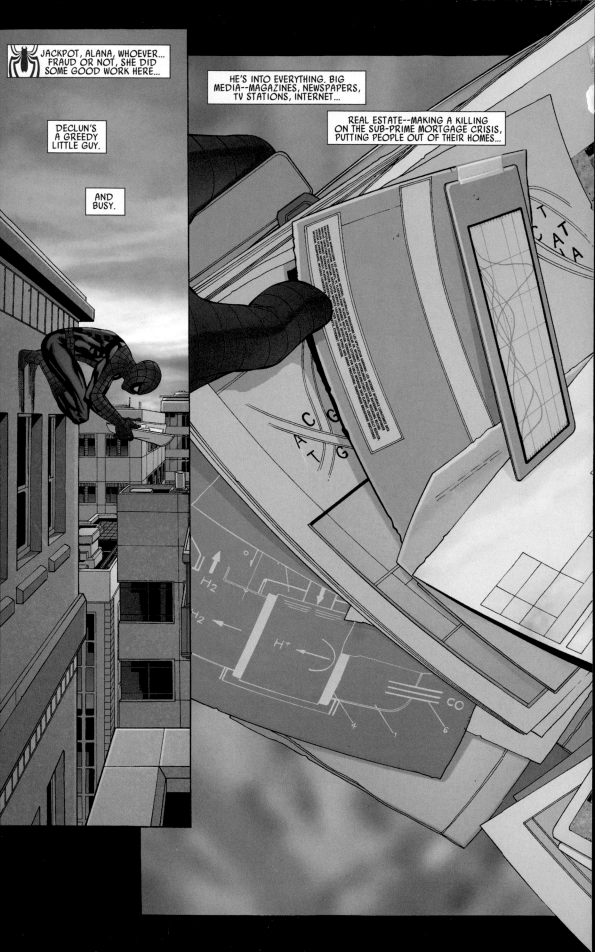

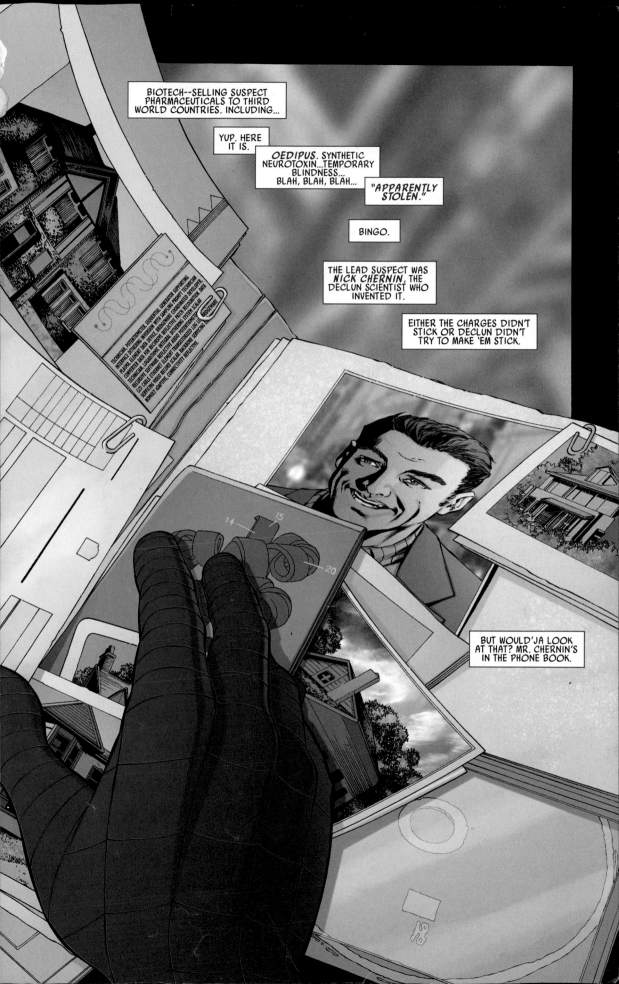

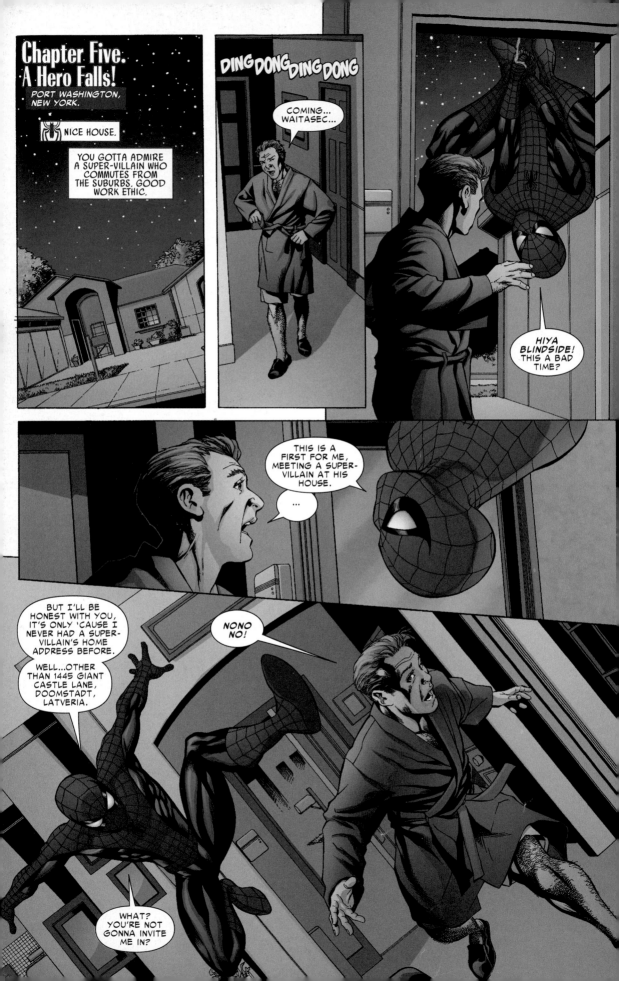

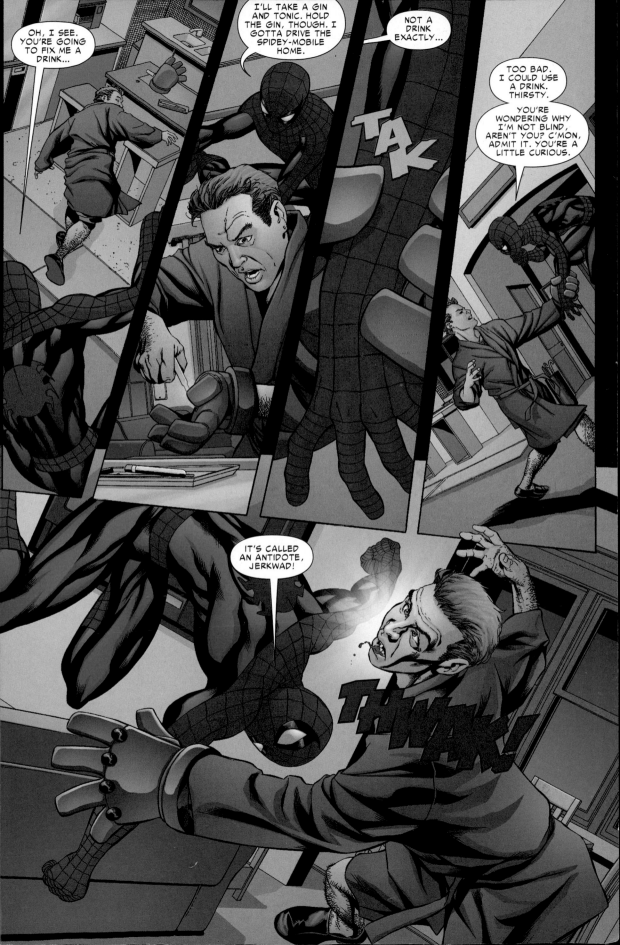

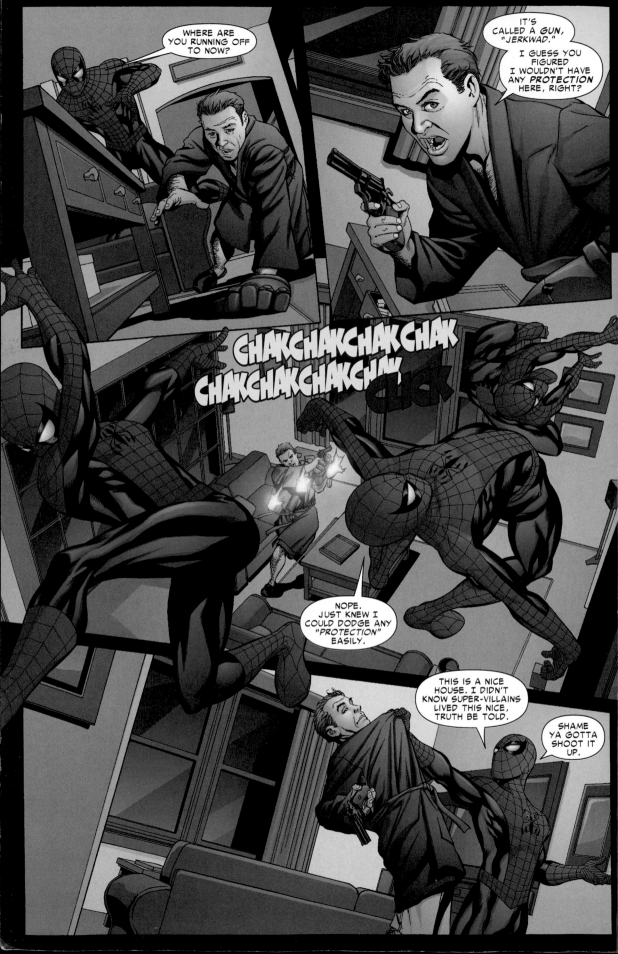

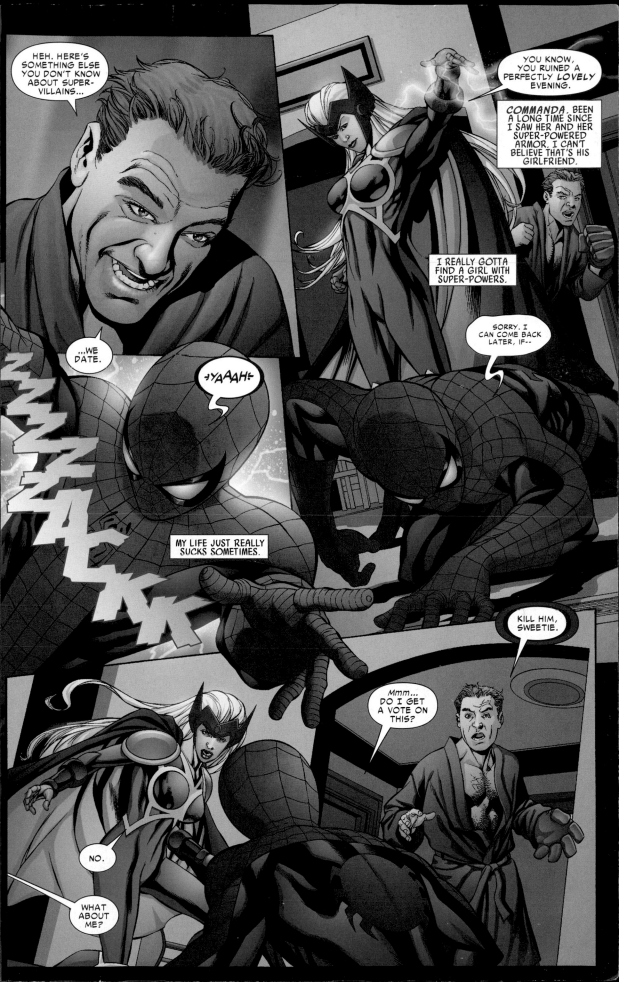

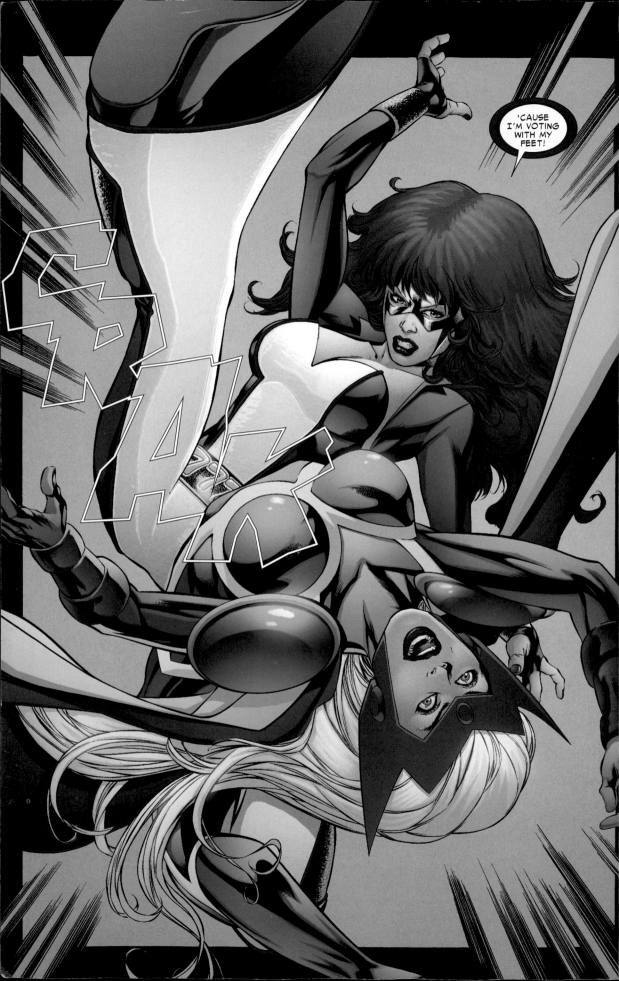

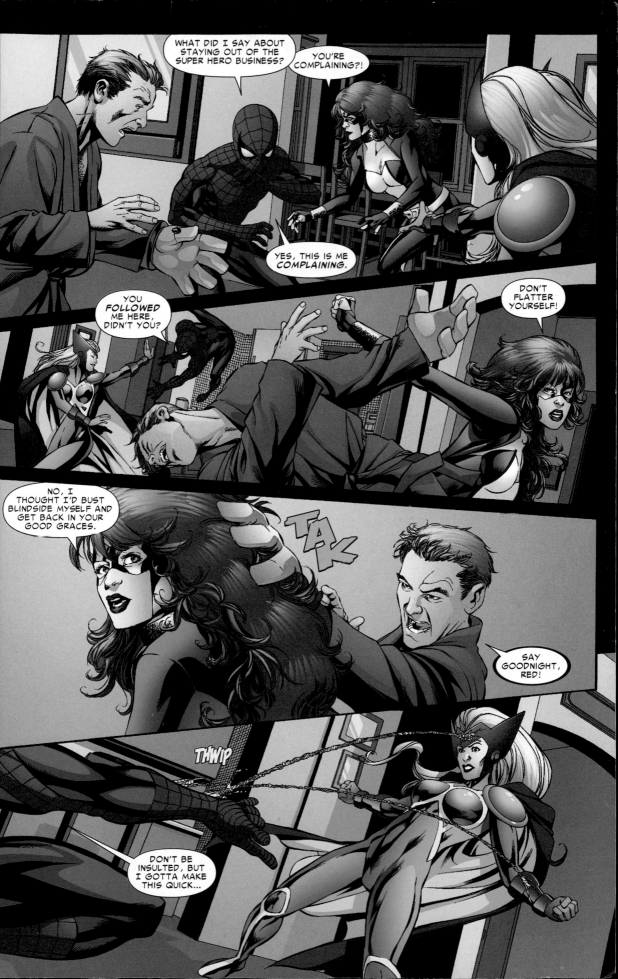

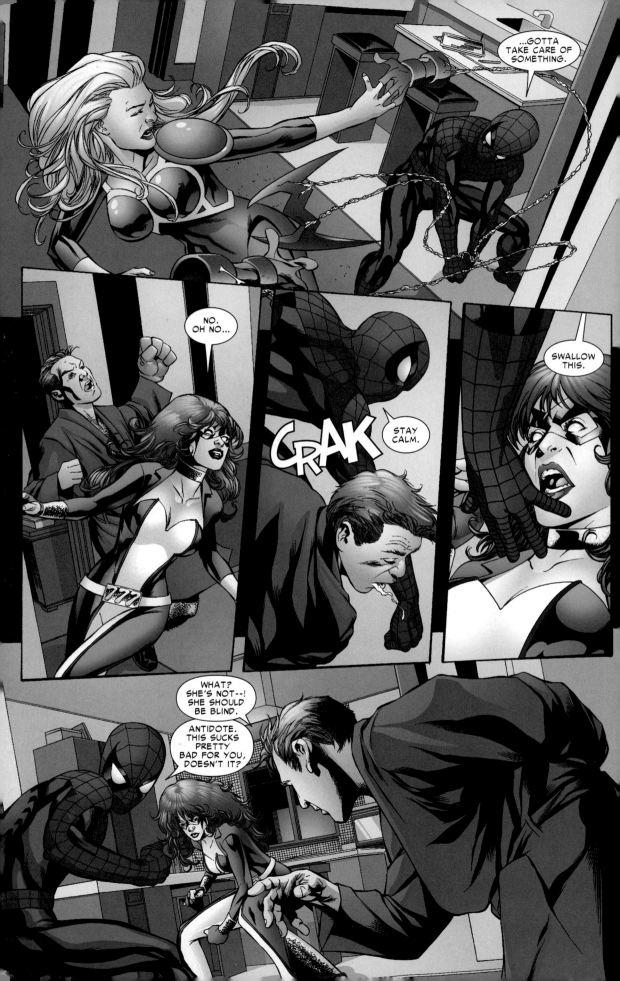

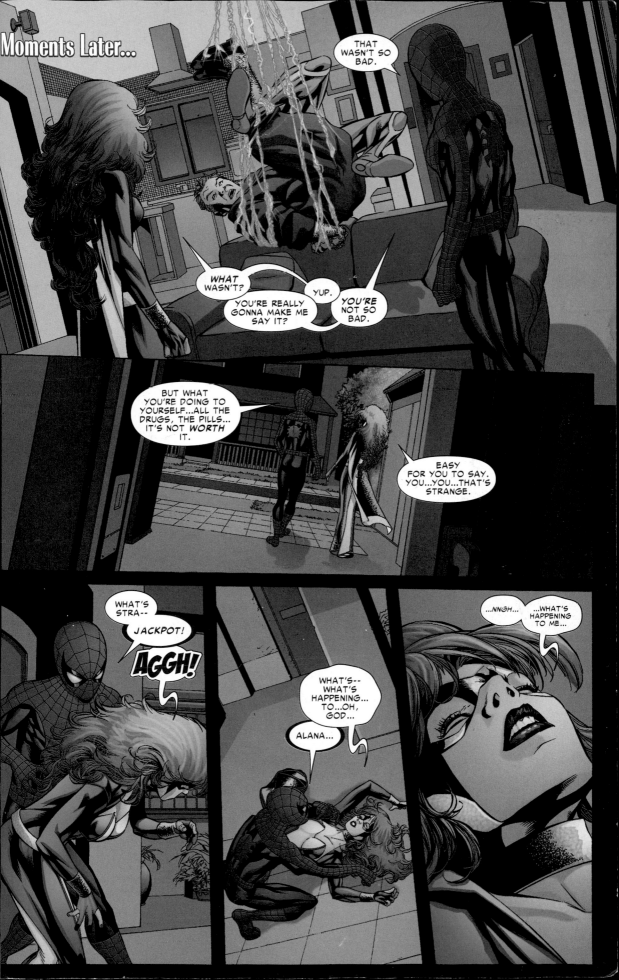

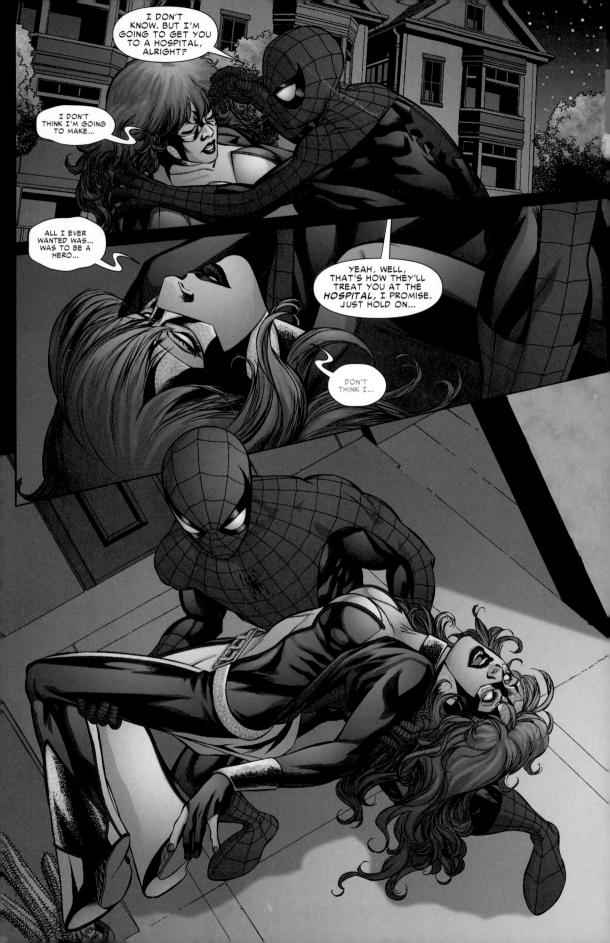

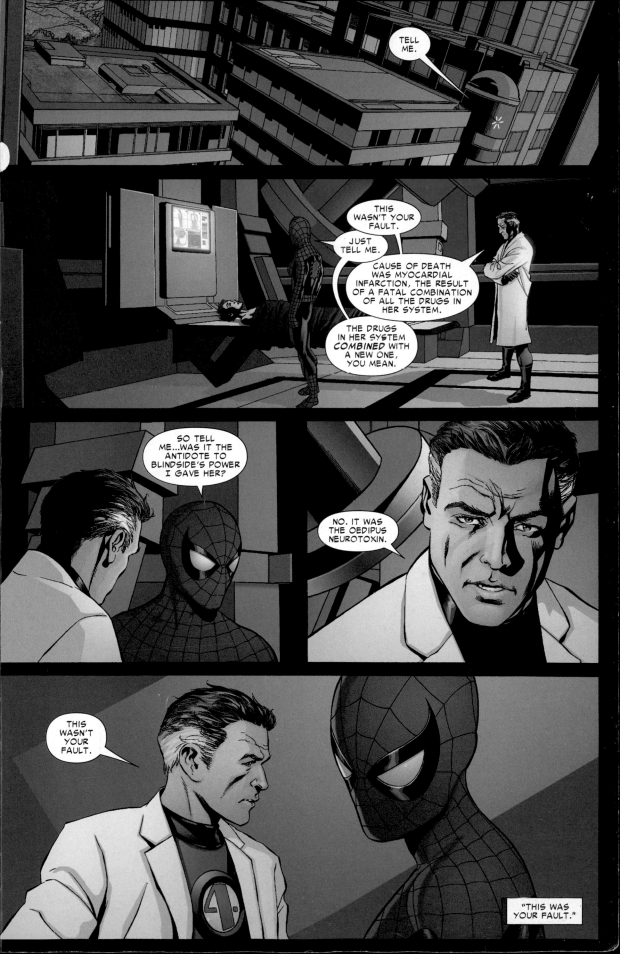

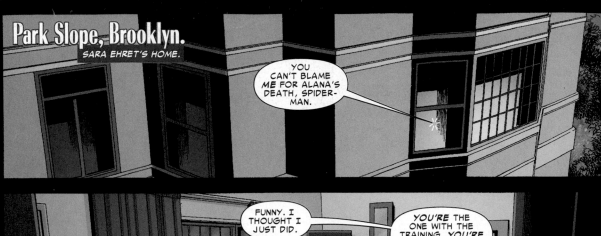

YOU CAN'T BLAME *ME* FOR ALANA'S DEATH, SPIDER-MAN.

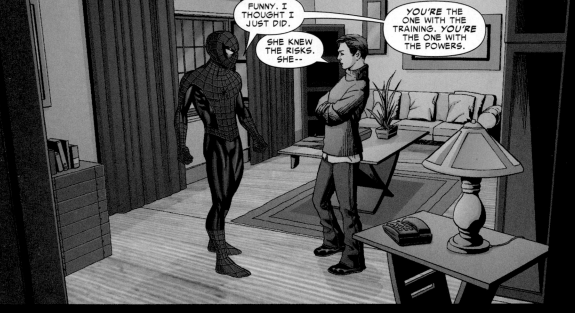

FUNNY. I THOUGHT I JUST DID.

SHE KNEW THE RISKS. SHE--

YOU'RE THE ONE WITH THE TRAINING. *YOU'RE* THE ONE WITH THE POWERS.

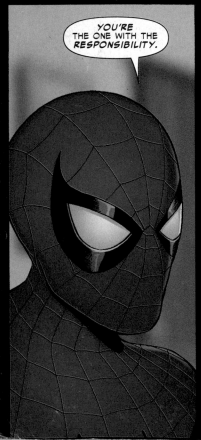

YOU'RE THE ONE WITH THE *RESPONSIBILITY.*

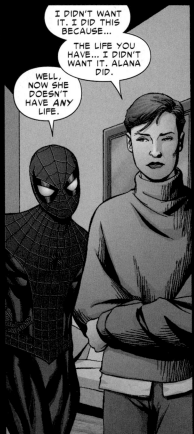

I DIDN'T WANT IT. I DID THIS BECAUSE...

THE LIFE YOU HAVE... I DIDN'T WANT IT. ALANA DID.

WELL, NOW SHE DOESN'T HAVE *ANY* LIFE.

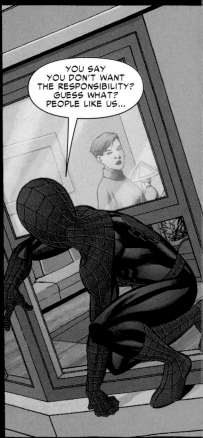

YOU SAY YOU DON'T WANT THE RESPONSIBILITY? GUESS WHAT? PEOPLE LIKE US...

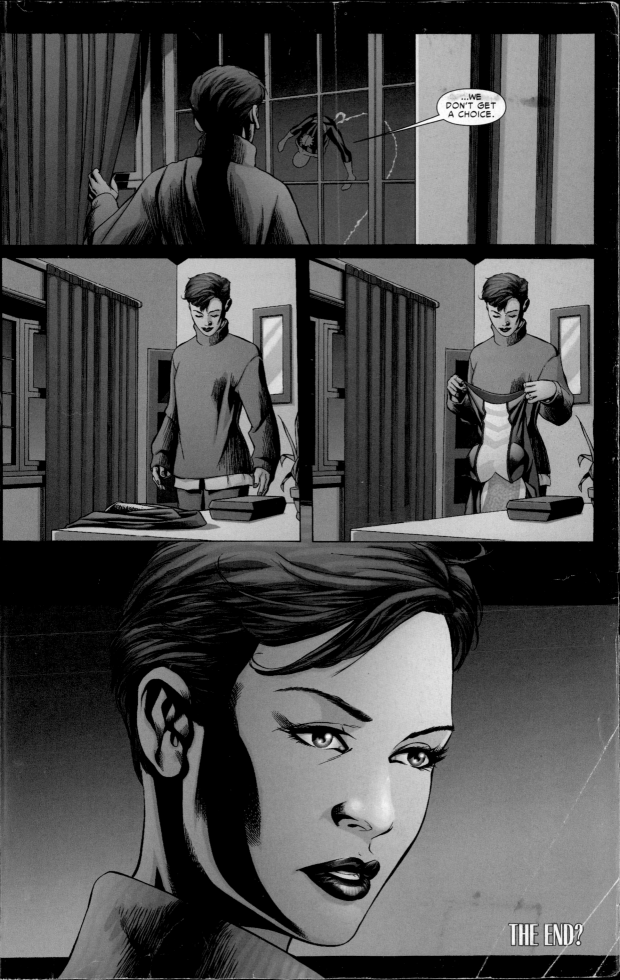

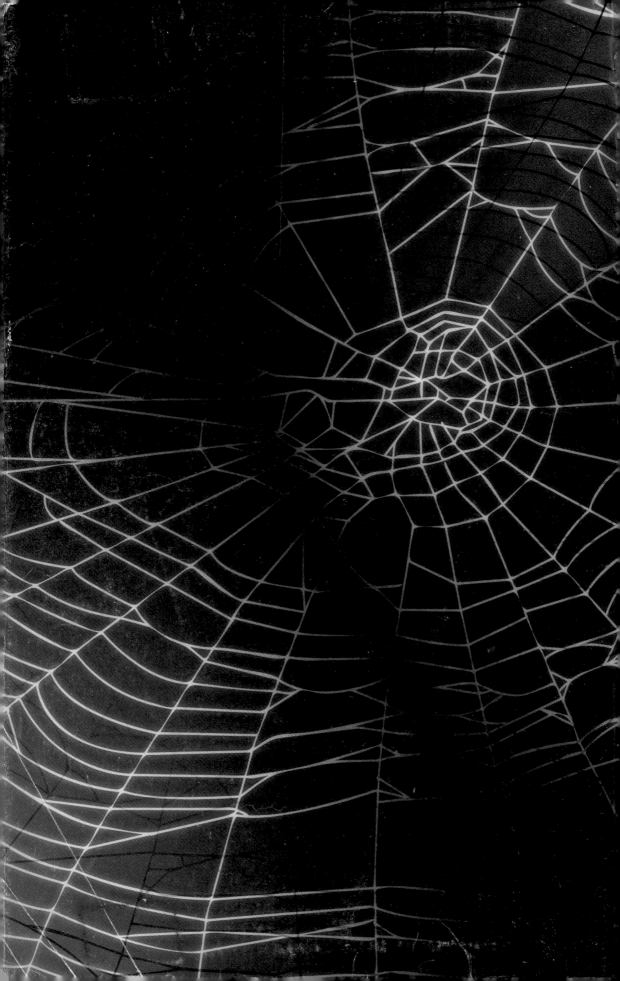